CONTEMPORARY STUDIES ON RELATIONSHIPS, HEALTH, AND WELLNESS

Close relationships are a vital part of people's daily lives; thus family members, friends, and romantic partners play an integral role in people's health and well-being. Understanding the ways in which close relationships both shape and reflect people's health and wellness is an important area of inquiry. Showcasing studies from various disciplines that are on the cutting edge of research exploring the interdependence between health and relationships, this collection highlights several relationship processes that are instrumental in the maintenance of health and the management of illness, including interpersonal influence, information management, uncertainty, social support, and communication. Although the existing health literature is rich with knowledge about individual and ecological factors that are influential in promoting certain health behaviors, the relationship scholars featured in this volume have much to contribute in terms of documenting the interpersonal dynamics that are involved in experiences of health and illness.

Jennifer A. Theiss is a professor in the Department of Communication and a Chancellor's Scholar at Rutgers University, New Jersey. She has published two books and more than fifty empirical articles and book chapters on communication and relationships.

Kathryn Greene is a professor in the Department of Communication at Rutgers University, New Jersey. She has published more than 100 articles and chapters on health communication, focusing on communication processes in preventing illness as well as maintaining health in close relationships.

Advances in Personal Relationships

Christopher R. Agnew
Purdue University

John P. Caughlin
University of Illinois at Urbana-Champaign

C. Raymond Knee
University of Houston

Terri L. Orbuch
Oakland University

Although scholars from a variety of disciplines have written and conversed about the importance of personal relationships for decades, the emergence of personal relationships as a field of study is relatively recent. *Advances in Personal Relationships* represents the culmination of years of multidisciplinary and interdisciplinary work on personal relationships. Sponsored by the International Association for Relationship Research, the series offers readers cutting-edge research and theory in the field. Contributing authors are internationally known scholars from a variety of disciplines, including social psychology, clinical psychology, communication, history, sociology, gerontology, and family studies. Volumes include integrative reviews, conceptual pieces, summaries of research programs, and major theoretical works. *Advances in Personal Relationships* presents first-rate scholarship that is both provocative and theoretically grounded. The theoretical and empirical work described by authors will stimulate readers and advance the field by offering new ideas and retooling old ones. The series will be of interest to upper-division undergraduate students, graduate students, researchers, and practitioners.

Other Books in the Series

Attribution, Communication Behavior, and Close Relationships
Valerie Manusov and John H. Harvey, editors

Stability and Change in Relationships
Anita L. Vangelisti, Harry T. Reis, and Mary Anne Fitzpatrick, editors

Understanding Marriage: Developments in the Study of Couple Interaction
Patricia Noller and Judith A. Feeney, editors

Growing Together: Personal Relationships across the Lifespan
Frieder R. Lang and Karen L. Fingerman, editors

Communicating Social Support
Daena J. Goldsmith

Communicating Affection: Interpersonal Behavior and Social Context
Kory Floyd

Changing Relations: Achieving Intimacy in a Time of Social Transition
Robin Goodwin

Feeling Hurt in Close Relationships
Anita L. Vangelisti, editor

Romantic Relationships in Emerging Adulthood
Frank D. Fincham and Ming Cui, editors

Responding to Intimate Violence against Women: The Role of Informal Networks
Renate Klein

Social Influences on Romantic Relationships: Beyond the Dyad
Christopher R. Agnew, editor

Positive Approaches to Optimal Relationship Development
C. Raymond Knee and Harry T. Reis, editors

Personality and Close Relationship Processes Stanley O. Gaines, Jr.

The Experience and Expression of Uncertainty in Close Relationships
Jennifer A. Theiss

Contemporary Studies on Relationships, Health, and Wellness

Edited by

Jennifer A. Theiss

Rutgers University, New Jersey

Kathryn Greene

Rutgers University, New Jersey

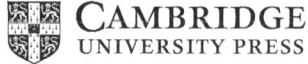

CAMBRIDGE
UNIVERSITY PRESS

University Printing House, Cambridge CB2 8BS, United Kingdom

One Liberty Plaza, 20th Floor, New York, NY 10006, USA

477 Williamstown Road, Port Melbourne, VIC 3207, Australia

314-321, 3rd Floor, Plot 3, Splendor Forum, Jasola District Centre, New Delhi - 110025, India

79 Anson Road, #06-04/06, Singapore 079906

Cambridge University Press is part of the University of Cambridge.

It furthers the University's mission by disseminating knowledge in the pursuit of
education, learning and research at the highest international levels of excellence.

www.cambridge.org
Information on this title: www.cambridge.org/9781108412285
DOI: 10.1017/9781108304344

© Cambridge University Press 2019

First published 2019
First paperback edition 2020

A catalogue record for this publication is available from the British Library

Library of Congress Cataloging in Publication data
NAMES: Theiss, Jennifer, editor. | Greene, Kathryn, editor.
TITLE: Contemporary studies on relationships, health, and wellness / edited by Jennifer
A. Theiss, Kathryn Greene.
OTHER TITLES: Advances in personal relationships (Cambridge, England)
DESCRIPTION: Cambridge, United Kingdom ; New York, NY : University Printing House, 2019. |
Series: Advances in personal relationships | Includes bibliographical references and index.
IDENTIFIERS: LCCN 2018026129 | ISBN 9781108419864 (hardback : alk. paper)
SUBJECTS: | MESH: Attitude to Health | Interpersonal Relations | Social Support
CLASSIFICATION: LCC RA776 | NLM W 85 | DDC 613–dc23
LC record available at https://lccn.loc.gov/2018026129

ISBN 978-1-108-41986-4 Hardback
ISBN 978-1-108-41228-5 Paperback

This book is dedicated to our many current and former doctoral advisees who inspire us to continue working to improve the health and relationships of others.

In memory of Zhanna Bagdasarov and John Leustek.

CONTENTS

FIGURES

TABLES

CONTRIBUTORS

LINDSAY SUSAN ALOIA, *University of Arkansas*

SMITA C. BANERJEE, *Memorial Sloan Kettering*

WENDY C. BIRMINGHAM, *Brigham Young University*

TRICIA J. BURKE, *Texas State University*

AMANDA CARPENTER, *Fors Marsh Group*

DANIELLE CATONA, *University of Delaware*

MARIA G. CHECTON, *College of St. Elizabeth*

SKYE CHERNICHKY-KARCHER, *Purdue University*

ERICA COGLAND, *The College of New Jersey*

BRITTANI CROOK, *The University of Texas at Austin*

AMY L. DELANEY, *Millikin University*

BRANDI N. FRISBY, *University of Kentucky*

PATRICIA E. GETTINGS, *Indiana University Southeast*

KATHRYN GREENE, *Rutgers University*

STEPHEN M. HAAS, *University of Cincinnati*

CHRISTINA J. HARRIS, *University of Kentucky*

MARIE C. HAVERFIELD, *Veterans Administration of Menlo Park, CA*

TERESA KEELER, *Kean University*

JOHN LEUSTEK, *The College of New Jersey*

RUTH MANNA, *Memorial Sloan Kettering*

JACOB M. MATIG, *University of Kentucky*

CAITLIN MCNAIR, *The College of New Jersey*

KEELIN MORAN, *The College of New Jersey*

ERIN NELSON, *Concordia University, Irvine*

PATRICIA A. PARKER, *Memorial Sloan Kettering*

ASHLEY K. RANDALL, *Arizona State University*

MAIJA REBLIN, *Moffitt Cancer Center*

EMILY SCHEINFELD, *The University of Texas at Tyler*

KELI STEUBER-FAZIO, *The College of New Jersey*

ANNE M. STONE, *Rollins College*

CHUN TAO, *Arizona State University*
JENNIFER A. THEISS, *Rutgers University*
CASEY J. TOTENHAGEN, *University of Alabama*
MARIA K. VENETIS, *Purdue University*

ACKNOWLEDGMENTS

The idea for this volume of research began percolating at a mini-conference on Relationships, Health, and Wellness that was held at Rutgers University in the summer of 2015. Most of the chapters in this volume began as papers that were presented at that interdisciplinary conference. We decided to assemble some of the best research from the conference into a volume that would showcase the leading research on relationships and health from various fields of study. We are grateful to the International Association for Relationship Research and the School of Communication and Information at Rutgers University for co-sponsoring the mini-conference that inspired this collection of studies. Without their generous support, this volume would not have been possible.

We are also grateful to the editorial board of the Advances in Personal Relationships book series for seeing the merit in this project and including it in the series. The board provided valuable feedback on our initial proposal that helped strengthen the content and organization of this volume. In addition, we are grateful to Cambridge University Press for publishing this collection, and especially thank our gracious and patient editor, Janka Romero.

Our appreciation also goes to the contributors whose research is included in this volume. These scholars are conducting thoughtful, ambitious, and impactful research on health and relationships that has significant theoretical and pragmatic implications for people's relationships, health, and wellness. We feel fortunate that they were willing to contribute their research to this important volume. We also wish to thank Shuktara Das, Allyson C. Bontempo, and Deborah B. Yoon for their help in proofreading and copy-editing all of the chapters.

Finally, as scholars of communication and relationships, we are also mindful of the myriad ways that our friends and loved ones provide implicit and explicit support of our personal goals. Therefore, we extend our heartfelt gratitude to our countless friends and family members, especially our spouses Kevin and Gaby, for all of the big and small ways in which they have supported us in this endeavor.

Introduction: The Interdependent Influence among Relationships, Health, and Wellness

JENNIFER A. THEISS AND KATHRYN GREENE

In recent years, there has been an explosion of research across a variety of disciplines investigating the individual, interpersonal, and ecological factors that are responsible for enhancing or undermining people's health and well-being. Scholars have invested considerable effort in exploring the best strategies for addressing health issues, such as discouraging unhealthy behaviors, promoting healthy lifestyles, improving encounters between patients and health care practitioners, developing community-based health initiatives, and addressing health disparities. An equally important yet understudied aspect of health behavior is the role of close relationships in promoting well-being and managing illness. Close relationships are a vital part of people's daily lives and lived experiences; thus, family members, friends, and romantic partners often play an integral role in people's health and well-being. On the one hand, close relationships have the potential to shape people's health behavior in both positive and negative ways. For example, friends and loved ones may facilitate a healthier lifestyle by encouraging a proper diet and exercise, or they could contribute to poorer health by suggesting, modeling, or reinforcing unhealthy habits, such as the excessive use of alcohol or other drugs. On the other hand, close relationships can also be affected by the health or illness of one or both partners. For instance, when illness strikes, individuals typically turn to their close relationships for support and comfort, which has the potential to bring partners closer together or to strain the relationship with increased uncertainty, goal disruptions, and threats to longevity. Thus, understanding the ways in which close relationships both shape and reflect people's health and wellness is an important area of inquiry.

This volume showcases studies from various disciplines that are on the leading edge of research exploring the interdependence between health and relationships, including scholarship from the fields of communication, counseling, health services, human development and family studies, public health, and psychology. The research included in this volume highlights several relationship processes that are instrumental in the maintenance of health and the management of illness, including interpersonal influence, information management, uncertainty, social support, and communication. Although the existing health literature is rich with knowledge about individual and ecological factors that are influential in promoting certain health behaviors, relationship scholars have much to contribute in terms of documenting the interpersonal dynamics that are involved in experiences of health and illness. This introduction begins with an overview of the existing trends in the literature on health and illness, followed by a description of the core relationship processes that are influential in health contexts, and an overview of the chapters in this volume.

TRENDS IN THE LITERATURE ON HEALTH AND WELLNESS

There is a robust literature that examines conditions associated with health and wellness. Existing research on health and wellness tends to focus on prevention campaigns and strategies for promoting individual health behavior, strategies for enhancing communication between patients and health care practitioners, the impacts of social and environmental factors on health disparities, and program or policy recommendations for addressing inequalities. An overview of these programs of research reveals important discoveries that have been instrumental in promoting health and wellness for individuals and their communities.

One important goal of existing health research has been to identify features of health messages that can change people's attitudes, perceived norms, and behaviors with regard to health issues. Drawing heavily on the literature on persuasion and social influence, these studies aim to improve people's knowledge and awareness of a particular health issue, shift their attitudes about a health issue, increase their intention to adopt healthy behaviors, and improve the likelihood that they will actually engage in healthier behaviors (e.g., Atkin, 2001; Logan, 2008). Countless studies have demonstrated the utility of broad-based media campaigns for targeting individuals' attitudes, beliefs, and behaviors with regard to a variety of health issues, including smoking cessation, cancer screenings, and drug prevention, to name a few (e.g., Noar, 2006). Although this line of research focuses mostly on the persuasive features of mass messages that are most effective at altering people's health behaviors, some studies have also considered the potential for individual influences on health behavior, such as the benefits of having a workout buddy (e.g., Wing & Jeffrey, 1999), the influence of friends and romantic partners on cigarette smoking (e.g., Etcheverry & Agnew, 2008), and spousal influence on the intent to obtain cancer screenings (e.g., Manne, Kashy, Weinberg, Boscarino, & Bowen, 2012).

Another prominent area of health research focuses on the health care system and features of communication between patients and health care practitioners that promote both patient satisfaction and patient compliance (e.g., with medication or exercise recommendations). Research indicates that effective patient–practitioner communication can encourage patients to acknowledge health problems, resolve their symptoms, understand treatment options, and adhere to a treatment plan (Haskard Zolnierek & DiMatteo, 2009; Stewart, 1995). Unfortunately, health care providers face a number of barriers to effective patient interactions, including pressure from insurance companies for shorter office visits, patient linguistic and cultural differences, and patients' abilities to access health information online. Each of these features, separately and in combination ultimately undermine health care providers' ability to communicate effectively and encourage health behavior change (Travaline, Ruchinskas, & D'Alonzo, 2005). A primary goal of this research, then, is to identify the features of patient–practitioner interaction that are most effective for promoting healthy outcomes for patients and increasing satisfaction with the health care experience.

A third prevalent area of health research considers the environmental and social factors that contribute to health disparities. There is a substantial body of literature indicating that individuals from racial and ethnic minority groups receive lower quality health care and experience worse health outcomes than individuals from majority groups (e.g., Collins, Hall, & Neuhaus, 1999). Studies also suggest that both urban communities and rural communities may lack access to sufficient health care services (e.g., Hartley, 2004). Consequently, an important goal of health research is to develop public policies that can reduce sociocultural inequalities in the availability and quality of health services (Arblaster et al., 1996).

Although each of these three research trends have produced findings that have improved individual health behavior and institutional health care practices, they tend to overlook the crucial role that close relationships play in promoting or sometimes undermining healthy outcomes. To date, close relationships have been an understudied aspect of health research. The studies included in this volume aim to address this shortcoming in the literature and highlight relationship processes that are influential in promoting health and wellness.

CLOSE RELATIONSHIPS CAN SHAPE AND REFLECT HEALTH AND WELLNESS

Given that close relationships are ubiquitous aspects of people's daily lives, they are heavily involved in people's experiences of health and wellness. Relationship processes can both shape and reflect personal health conditions. Much of the existing research on health and relationships focuses on the ways in which health or illness can affect the quality of relationships in terms of communication, intimacy, support, relationship satisfaction, and commitment (e.g., Lewis et al., 2006). Unexpected diagnoses and health conditions strain relationships by introducing stressful circumstances that can promote uncertainty or compromise interdependence (e.g., Goldsmith, 2009; Miller, 2012; Steuber & Solomon, 2008; Stone & Jones, 2009; Weber & Solomon, 2008). In addition, relationship partners and families are often forced to consider a number of issues related to health diagnoses, such as making treatment decisions, navigating social or environmental barriers to health care, including, but not limited to, draining financial resources or managing end-of-life care, that can introduce stress, conflict, or disagreement between relationship partners.

In contrast, other programs of research have considered the ways in which close personal relationships can be influential in shaping health outcomes for individuals. In general, participating in close relationships increases longevity and contributes to well-being through increased satisfaction, happiness, and involvement (e.g., Loving & Slatcher, 2013). There are also many specific ways in which friends, family members, and romantic partners can bolster one's personal health, in terms of encouraging exercise, healthy eating habits, regular doctor visits, and other healthy choices (e.g., Burke, Randall, Corkery, Young, & Butler, 2012; Homish & Leonard, 2008; Theiss, Carpenter, & Leustek, 2016). On the other hand, studies also show that features of close relationships can be detrimental to partners' physical health (Wu & Hart, 2002). For example, heightened conflict, demand/withdraw patterns, and hurtful communication have all been associated with physical outcomes of increased blood pressure, higher stress hormones, and lower immune system functioning (e.g., Heffner et al., 2006; Malis & Roloff, 2006; Priem & Solomon, 2011). This evidence suggests that relationship partners and their interactions can shape personal health and well-being.

RELATIONSHIP PROCESSES THAT ARE RELEVANT TO HEALTH AND WELLNESS

Although there are myriad ways in which close relationships can shape and reflect health behavior, the chapters in this volume point to five relationship processes that are particularly influential in health contexts. Specifically, the research in this volume is organized into five sections that reflect features of relationships that share a reciprocal influence with health and wellness: (a) interpersonal influence, (b) information management, (c) uncertainty, (d) social support, and (e) communication patterns.

Part I of this volume highlights research on interpersonal influence in health contexts. Interdependence models of close relationships suggest that relationship partners exert influence on one another in ways that can facilitate or undermine goal achievement (e.g., Berscheid, 1983; Rusbult & Buunk, 1993; Solomon, Knobloch, Theiss, & McLaren, 2016). In health contexts, relationship partners can attempt to influence their partner's health behavior in a variety of ways. The first chapter in this volume by Birmingham and Reblin, examines the ways in which spouses of individuals with a family history of colorectal cancer attempt to influence their partner to adopt healthy lifestyle changes and adhere to cancer screenings in an effort to prevent or forestall the onset of a cancer diagnosis. In Chapter 2, Haas explores the degree of involvement or influence that romantic partners in male same-sex couples have with regard to certain health behaviors and decision-making, especially involving decisions to disclose one's sexual identity to a health care provider. In Chapter 3, Burke examines romantic partner influence in diet and exercise behaviors and the ways that perceived social control interacts with maintenance behaviors to predict relationship satisfaction. As a set, these studies point to the ways in which interpersonal influence can be both beneficial and detrimental to people's health behavior.

Another interpersonal process that is highly salient for individuals facing a health condition involves decisions regarding information management. One consideration is how much information about their health condition individuals feel comfortable sharing with other people in their social network. The literature on disclosure (Greene, 2009) and privacy management (Petronio, 2002) highlights factors that shape people's decisions to share or conceal information about their health. Another important consideration is how much information about a health condition individuals want to know. The uncertainty management literature suggests that certain conditions may motivate individuals to seek or avoid information about their health (e.g., Afifi & Weiner, 2004; Brashers, 2007). Thus, the studies presented in Part II of this volume address issues related to information management in health contexts. In Chapter 4, Leustek and Theiss focus on privacy motivations by examining the topics that individuals with type 2 diabetes avoid discussing with their romantic partner. In Chapter 5, Venetis, Gettings, and Chernichky focus on sharing information in their study of the strategies that people use to disclose a mental health condition to close friends. Finally, in Chapter 6, Scheinfeld, Nelson, and Crook explore the ways that parents seek information about healthy diet and exercise and the strategies they employ to communicate that information to their children. Taken together, these studies highlight the complexities surrounding people's decisions to seek, share, or withhold information about their health.

Part III of this volume focuses on the uncertainties that arise for individuals and in their relationships when confronted with health issues. There is an extensive literature on the causes and consequences of uncertainty in relationships and in response to unexpected life events (Theiss, 2018). The ambiguity that people sometimes experience with regard to health diagnoses is reflected in illness uncertainty, which involves questions about one's symptoms, treatment, prognosis, and long-term health outcomes (e.g., Mishel, 1990). Uncertainty about health or illness can motivate people to either seek information that will provide greater certainty and clarity about their situation, or avoid information that might reveal uncomfortable or undesirable realities (Brashers, 2007). Beyond the uncertainties people may experience with regard to their health, the diagnosis of illness can also elicit questions about the impact that health problems might have on relationship quality or functioning (Solomon et al., 2016). The chapters in this section consider the implications of both illness uncertainty and relational uncertainty. In Chapter 7, Catona studies the ways in which coping with a spouse's Alzheimer's disease can give rise to relational uncertainty and interfere with personal goals and routines. In Chapter 8, Keeler examines the uncertainties that arise for adult children who are co-managing care for an aging parent and the information management strategies they employ to coordinate their actions. Shifting focus to illness uncertainty in Chapter 9, Carpenter, Greene, Checton, and Catona consider how uncertainty about a cardiac condition influences people's decisions to share information about their condition with their spouse. Finally, in Chapter 10, Frisby, Matig, and Harris examine the questions that children grapple with following the death of a parent and the uncertainties that surviving parents encounter with regard to helping their children cope with grief and loss. Thus, these chapters highlight the prevalence of uncertainty in health contexts and the effects it has on close relationships.

Part IV of this book focuses on the role of social support in managing health and wellness. Close relationships are a valuable resource for individuals coping with a stressful health condition. In close relationships, family members, friends, and romantic partners can share in the burden of managing conditions and outcomes of illness (Lyons, Mickelson, Sullivan, & Coyne, 1998). On the one hand, individuals may benefit from the support and comfort they receive from a relationship partner who is willing to share the load of managing and treating a health diagnosis. On the other hand, providing support in the context of illness can introduce unwanted stress and burden for individuals and in their relationships. The chapters in this section highlight some of the benefits and challenges associated with receiving and providing social support in the context of health and wellness. Chapter 11, by Tao, Randall, and Totenhagen, explores the ways that same-sex couples support one another in the face of stress and depressive symptoms associated with potential rejection from family members. In Chapter 12, Steuber-Fazio, Moran, McNair, and Cogland describe the stressors that arise for husbands when dealing with a wife's postpartum depression and the ways that they solicit support from social networks to help cope with uncertainty in this context. Finally, in Chapter 13, Banerjee, Manna, and Parker examine the patient–provider relationship and the strategies that oncology nurses use to convey sensitivity and support to patients who are confronted with a serious health condition. The studies in this section point to the ways that close relationships can be the source of incredible support, but also tremendous stress, when sharing in the maintenance of health and wellness.

The final section of this volume highlights the various communication patterns that are employed in close relationships in various health contexts. Two of the studies in this section focus on the communication dynamics in families, especially parent–child communication patterns, that have implications for health outcomes in the family. For example, in Chapter 14, Haverfield and Theiss examine the family communication patterns in families of parents coping with alcoholism that set the stage for social adjustment and psychological well-being for adult children of alcoholics. Similarly, in Chapter 15, Aloia and Stone describe the ways that childhood exposure to verbal aggression in the family can buffer against the stress of being a caregiver for ailing parents during adulthood. Going beyond the family context, Chapter 16, by Delaney, examines the impact that depressive symptoms can have on people's communication about sexual intimacy with a romantic partner. Collectively, these studies highlight the ways in which communication patterns can both shape and reflect the ways people navigate health and wellness in their families and close relationships.

CONCLUSION

Relationships and health are intertwined in complex and nuanced ways. Conditions in families and close relationships can shape the way that people respond to various health conditions and they can be shaped by the unexpected diagnosis of illness. In many ways, close relationships serve as a safe haven, a source of support and encouragement for those who are coping with illness or attempting a healthier lifestyle. In contrast, coping with illness or managing one's health behavior can present a number of threats and challenges to people's close relationships. This volume shines a light on interpersonal influence, information management, uncertainty, social support, and communication patterns as five processes inherent to close relationships that are particularly influential in health contexts. Studying the antecedents and outcomes of these processes can provide important insights for positioning close relationships to have a positive influence on people's health and wellness.

REFERENCES

Afifi, W. A., & Weiner, J. L. (2004). Toward the theory of motivated information manage-ment. *Communication Theory, 14*, 167–190. doi: 10.1111/j.1468-2885.2004.tb00310.x

Arblaster, L., Lambert, M., Entwistle, V., Forster, M., Fullerton, D., Sheldon, T., & Watt, I. A. (1996). Systematic review of the effectiveness of health service interven-tions aimed at reducing inequalities in health. *Journal of Health Services Research & Policy, 1*, 93–103.

Atkin, C. K. (2001). Theory and principles of media health campaigns. In R. E. Rice & C. K. Atkin (Eds.), *Public communication campaigns* (3rd ed., pp. 49–68). Thousand Oaks, CA: SAGE.

Berscheid, E. (1983). Emotion. In H. H. Kelley, E. Berscheid, A. Christensen, J. H. Harvey, T. L. Huston, G. Levinger, . . . D. R. Peterson (Eds.), *Close relationships* (pp. 110–168). New York, NY: Freeman.

Brashers, D. E. (2007). A theory of communication and uncertainty management. In B. B. Whaley & W. Samter (Eds.), *Explaining communication: Contemporary theories and exemplars* (pp. 201–218). Mahwah, NJ: Lawrence Erlbaum Associates.

Burke, T. J., Randall, A. K., Corkery, S. A., Young, V. J., & Butler, E. A. (2012). "You're going to eat that?" Relationship processes and conflict among mixed-weight cou-ples. *Journal of Social and Personal Relationships, 29*, 1109–1130. doi: 10.1177/0265407512451199

Collins, K. S., Hall, A., & Neuhaus, C. (1999). *U.S. minority health: A chartbook.* New York, NY: Commonwealth Fund.

Etcheverry, P. E., & Agnew, C. R. (2008). Romantic partner and friend influences on young adult cigarette smoking: Comparing close others' smoking and injunctive norms over time. *Psychology of Addictive Behaviors, 22*, 313–325. doi: 10.1037/0893-164X.22.3.313

Goldsmith, D. J. (2009). Uncertainty and communication in couples coping with serious illness. In T. D. Afifi & W. A. Afifi (Eds.), *Uncertainty, information manage-ment, and disclosure decisions: Theories and applications* (pp. 203–225). New York, NY: Routledge.

Greene, K. (2009). An integrated model of health disclosure decision making. In T. D. Afifi & W. A. Afifi (Eds.), *Uncertainty, information management, and disclosure decisions: Theories and applications* (pp. 226–253). New York, NY: Routledge.

Hartley, D. (2004). Rural health disparities, population health, and rural culture. *American Journal of Public Health, 94*, 1675–1678. doi: 10.2105/AJPH.94.10.1675

Haskard Zolnierek, K. B., & DiMatteo, M. R. (2009). Physician communication and patient adherence to treatment: A meta-analysis. *Medical Care, 47*, 826–834. doi: 10.1097/MLR.0b013e31819a5acc

Heffner, K. L., Loving, T. J., Kiecolt-Glaser, J. K., Himawan, L. K., Glaser, R., & Malarkey, W. B. (2006). Older spouses' cortisol responses to marital conflict: Associations with demand/withdraw communication patterns. *Journal of Behavioral Medicine, 29*, 317–325. doi: 10.1007/s10865-006-9058-3

Homish, G. G., & Leonard, K. F. (2008). Spousal influence on general health behaviors in a community sample. *American Journal of Health Behavior, 32*, 754–763. doi: 10.5993/AJHB.32.6.19

Lewis, M. A., McBride, C. M., Pollak, K. L., Puleo, E., Butterfield, R. M., & Emmons, K. M. (2006). Understanding health behavior change among couples:

An interdependence and communal coping approach. *Social Science and Medicine*, 62, 1369–1380. doi: 10.1016/ j.socscimed.2005.08.006

Logan, R. A. (2008). Health campaign research. In M. Bucchi & B. Trench (Eds.), *Handbook of public communication of science and technology* (pp. 77–92). New York, NY: Routledge.

Loving, T. J., & Slatcher, R. (2013). Romantic relationships and health. In J. Simpson & L. Campbell (Eds.), *The Oxford handbook of close relationships* (pp. 617–637). New York, NY: Oxford University Press.

Lyons, R. F., Mickelson, K., Sullivan, J. L., & Coyne, J. C. (1998). Coping as a communal process. *Journal of Social and Personal Relationships*, 15, 579–605. doi: 10.1177/0265407598155001

Malis, R. S., & Roloff, M. E. (2006). Features of serial arguing and coping strategies: Links with stress and well-being. In R. M. Dailey & B. A. LePoire (Eds.), *Applied interpersonal communication matters: Family, health, and community relations* (pp. 39–65). New York, NY: Peter Lang.

Manne, S., Kashy, D., Weinberg, D. S., Boscarino, J. A., & Bowen, D. J. (2012). Using the interdependence model to understand spousal influence on colorectal cancer screening intentions: A structural equation model. *Annals of Behavioral Medicine*, 43, 320–329. doi: 10.1007/s12160-012-9344-y

Miller, L. E. (2012). Sources of uncertainty in cancer survivorship. *Journal of Cancer Survivorship*, 6, 431–440. doi: 10.1007/s11764-012-0229-7

Mishel, M. H. (1990). Reconceptualization of uncertainty in illness theory. *Image: Journal of Nursing Scholarship*, 22, 256–262. doi: 10.1111/j.1547-5069.1990.tb00225.x

Noar, S. M. (2006). A 10-year retrospective of research in health mass media campaigns: Where do we go from here? *Journal of Health Communication*, 11, 21–42. doi: 10.1080/10810730500461059

Petronio, S. (2002). *Boundaries of privacy: Dialectics of disclosure*. Albany, NY: SUNY Press.

Priem, J. S., & Solomon, D. H. (2011). Relational uncertainty and cortisol responses to hurtful and supportive messages from a dating partner. *Personal Relationships*, 18, 198–223. doi: 10.1111/j.1475-6811.2011.01353.x

Rusbult, C. E., & Buunk, B. P. (1993). Commitment processes in close relationships: An interdependence analysis. *Journal of Social and Personal Relationships*, 10, 175 204. doi: 10.1177/0265407593301000202

Solomon, D. H., Knobloch, L. K., Theiss, J. A., & McLaren, R. M. (2016). Relational turbulence theory: Explaining variation in subjective experiences and communication within romantic relationships. *Human Communication Research*, 42, 507–532. doi: 10.1111/hcre.12091

Steuber, K. R., & Solomon, D. H. (2008). Relational uncertainty, partner interference, and infertility: A qualitative study of discourse within online forums. *Journal of Social and Personal Relationships*, 25, 831–855. doi: 10.1177/0265407508096698

Stewart, M. A. (1995). Effective physician-patient communication and health outcomes: A review. *Canadian Medical Association Journal*, 15, 1423–1433.

Stone, A. M., & Jones, C. L. (2009). Sources of uncertainty: Experiences of Alzheimer's disease. *Issues in Mental Health Nursing*, 30, 677–686. doi: 10.1080/01612840903046354

Theiss, J. A. (2018). *The experience and expression of uncertainty in close relationships*. Cambridge: Cambridge University Press.

Theiss, J. A., Carpenter, A. M., & Leustek, J. (2016). Partner facilitation and partner interference in individuals' weight loss goals. *Qualitative Health Research, 26,* 1318–1330. doi: 10.1177/1049732315583980

Travaline, J. M., Ruchinskas, R., & D'Alonzo, G. E. (2005). Patient-physician communication: Why and how? *The Journal of the American Osteopathic Association, 105,* 13–18.

Weber, K. M., & Solomon, D. H. (2008). Locating relationship and communication issues among stressors associated with breast cancer. *Health Communication, 23,* 548–559. doi: 10.1080/10410230802465233

Wing, R. R., & Jeffrey, R. W. (1999). Benefits of recruiting participants with friends and increasing social support for weight loss and maintenance. *Journal of Consulting and Clinical Psychology, 67,* 132–138. doi: 10.1037/0022-006X.67.1.132

Wu, Z., & Hart, R. (2002). The effects of marital and nonmarital union transition on health. *Journal of Marriage and Family, 64,* 420–432. doi: 10.1111/j.1741-3737.2002.00420.x

PART I

INTERPERSONAL INFLUENCE IN HEALTH AND RELATIONSHIPS

1

Differences in Perceptions of Spousal Influence and Family Communication in Cancer Risk-Reducing Behaviors

WENDY C. BIRMINGHAM AND MAIJA REBLIN

Cancer is the second most common cause of death in the United States, accounting for nearly one of every four deaths, according to the American Cancer Society (ACS, 2016). Although cancer treatments have been greatly improved, the ACS estimated that in 2017, just over 600,000 Americans died of cancer (ACS, 2017). An important risk factor for many cancers is family history. Having a first-degree relative (FDR; i.e., parent, siblings, children) who was diagnosed with cancer such as breast, colorectal, or prostate cancer increases the likelihood of developing the disease. For colorectal cancer (CRC), a family history of CRC is one of the strongest risk factors for the disease, with estimations indicating that inheritance plays a role in up to 25% of CRC cases (Kerber, Neklason, Samowitz, & Burt, 2005; Potter, 1999). Those with an FDR with CRC have a two- to fourfold increased risk of CRC compared to the general population, and having two or more relatives with CRC increases the risk three- to sixfold over that of the general population (Burt, DiSario, & Cannon-Albright, 1995; Fuchs et al., 1994).

Despite this increased risk, there is much that individuals with a family history of CRC can do to avoid a cancer diagnosis of their own. Screening procedures, such as colonoscopy, can identify precancerous polyps; removing these polyps can markedly decrease CRC incidence (Winawer et al., 1993) and reduce mortality (Jarvinen et al., 2000; Renkonen-Sinisalo, Aarnio, Mecklin, & Jarvinen, 2000). Lifestyle choices, including quitting smoking, eating a healthy diet, and limiting alcohol, as well as getting regular physical exercise and maintaining a healthy weight, can also reduce risk (ACS, 2016; Aran, Victorino, Thuler, & Ferreira, 2016; Song & Giovannucci, 2016). The links between diet, weight, and exercise and colorectal cancer are some of the strongest for any type of cancer, and most cases of CRC can be prevented by screening (Winawer et al., 1993) and engaging in healthy lifestyle behaviors (Gingras & Beliveau, 2011).

THE IMPORTANCE OF SOCIAL RELATIONSHIPS

Although the link between healthy behaviors and reducing one's risk for CRC and other cancers (e.g., breast cancer) is well established, many individuals at increased risk fail to engage in them. One key factor that may explain why some engage in risk-reducing behaviors and others do not is the presence of supportive others who encourage healthier decisions. A robust body of evidence indicates that supportive relationships protect individuals from various causes of morbidity and mortality (Holt-Lunstad, Smith, & Layton, 2010; Reblin & Uchino, 2008; Robles & Kiecolt-Glaser, 2003; Robles, Slatcher, Trombello, & McGinn, 2013). Such relationships may be acting through several pathways to affect health, including indirect ones (Robles, 2014). Relationships can act on biological mediators of health, including cardiovascular, neuroendocrine, and immune pathways, with more supportive relationships showing a protective effect against stress. Interactions within a relationship may influence one's emotion regulation by encouraging either hostility, which can have a detrimental effect on health (Smith et al., 2011; Smith, Uchino, Bosch, & Kent, 2014), or emotional disclosure, which can improve health (Pennebaker, 1995). Close relationships can also activate role scripts and instill norms, such as obligation and responsibility for one's family members (Umberson, 1987; Waite, 1995). For instance, the sense of responsibility toward one's partner may lead married individuals to avoid risky behaviors, such as problem drinking, smoking, or drug use (Nock, 1998). Even the anticipation of taking on the spousal role can alter one's less-than-desirable behaviors to more socially acceptable ones (Arocho & Kamp Dush, 2016; Bachman, Wadsworth, O'Malley, Johnson, & Schulenberg, 1997; Miller-Tutzauer, Leonard, & Windle, 1991). Supportive influence from network members has also been associated with disease risk–reducing behaviors, including smoking cessation and adherence to medical regimens such as medication (Ma, 2016), preventative health-related behaviors such as cancer screening (Brittain & Murphy, 2015), and health protective behaviors such as seat belt use (Habib et al., 2010) and less risky driving (Sarma, Carey, Kervick, & Bimpeh, 2013).

Relationships can also affect specific health behaviors more directly. Important others can provide important modeling of behavior, or exert control over health behavior. For example, a husband may choose to schedule a colonoscopy because his wife has done so (modeling), or a wife may simply make the appointment for her husband (control). Both of these types of influence can lead to changes in health behavior.

However, behavior one spouse uses to influence or promote healthier behaviors may not be visible to the other spouse. Bolger, Zuckerman, and Kessler (2000) found that spouses do not always recognize the support provided by their partner, and this may be advantageous. Spouses whose partner provided invisible practical support (e.g., advice, suggestions of course of action, offers of direct assistance without the recognition by the other spouse as support) had reduced levels of anxiety and increased levels of self-efficacy (Howland & Simpson, 2010). In fact, recipients of invisible support experienced the largest decline in negative emotion and the greatest increase in self-efficacy (Howland & Simpson, 2010). This is important, as increased self-efficacy has been associated with cancer risk–reducing behaviors, such as reducing alcohol consumption (Oei & Burrow, 2000), smoking cessation (Baldwin et al., 2006), and adopting and maintaining physical activity (Strachan, Woodgate, Brawley, & Tse, 2005).

CANCER SCREENING DECISION-MAKING

Research has clearly shown that supportive relationships can influence health behaviors, but little is known about spousal influence in cancer screening decision-making, and less is known regarding spousal influence on risk-reducing behaviors. In a pilot study comprising 23 men at familial risk for prostate cancer (Birmingham et al., 2013), our data indicated that men at increased risk for prostate cancer rated their spouse as more influential in lifestyle (diet, exercise) and screening decision-making than their physicians (Birmingham et al., 2012). This is particularly informative as, traditionally, the primary predictor of screening behavior is provider recommendation (Seeff et al., 2004; Ye, Xu, & Aladesanmi, 2009). Additionally, as part of a larger study, Birmingham, Boonyasiriwat, Schwart, Edwards, and Kinney (2013) assessed levels of family and spousal influence ("Generally speaking, I want to do what my family or spouse think I should do.") and levels of spousal communication ("How much do you talk about having a colonoscopy with your spouse?") in 208 males and 288 females with a familial history of CRC. Most participants were high in spousal influence (SI: males = 68%; females = 64%), yet only 11% of high-SI males and 22% of high-SI females reported high levels of communication with their spouse regarding colonoscopy and, overall, regardless of SI, only 13.3% of at-risk individuals reported high levels of communication with their spouse (Birmingham et al., 2013). This is problematic, as a spouse cannot exert a direct influence on one's partner if couples are not communicating about risk-reducing behaviors.

There is some literature that suggests that increased social influence and family support for screening (Stimpson, Wilson, Watanabe-Galloway, & Peek, 2012; Ye, Williams, & Xu, 2009) and lower levels of social isolation (Ye et al., 2009) are associated with increased CRC screening. However, much of the work on social relationships has focused on the broader concept of marital status on cancer screening behavior (Beydoun & Beydoun, 2008; Husaini et al., 2001; Keating, O'Malley, Murabito, Smith, & Christakis, 2011;

Stimpson et al., 2012). Some work focusing on the specific influence of spouses found evidence that spouses and family members have an influence on prostate cancer screening decision-making (Shaw, Scott, & Ferrante, 2013). Couples have been shown to have interdependent attitudes about cancer screening, and these attitudes have been linked to screening intentions. Screening intention was also linked to whether partners had discussed screening with each other (Manne, Kashy, Weinberg, Boscarino, & Bowen, 2012). In qualitative interviews, spouses reported using indirect and direct means to influence CRC screening. Direct spousal effect themes included leadership, persuasion, and partnership, which are the types of social control described earlier. Indirect spousal effects, such as companionship, support, and peer socialization, were also identified as strategies to encourage general health behaviors, but were applied to CRC screening (Manne, Etz et al., 2012). While this work creates an important link between relationship processes, including communication and cancer screening, there is little work studying actual conversations between couples regarding risk-reducing health behavior choices looking at both visible and invisible influences. Thus, the primary goal of this project was to examine the effect of spousal influence, both visible and invisible, on cancer screening decision-making and on risk-reducing lifestyle and health behaviors.

METHOD

Participants

As part of a broader pilot study, we recruited 16 individuals who had an FDR with a CRC diagnosis and their spouse (N = 32). All participants were recruited through newspaper advertisements from the community and through medical and radiation oncology clinics at a National Cancer Institute (NCI)-designated cancer center. Physicians within the clinics recommended CRC patients and interested patients gave consent to be contacted. Study personnel met with the patient following his or her office visit/procedure, explained the study, and requested permission to contact the patient's eligible FDRs. Potentially eligible FDRs were sent an introductory letter, a consent cover letter, and a permission to contact form. Once FDRs returned the forms, study personnel contacted them to provide additional information, answer questions, ascertain eligibility, and obtain consent from both the FDR and the spouse. Eligible participants were married couples with one member of the couple as an FDR at least 45 years of age, and without a personal history of cancer except nonmelanoma skin cancer. Spouses were not restricted by age or family cancer history.

Procedures

Participants (FDRs and their spouse) arrived at the laboratory, study personnel conducted the required consent processes, and the participants completed demographic information and self-reported health and marital quality surveys, surveys of spousal influence on risk-reducing behaviors, and health behavior questionnaires. Following completion of the questionnaire, a licensed American Board of Genetic Counseling certified counselor delivered a semipersonalized evaluation of CRC risk for the FDR and discussed modifiable risk prevention strategies for both spouses (NCI, n.d.). After the genetic counseling information session, the couple participated in an audio- and video-recorded semistructured discussion task in which they were asked to discuss the lifestyle choices they have taken or could take to reduce CRC risk for the FDR. The average discussion time was 7 minutes, with discussions ranging from approximately 4 minutes to approximately 10 minutes. All sessions were subsequently transcribed verbatim by a study personnel member and verified by a second study personnel member. Details from the discussion task are discussed elsewhere (Reblin, Birmingham, Kohlmann, & Graff, 2018). This study was approved by university Institutional Review Boards.

Measures

Demographic assessment. A demographic sheet utilized in our laboratory was used to assess standard variables including age, income, education, occupational status, and Hollingshead classification (Hollingshead, 1975).

Health behavior assessments. A standardized health behavior questionnaire provided information on the following potential health-related variables: medication use, exercise habits, smoking habits, alcohol consumption, and caffeine intake.

Social control. We assessed spousal influence with an adapted version of the Social Control Assessment Tactics Scale (Lewis, Butterfield, Darbes, & Johnston-Brooks, 2004), which provides a more comprehensive assessment of social control/social influence tactics (i.e., spouse making structural changes that facilitate behavior change). Our data demonstrated adequate internal consistency ($\alpha = 0.77$). FDRs were asked if their spouse influences/encourages them to change any of 14 designated health behaviors (e.g., "To drink less alcohol?"; "To get more sleep?"). Ten items assessed spousal efforts to influence/encourage the FDR to initiate or increase healthy behaviors. Four items assessed spousal efforts to influence/encourage participants to discontinue or decrease unhealthy behavior.

Spousal and family influence and communication. We assessed levels of spousal and family influence with a single-item scale developed by the researchers: "Generally speaking, I want to do what my family or spouse think I should do." Levels of spousal communication were assessed using four items, such as, "How much do you talk about having a colonoscopy with your spouse?" The current measure was expanded from the two-item measure of family support (Manne et al., 2002, 2003) to assess more aspects of family influence and normative influence (i.e., whether one wants to comply with what the family wants). All items were rated on a 5-point Likert scale (1–5, *Strongly Agree* to *Strongly Disagree*). Our data demonstrated adequate internal reliability (α = 0.77).

Worry about colorectal cancer. The McCaul Brief Worry Scale (McCaul, n. d.) is a three-item scale designed to measure both the intensity and the frequency of worry about colorectal cancer. For the present study, the McCaul scale (n.d.) was modified to assess both FDR and spouse worry, and included the following: "How worried are you about [your spouse] getting colorectal cancer?"; "How bothered are you by thinking about [your spouse] getting colorectal cancer?"; "During the last week, how often have you worried about [your spouse] getting colorectal cancer?" Each item was answered on a 5-point scale that ranges from *Not at All* to *Extremely*. Similar to previous research (Jensen, Bernat, Davis, & Yale, 2010), this scale showed good internal reliability in our data (Cronbach's α = 0.78).

Analysis

Descriptive analysis of questionnaire items was conducted using SPSS 23. Frequencies, percentages, and measures of central tendency were calculated. Communication discussion task conversations were transcribed and coded using NVivo software (QSR International, 2010). Themes were identified using a grounded theory approach (Charmaz, 2008; Glaser & Strauss, 1967), allowing codes, concepts, and categories to emerge from the data. Our approach consisted of open coding of the data and organizing the data into segments based on key words and concepts to form categories and to identify patterns and major themes in the discussion narratives. Transcripts were coded by consensus by trained research staff.

Results

Participants were all legally married and living with their spouse. The mean number of years married was 22.28 (*SD* = 12.28), with a range of 5 years to 45 years. FDRs (*n* = 16) were 45 to 66 years of age (*M* = 57, *SD* = 6.03). Spouses (*n* = 16) were 39 to 70 years of age (*M* = 58.25, *SD* = 7.99). Most participants were white (91%), had at least some college education (90%), and all who reported income had an income of more than \$40,000. We also examined health practices and found that most (both FDRs and spouses) had an FDR diagnosed with some form of cancer (84%). Only one participant reported being a smoker, and body mass index (BMI) ranged from 19.17 to 36.18 (M = 26.82, SD = 4.75). Mean reported weekly hours of exercise was 2.48 (SD = 4.75), of sleep was 47.13 (SD = 7.05), and of weekly alcoholic drinks consumed was 1.35 (SD = 2.71). Only three participants reported drinking eight or more alcoholic drinks per week.

Cancer Worry

We found intensity of cancer worry to be moderate to high in both FDRs and their spouse. Most FDRs (69%) reported being worried about getting CRC, and most spouses (81.4%) reported being worried about their at-risk partner being diagnosed with CRC. We examined the effect of worry on levels of spousal influence and found that higher worry intensity was associated with higher reported levels of influence (B = 1.78 p = 0.03).

Family and Spousal Influence and Communication

We looked at how receptive FDRs were to family influence with a single item: "Generally speaking I want to do what my family or spouse think I should do." Most FDRs agreed or strongly agreed they wanted to do what their spouse or family wanted them to do (56.3%), with 31.3% neither agreeing nor disagreeing. Spouses of FDRs mostly agreed or strongly agreed (68.8%) that they believed their partner wants to do what his or her family or spouse thinks he or she should do. We next asked about family communication regarding CRC screening. There were differences in the perceptions of FDRs and those of spouses regarding the amount of family communication between FDRs and their children and siblings. FDRs who reported they had at least one brother either did not talk about colonoscopy at all (54%), or talked about it a lot (45%). No FDRs reported talking "a little" or "some" with brothers, while more than 30% of spouses reported their at-risk partner talked "a little" or "some" with brothers and only 7% reported their at-risk partner talked "a lot" with brothers. FDRs and spouses were fairly similar in their reports of talking "a lot" about colonoscopy with each other (25% and 18.8% respectively); however, most FDRs did not actively talk with their children (43.8% "not at all"; 12.5% "a little") and spouses mostly agreed (37% and 18.8%, respectively). Of those FDRs who reported they had a sister, 33.3% did not discuss colonoscopy "at all" with sisters, 13% "a little" with sisters, and 53.3% discussed it "some" or "a lot" with sisters. Spouses believed their partner discussed colonoscopy with his or her sisters "some" (18.8%), but never "a lot."

When FDRs were asked about influence from their spouse regarding health practices or behaviors, we found clear differences in the perspectives of FDRs and their spouse. When asked about cancer risk–reducing behaviors such as cancer screening behavior, only 6.3% of FDRs reported their spouse encouraged them to do self-examinations such as checking skin for irregularities or breasts for lumps or other changes (for women), yet 18.8% of spouses reported encouraging their partner to do self-examination. Fifty percent of FDRs reported their spouse encouraged them to eat healthy food and to visit the doctor regularly. Yet, 62.5% of spouses reported encouraging their partner to eat healthy food and 61.5% reported encouraging their partner to visit the doctor regularly. Less than half (43.8%) of FDRs reported their spouse encouraged them to take better care of themselves, while 62.5% of spouses said they encourage their at-risk partner (FDR) to take better care of themselves. Only 37.5% of FDRs reported their spouse encouraged them to get adequate exercise, while 52.8% of spouses reported encouraging their partner to get adequate exercise. Of the FDRs, 37.5% reported their spouse encouraged them to get their age-appropriate cancer screenings (including colonoscopy), while 50% of spouses reported that they did encourage their at-risk partner (FDR) to get their age-appropriate cancer screenings. When we examined more general risk-reducing behaviors, few FDRs reported their spouse encouraged them to take more time to relax (25%) or to get enough sleep (25%); 53.8% of spouses reported encouraging their at-risk partner (FDR) to take time to relax, and 62.9% reported encouraging their partner to get enough sleep. Most FDRs reported their spouse did not encourage seatbelt use (12.5%), and 37.5% reported their spouse encouraged them to drive slower; 25% of spouses indicated they encouraged seatbelt use, and 31.3% reported they encouraged slower driving.

Communication Themes

When we assessed actual verbal communication, two major themes arose: active engagement in health behaviors and lack of engagement in health behaviors. Both themes were equally prevalent. Active engagement included mentioning health behaviors already incorporated into couples' lifestyles as well as problem-solving ways to include new health behaviors. All couples mentioned diet and exercise as areas they did actively engage in or problem-solved. One FDR stated, "I certainly eat differently, way different than I did when you met me. Way better. I didn't have fresh squash and fresh tomatoes, you know?" Other FDRs also noted spousal influence for eating behavior, "You bug me to eat better, lose weight. That's good. You've allowed me to go to the gym in the mornings when you're taking the kids to school so that's helped," and problem-solving physical exercise, "One more thing to consider is a stationary bike … if we had something—an additional piece we'd have a variety, switch off." Spouses also discussed active engagement or problem-solving.

I think just our healthy food choices is [sic] important because if you wanted to eat crappy all the time, or I wanted to eat crappy all the time, that would be bad. So we balance each other, we both kind of actively choose healthy foods, even when we are out and about and we enjoy doing things together. So that makes being active easier because we make time for each other and we make time to do it. We both are prioritizing it.

However, there were many missed opportunities, and even encouragement to avoid engaging in healthier behaviors. This often involved justification about why the things they did were not "that bad," or minimizing the importance of consistent healthy eating and exercise. One FDR stated, "But I'm not going to go with the whole wheat bread. I'm sorry." FDRs also justified not exercising, "It's like we can't even find time to exercise because of what we're up against right now." Spouses also justified poor eating, "The only time we eat [unhealthy cold cuts] is on the weekends," while some FDRs negated behavior changes as immediately important, "I can always make lifestyle changes."

Interestingly, some of the justification for avoiding healthier behaviors may have been due to more accurate perceptions of risk based on the genetic counseling session. Despite the high degree of worry expressed in the worry questionnaire, and an increased level of risk compared to the general population, couples expressed lower amounts of worry in the discussions after the genetic counseling session. One spouse stated, "My worry is fairly low. Because you've gotten the colonoscopy ... we were both clean. We know now to go every five years and [CRC is] never gonna jump out ... against you." One FDR also noted a lack of worry: "I don't feel that either of us is at [such] an elevated risk that it should be a concern," while another FDR reported, "Talking to [the genetic counselor] made me feel better about my risk."

DISCUSSION

Marriage has been associated with health benefits, and one mechanism by which marriage impacts health may be the support and influence that spouses exert on their partner's health-relevant and risk-reducing behaviors, although this influence might not always be visible to the recipient. We examined both FDR perceptions of their spouse's influence and spousal reports of their influence on their partner's risk-reducing behavior in 16 couples in which the partner had a family history of CRC. The couples were provided important information about the at-risk partner's risk during a genetic counseling risk assessment session, and were given semipersonalized risk-reducing information. Because family history of CRC increases one's risk of being diagnosed, it is especially important these individuals practice risk-reducing lifestyle behaviors and adhere to screening recommendations.

Influence on Healthier Lifestyle Behavior

We assessed FDRs to determine the amount of influence their spouse exerted to encourage behaviors related to cancer risk-reducing behaviors as well as to general overall health behaviors. We also assessed spouses' reports of the influence they exerted to encourage these same healthy behaviors in their at-risk partner. We found that FDRs perceived their spouse was influencing them in some behaviors, and that spouses also perceived they were influencing their partner, but this influence was not perceived as being at the same level. More than twice as many spouses reported encouraging partner relaxation and adequate sleep than their at-risk partner reported.

One possibility is that spouses are encouraging behavior, or even providing support and encouragement, for those risk-reducing behaviors of which FDRs are not aware. For instance, spouses may be preparing healthier meals, and thus "encouraging" healthier eating. Or, a spouse may make the appointment for a doctor visit, but if this is a typical behavior pattern in a long-term relationship, then the FDR may not perceive this as encouragement, while the spouse does. The social support literature argues that the best form of received support may be those acts that are not actually noticed by the recipient (Bolger et al., 2000), and certainly FDRs do not appear to be noticing the influence toward healthier behaviors that their spouse is reporting to provide. This is particularly interesting, as social support researchers have speculated that *perceptions* of available support may be the component related to the positive outcomes associated with social support, while the actual *receipt* of support can have negative impacts such as loss of self-esteem, feelings of indebtedness, or incompetence (Bolger & Amarel, 2007; Newsom, 1999). However, in cases in which the received support is invisible to the recipient, the individual can benefit from the received support while not suffering the diminished self-esteem that may be experienced when having to rely on another for support (Bolger & Amarel, 2007; Uchino, 2004). Invisible influence may act in the same manner as invisible support-giving. Influence that is not perceived by the receiving partner may increase the receiving partner's efficacy, such that the partner performs the healthy behavior without recognizing the spouse's influence and thus feels a sense of accomplishment for the healthy choices made.

Applying the concept of invisible support to influence between partners, if a spouse's encouragement of healthier behaviors is "under the radar," the at-risk partner may not experience the negative emotions often associated with feeling controlled by their spouse. In fact, such control can often be perceived as nagging. Nagging, or attempts to control another's behavior (e.g., social control), has been associated with resentment and anger (Lewis & Rook, 1999; Tucker & Anders, 2001) and even reactance, leading to worse rather than better health behavior (Hughes & Gove, 1981; Lewis & Rook, 1999). The influencing spouse may even, in order to continue to be perceived as a "good guy," not challenge and may actually support poor health behaviors. Spouses may even refrain from attempting to exert influence toward healthy behavior to eliminate the likelihood of their partner attempting to exert influence on their own behavior.

There are few health behaviors that do not have an interdependent effect on married couples. Often, households have shared groceries and/or meals, impacting diet, and use of shared leisure time may impact a couple's exercise habits (i.e., shared hobbies may be active or sedentary). Because of this, spouses advocating for change must also be willing to change themselves. Although a family decision and commitment to improve health behavior may be an important factor in success (Gallagher et al., 2013; Hindle & Carpenter, 2011; Kiernan et al., 2012), there are often barriers to change established patterns that require something dramatic to remove.

Influence on Cancer Screening Behavior

For these couples, an increased risk of CRC based on family history should have made salient the importance of engaging in cancer-specific risk-reducing behaviors, particularly adhering to cancer screening and self-examination guidelines. FDRs in the present study were mostly in the age bracket for yearly or bi-yearly mammograms (for women) and for physician discussion regarding prostate cancer testing (for men; ACS, 2016). Additionally, women, in general, should perform breast examinations monthly (ACS, 2016), and although regular testicular self-exams have not been studied enough for the ACS to make recommendations on exam regularity, some doctors recommend that all men perform monthly testicular self-exams (ACS, 2016). As such, we were particularly interested in the reports of spousal influence on cancer self-examinations and age-appropriate cancer screening, and were surprised by the low rates of encouragement reported by both FDRs and spouses.

Both FDRs and spouses reported high levels of cancer worry intensity at baseline, yet just over one-third of FDRs reported influence from their spouse to get their age-appropriate cancer screenings, which would include CRC screening, and less than 7% of FDRs reported influence from their spouse to do self-exams. It may certainly be that FDRs were very compliant about self-examinations and cancer screening, so the spouse did not feel the need to encourage or influence them; however, the fact that almost three times the number of spouses reported they *did* encourage self-examinations, and half of spouses reported influencing age-appropriate cancer screenings, indicate that

FDRs may not be as adherent to self-exam and screening recommendations as FDRs believe. Additionally, during the discussions that followed the genetic counseling session, most couples indicated that they were less worried about the FDR's CRC risk. This may be due to the genetic counseling session that outlined actual risk, which may have counteracted inflated perceptions of risk that often accompany the way individuals view cancer (Patterson, 1989). Fear is one factor that has been shown to reliably influence individuals' behavior (Witte & Allen, 2000), and although unwarranted fear and worry can be detrimental in many ways, it can also encourage adherence to health behaviors.

Limitations

The current findings from our small pilot sample may not generalize beyond the largely Caucasian and middle- and upper-middle-class populations studied here. Additionally, FDR and spousal reports of low encouragement for age-appropriate screenings and self-examinations may have been a result of prior guideline adherence. Finally, our couple discussion period was fairly short; however, allowing for a longer discussion may yield more in-depth data on influence between FDRs and their spouse.

Implications

The results of this study suggest that spouses can and do exert influence on their at-risk partner's (FDR) lifestyle and general health behaviors, but that their at-risk partner may be unaware of their efforts. Additionally, despite evidence that spouses did support each other's diet and exercise behaviors, not all of these behaviors were beneficial, nor did spouses consistently choose to exert this influence. This suggests that while spousal behavior can be a powerful predictor of partner behavior, this relationship can be much more complex. The challenge of conducting dyadic research on health behavior is that not only are more individuals involved, but often the whole is greater than the sum of its parts. We must consider individual perceptions, attitudes, and decisions; the strategies individuals use to convey these attitudes to each other; and the co-constructed reality that emerges. While spousal influence has the potential to be a profound tool in increasing health behaviors, future research needs to be done to examine the process of spousal influence in real interactions to determine when spouses choose to exert influence, the type of influence strategies they use, and to what effect.

REFERENCES

American Cancer Society (ACS). (2017). *Cancer facts & figures*. Atlanta, GA: American Cancer Society.

Aran, V., Victorino, A. P., Thuler, L. C., & Ferreira, C. G. (2016). Colorectal cancer: Epidemiology, disease mechanisms and interventions to reduce onset and mortality. *Clinical Colorectal Cancer, 15*, 195–203. doi: 10.1016/j.clcc.2016.02.008

Arocho, R., & Kamp Dush, C. M. (2016). Anticipating the "ball and chain"? Reciprocal associations between marital expectations and delinquency. *Journal of Marriage and Family, 78*, 1371–1381. doi: 10.1111/jomf.12328

Bachman, J., Wadsworth, K. N., O'Malley, P. M., Johnson, L. D., & Schulenberg, J. E. (1997). *Smoking, drinking, and drug use in young adulthood*. Mahwah, NJ: Lawrence Erlbaum Associates.

Baldwin, A. S., Rothman, A. J., Hertel, A. W., Linde, J. A., Jeffery, R. W., Finch, E. A., & Lando, H. A. (2006). Specifying the determinants of the initiation and maintenance of behavior change: An examination of self-efficacy, satisfaction, and smoking cessation. *Health Psychology, 25*, 626–634. doi: 10.1037/0278-6133.25.5.626

Beydoun, H. A., & Beydoun, M. A. (2008). Predictors of colorectal cancer screening behaviors among average-risk older adults in the United States. *Cancer Causes and Control, 19*, 339–359. doi: 10.1007/s10552-007-9100-y

Birmingham, W. C., Agarwal, N., Bishoff, J., Kohlmann, W., Aspinwall, L., Dechet, C., & Kinney, A. (2012). *Genetic prostate cancer risk assessment: Determining knowledge, attitudes and intentions in patients and providers*. Paper presented at the Annual Meeting of the American Society of Preventive Oncology, Washington, DC.

Birmingham, W. C., Agarwal, N., Kohlmann, W., Aspinwall, L. G., Wang, M., Bishoff, J., . . . Kinney, A. Y. (2013). Patient and provider attitudes toward genomic testing for prostate cancer susceptibility: A mixed method study. *BMC Health Services Research, 13*, 279. doi: 10.1186/1472-6963-13-279

Birmingham, W. C., Boonyasiriwat, W., Schwartz, M., Edwards, S., & Kinney, A. Y. (2013). *"Is anybody talking?" Spousal communication and influence on colorectal cancer screening in at-risk individuals*. Paper presented at the American Psychological Society, Miami, FL.

Bolger, N., & Amarel, D. (2007). Effects of social support visibility on adjustment to stress: Experimental evidence. *Journal of Personality and Social Psychology, 92*, 458–475. doi: 10.1037/0022-3514.92.3.458

Bolger, N., Zuckerman, A., & Kessler, R. C. (2000). Invisible support and adjustment to stress. *Journal of Personality and Social Psychology, 79*, 953–961. doi: 10.1037/0022-3514.79.6.953

Brittain, K., & Murphy, V. P. (2015). Sociocultural and health correlates related to colorectal cancer screening adherence among urban African Americans. *Cancer Nursing, 38*, 118–124. doi: 10.1097/ncc.0000000000000157

Burt, R. W., DiSario, J. A., & Cannon-Albright, L. (1995). Genetics of colon cancer: Impact of inheritance on colon cancer risk. *Annual Review of Medicine, 46*, 371–379. doi: 10.1146/annurev.med.46.1.371

Charmaz, K. (2008). Grounded Theory as an emergent method. In S. N. Hesse-Biber & P. Leavy (Eds.), *The handbook of emergent methods* (pp. 155–170). New York, NY: Guilford Press.

Fuchs, C. S., Giovannucci, E. L., Colditz, G. A., Hunter, D. J., Speizer, F. E., & Willet, W. C. (1994). A prospective study of family history and the risk of colorectal cancer. *New England Journal of Medicine, 331,* 1669–1674. Retrieved from: www .nejm.org.

Gallagher, P., Yancy, W. S., Jr., Jeffreys, A. S., Coffman, C. J., Weinberger, M., Bosworth, H. B., & Voils, C. I. (2013). Patient self-efficacy and spouse perception of spousal support are associated with lower patient weight: Baseline results from a spousal support behavioral intervention. *Psychology, Health & Medicine, 18,* 175–181. doi: 10.1080/13548506.2012.715176

Gingras, D., & Beliveau, R. (2011). Colorectal cancer prevention through dietary and lifestyle modifications. *Cancer Microenvironment, 4,* 133–139. doi: 10.1007/s12307-010-0060-5

Glaser, B. G., & Strauss, A. L. (1967). *The discovery of grounded theory: Strategies for qualitative research.* Chicago, IL: Aldine.

Habib, R. R., Hamdan, M., Al-Sahab, B., Tamim, H., Mack, A., & Afifi, R. A. (2010). The influence of parent-child relationship on safety belt use among school children in Beirut. *Health Promotion International, 25,* 403–411. doi: 10.1093/heapro/daq038

Hindle, L., & Carpenter, C. (2011). An exploration of the experiences and perceptions of people who have maintained weight loss. *Journal of Human Nutrition and Dietetics, 24,* 342–350. doi: 10.1111/j.1365-277X.2011.01156.x

Hollingshead, A. B. (1975). *Four factor index of social position.* Unpublished manuscript, Yale University, New Haven, CT.

Holt-Lunstad, J., Smith, T. B., & Layton, J. B. (2010). Social relationships and mortality risk: A meta-analytic review. *PLoS Medicine, 7*(7), e1000316. doi: 10.1371/journal. pmed.1000316

Howland, M., & Simpson, J. A. (2010). Getting in under the radar: A dyadic view of invisible support. *Psychological Science, 21,* 1878–1885. doi: 10.1177/0956797610388817

Hughes, M., & Gove, W. R. (1981). Living alone, social integration, and mental health. *American Journal of Sociology, 87,* 48–74. doi: 10.1086/227419

Husaini, B. A., Sherkat, D. E., Bragg, R., Levine, R., Emerson, J. S., Mentes, C. M., & Cain, V. A. (2001). Predictors of breast cancer screening in a panel study of African American women. *Women and Health, 34,* 35–51. doi: 10.1300/J013v34n03_03

Jarvinen, H. J., Aarnio, M., Mustonen, H., Aktan-Collan, K., Aaltonen, L. A., Peltomaki, P., . . . Mecklin, J. P. (2000). Controlled 15-year trial on screening for colorectal cancer in families with hereditary nonpolyposis colorectal cancer. *Gastroenterology, 118,* 829–834. doi: 10.1016/S0016-5085(00)70168-5

Jensen, J. D., Bernat, J. K., Davis, L. A., & Yale, R. (2010). Dispositional cancer worry: Convergent, divergent, and predictive validity of existing scales. *Journal of Psychosocial Oncology, 28,* 470–489. doi: 10.1080/07347332.2010.498459

Keating, N. L., O'Malley, A. J., Murabito, J. M., Smith, K. P., & Christakis, N. A. (2011). Minimal social network effects evident in cancer screening behavior. *Cancer, 117,* 3045–3052. doi: 10.1002/cncr.25849

Kerber, R. A., Neklason, D. W., Samowitz, W. S., & Burt, R. W. (2005). Frequency of familial colon cancer and hereditary nonpolyposis colorectal cancer (Lynch syndrome) in a large population database. *Familial Cancer, 4,* 239–244. doi: 10.1007/s10689-005-0657-x

Kiernan, M., Moore, S. D., Schoffman, D. E., Lee, K., King, A. C., Taylor, C. B., . . . Perri, M. G. (2012). Social support for healthy behaviors: Scale psychometrics and prediction of weight loss among women in a behavioral program. *Obesity, 20,* 756–764. doi: 10.1038/oby.2011.293

Lewis, M. A., Butterfield, R. M., Darbes, L. A., & Johnston-Brooks, C. (2004). The conceptualization and assessment of health-related social control. *Journal of Social and Personal Relationships*, 21, 669–687. doi: 10.1177/0265407504045893

Lewis, M. A., & Rook, K. S. (1999). Social control in personal relationships: Impact on health behaviors and psychological distress. *Health Psychology*, 18, 63–71. doi: 10.1037/0278–6133.18.1.63

Ma, C. (2016). A cross-sectional survey of medication adherence and associated factors for rural patients with hypertension. *Applied Nursing Research*, 31, 94–99. doi: 10.1016/j.apnr.2016.01.004

Manne, S., Etz, R. S., Hudson, S. V., Medina-Forrester, A., Boscarino, J. A., Bowen, D. J., & Weinberg, D. S. (2012). A qualitative analysis of couples' communication regarding colorectal cancer screening using the Interdependence Model. *Patient Education and Counseling*, 87, 18–22. doi: S0738-3991(11)00379-X [pii] 10.1016/j.pec.2011.07.012

Manne, S., Kashy, D., Weinberg, D. S., Boscarino, J. A., & Bowen, D. J. (2012). Using the interdependence model to understand spousal influence on colorectal cancer screening intentions: A structural equation model. *Annals of Behavioral Medicine*, 43, 320–329. doi: 10.1007/s12160-012-9344-y

Manne, S., Markowitz, A., Winawer, S., Guillem, J., Meropol, N. J., Haller, D., . . . Duncan, T. (2003). Understanding intention to undergo colonoscopy among intermediate-risk siblings of colorectal cancer patients: A test of a mediational model. *Preventive Medicine*, 36, 71–84. doi: 10.1006/pmed 2002.1122

Manne, S., Markowitz, A., Winawer, S., Meropol, N. J., Haller, D., Rakowski, W., . . . Jandorf, L. (2002). Correlates of colorectal cancer screening compliance and stage of adoption among siblings of individuals with early onset colorectal cancer. *Health Psychology*, 21, 3–15. doi: 10.1037/0278–6133.21.1.3

McCaul, K., & Goetz, P. W. (n.d.). Worry. Retrieved from: https://cancercontrol .cancer.gov/brp/research/constructs/worry.pdf

Miller-Tutzauer, C., Leonard, K. E., & Windle, M. (1991). Marriage and alcohol use: A longitudinal study of "maturing out." *Journal of Studies on Alcohol*, 52, 434–440. doi: 10.15288/jsa.1991.52.434.

National Cancer Institute, National Institutes of Health. (n.d.) *Colorectal cancer prevention* (PDQ). Retrieved from: http://www.cancer.gov/types/colorectal/ patient/colorectal-prevention-pdq

Newsom, J. T. (1999). Another side to caregiving: Negative reactions to being helped. *Current Directions in Psychological Science*, 8, 183–187. doi: 10.1111/1467–8721.00043

Nock, S. L. (1998). *Marriage in men's lives*. New York, NY: Oxford University Press.

Oei, T. P., & Burrow, T. (2000). Alcohol expectancy and drinking refusal self-efficacy: A test of specificity theory. *Addictive Behaviors*, 25, 499–507. Retrieved from: https:// www.ncbi.nlm.nih.gov/pubmed/10972442

Patterson, J. T. (1989). *The dread disease*. Cambridge, MA: Harvard University Press.

Pennebaker, J. W. (1995). Emotion, disclosure and health: An overview. In J. W. Pennebaker (Ed.), *Emotion, disclosure, & health* (pp. 3–10). Washington, DC: American Psychological Association.

Potter, J. D. (1999). Colorectal cancer: Molecules and populations. *Journal of the National Cancer Institute*, 91, 916–932. doi: 10.1093/jnci/91.11.916

Reblin, M., Birmingham, W. C., Kohlmann, W., & Graff, T. (2018). Support and negation of colorectal cancer risk prevention behaviors: Analysis of spousal discussions. *Psychology, Health & Medicine*, 23, 548–554. doi: 10.1080/ 13548506.2017.1381747

Reblin, M., & Uchino, B. N. (2008). Social and emotional support and its implication for health. *Current Opinion in Psychiatry, 21*, 201–205. doi: 10.1097/YCO.obo13e3282f3ad89

Renkonen-Sinisalo, L., Aarnio, M., Mecklin, J. P., & Jarvinen, H. J. (2000). Surveillance improves survival of colorectal cancer in patients with hereditary nonpolyposis colorectal cancer. *Cancer Detection and Prevention, 24*, 137–142. Retrieved from: www.sciencedirect.com/science/journal/0361090X

Robles, T. F. (2014). Marital quality and health: Implications for marriage in the 21st century. *Current Directions in Psychological Science, 23*(6), 427–432. doi: 10.1177/0963721414549043

Robles, T. F., & Kiecolt-Glaser, J. K. (2003). The physiology of marriage: Pathways to health. *Physiology and Behavior, 79*, 409–416. doi: 10.1016/S0031-9384(03)00160-4

Robles, T. F., Slatcher, R. B., Trombello, J. M., & McGinn, M. M. (2013). Marital quality and health: A meta-analytic review. *Psychological Bulletin, 140*, 140–187. doi: 10.1037/a0031859

Sarma, K. M., Carey, R. N., Kervick, A. A., & Bimpeh, Y. (2013). Psychological factors associated with indices of risky, reckless and cautious driving in a national sample of drivers in the Republic of Ireland. *Accident Analysis and Prevention, 50*, 1226–1235. doi: 10.1016/j.aap.2012.09.020

Seeff, L. C., Nadel, M. R., Klabunde, C. N., Thompson, T., Shapiro, J. A., Vernon, S. W., & Coates, R. J. (2004). Patterns and predictors of colorectal cancer test use in the adult U.S. population. *Cancer, 100*, 2093–2103. doi: 10.1002/cncr.20276

Shaw, E. K., Scott, J. G., & Ferrante, J. M. (2013). The influence of family ties on men's prostate cancer screening, biopsy, and treatment decisions. *American Journal of Men's Health, 7*, 461–471. doi: 10.1177/1557988313480226

Smith, T. W., Cribbet, M. R., Nealey-Moore, J. B., Uchino, B. N., Williams, P. G., Mackenzie, J., & Thayer, J. F. (2011). Matters of the variable heart: Respiratory sinus arrhythmia response to marital interaction and associations with marital quality. *Journal of Personality and Social Psychology, 100*, 103–119. doi: 10.1037/a0021136

Smith, T. W., Uchino, B. N., Bosch, J. A., & Kent, R. G. (2014). Trait hostility is associated with systemic inflammation in married couples: An actor-partner analysis. *Biological Psychology, 102*, 51–53. doi: 10.1016/j.biopsycho.2014.07.005

Song, M., & Giovannucci, E. (2016). Preventable incidence and mortality of carcinoma associated with lifestyle factors among white adults in the United States. *JAMA Oncology, 2*, 1154–1161. doi: 10.1001/jamaoncol.2016.0843.

Stimpson, J. P., Wilson, F. A., Watanabe-Galloway, S., & Peek, M. K. (2012). The effect of marriage on utilization of colorectal endoscopy exam in the United States. *Cancer Epidemiology, 36*, e325-332. doi: 10.1016/j.canep.2012.05.005

Strachan, S. M., Woodgate, J., Brawley, L. R., & Tse, A. (2005). The relationship of self-efficacy and self-identity to long-term maintenance of vigorous physical activity. *Journal of Applied Biobehavioral Research, 10*, 98–112. doi: 10.1111/j.1751–861.2005.tbo0006.x

Tucker, J. S., & Anders, S. L. (2001). Social control of health behaviors in marriage. *Journal of Applied Social Psychology, 31*, 467–485. doi: 10.1111/j. 1559–1816.2001.tbo2051.x

Uchino, B. N. (2004). *Social support and physical health: Understanding the health consequences of our relationships.* New Haven, CT: Yale University Press.

Umberson, D. (1987). Family status and health behaviors: Social control as a dimension of social integration. *Journal of Health and Social Behavior, 28*, 306–319. Retrieved from: http://journals.sagepub.com/loi/hsb

Waite, L. J. (1995). Does marriage matter? *Demography, 32*, 483–507. doi: 10.2307/2061670

Winawer, S. J., Zauber, A. G., Ho, M. N., O'Brien, M. J., Gottlieb, L. S., Sternberg, S. S., ... Stewart, E. T. (1993). Prevention of colorectal cancer by colonoscopic polypectomy. *New England Journal of Medicine, 329*, 1977–1981. doi: 10.1056/NEJM199312303292701

Witte, K., & Allen, M. (2000). A meta-analysis of fear appeals: Implications for effective public health campaigns. *Health Education and Behavior, 27*, 591–615. doi: 10.1177/109019810002700506

Ye, J., Williams, S. D., & Xu, Z. (2009). The association between social networks and colorectal cancer screening in American males and females: Data from the 2005 Health Information National Trends Survey. *Cancer Causes and Control, 20*, 1227–1233. doi: 10.1007/s10552-009-9335-x

2

Stigma, Heteronormative Passing with Health Care Providers, and Partner Health Involvement in Male Same-Sex Couples

STEPHEN M. HAAS

"On top of the fear of lesser care, there's a kind of a guilt – like I'm denying my own relationship because I'm afraid of something [stigma]. And then that makes me angry. So you're dealing with fear, shame, and anger, just all this stuff, and then you've got to worry because that person [provider] is not comfortable ... You have to act as a friend, and not their partner in the hospital room then, right? You can't be holding him, cuddling, and so on. Why would a friend do that?"

(Ryan)

Individuals who are lesbian, gay, bisexual, transgender, or questioning of their sexuality (LGBTQ) continue to experience social stigma, minority stress (Meyer, 1995, 2003), and negative health impacts in US society (Denton, Rostosky, & Danner, 2014; Hatzenbuehler, 2014; Institute of Medicine [IOM], 2011). Labeling someone a "fag," "queer," or "dyke," and phrases such as "That's so gay!" remain severe insults in US society (Nadal, 2013). Learning to adapt and live with social stigma is a basic survival skill for minority groups in societies (Rintamaki & Brashers, 2010). Studies have explored the experiences of LGBTQ persons within social contexts, such as in the workplace (Button, 2004; Spradlin, 1998), in the classroom (Malinksy, 1997), and within athletic teams (Miller, 1998). By and large, however, LGBTQ relationships have remained understudied in the relationship literature throughout the past 20 years (Haas & Whitton, 2015; Clark & Serovich, 1997; Duck & Wood, 1997). This study explores the areas of stigma, heteronormative passing behaviors in health care interactions, and partner health involvement by those in male same-sex romantic relationships, which has received sparse academic attention.

To begin, factors are highlighted that impact self-disclosure of sexual orientation and same-sex relationship status. The concepts of stigma and stigma avoidance (e.g., heteronormative passing behaviors) by LGBTQ persons also are reviewed. Then, findings on stigma, partner health involvement, and passing in health care settings are presented from a mixed-method data collection from long-term male same-sex couples (N = 61). The emergent findings illuminate several same-sex couple issues, such as how involved male partners are in each other's health and health care, and whether or not they are "out" to physicians as a gay male and as being in a long-term same-sex relationship. Also, reasons for enacting heterosexual passing behaviors with health care providers are described. Finally, health care implications of not disclosing sexual orientation or same-sex relationship status and a call for future research are discussed.

SELF-DISCLOSURE AND STIGMA

Decisions to self-disclose personal information are affected by both individual motivations and perceptions of potential reactions from others (Greene, 2009; Petronio, 2002). The relational risks and consequences of self-disclosing a personal characteristic or behavior that may be judged as inappropriate or socially undesirable may result in the attribution of stigma to individuals. Goffman (1963) defined *stigma* as a form of social rejection in which the stigmatized individual is "reduced in our minds from a whole and usual person to a tainted, discounted one" (p. 3) and in which a negatively valenced trait can overshadow other positive traits (p. 5). Stigma, then, taints identity presentation through negative assessments assigned to acts of self-disclosure and image management (Jackson & Mohr, 2016). For the stigmatized, the self may be coconstructed in such a way that the stigmatized characteristic becomes dominant and constrains other aspects of individuals' identities.

Stigma is rooted in communication and interaction with others. Stigmatized individuals may try to avoid being stigmatized if the negative characteristic is not immediately visible or identifiable; for example, with health conditions such as HIV/AIDS, Hepatitis C, autoimmune disorders, and more. *Communication competence*, which involves the "appropriateness and effectiveness" of one's communication skills within particular situations (Rubin, Rubin, & Jordan, 1997, p. 104) comes into play as individuals attempt to achieve their communicative goals and make decisions about which personal characteristics are relevant to a situation. Communication competence and social judgments of what is considered "normal" varies by context and group memberships (Rintamaki & Brashers, 2010). Link and Phelan (2001) defined *normal* as a "shared belief that a person ought to behave in a certain way at a certain time" (p. 81).

What is perceived as normal is often a taken-for-granted assumption within dominant cultural groups (Major & Eccleston, 2005). According to Gramsci (1971), *hegemony* is the process of maintaining the values and beliefs by a dominant group and subverting power and control of minority groups within the dominant culture. Thus, a cyclical process of power and control is established in which the dominant majority acts to disempower minority groups within hierarchical social structures. It is the degree to which the dominant social group is able to control social contexts that defines the majority power over minority groups. Not all minority groups or members may be equally affected by the majority's hegemony; rather, the power of the majority is in assigning negative valence and stigma to control specific contexts. Moreover, stigma is a value judgment that acts as an effective system of hierarchy to support the dominant group's values (Link & Phelan, 2001). Those in the majority reinforce behaviors as "normal" that are judged to be appropriate and communicatively competent within social contexts.

As punishment for lack of communicative competence in conforming to social norms, dominant groups stigmatize and reject minority group individuals. Assigned stigma acts as a further hindrance to minority group members' communicative competence and reinforces cyclical confirmation of stigma. Indeed, stigma is often tied to perceptions of mental health (Meyer, 1995, 2003). In 1973, homosexuality was removed from the American Psychiatric Association's list of mental illnesses, yet LGBTQ individuals continue to battle this stigma. Link and Phelan (2001) assert that stigma can only be enacted through power in conferring five negative components of stigma onto a minority group: (a) labeling, (b) stereotyping, (c) separation, (d) status loss, and (e) discrimination.

IMPRESSION MANAGEMENT, PASSING, AND OTHER ACTS OF STIGMA AVOIDANCE

For stigmatized groups, behavior-altering strategies may be employed to attempt to mask information or characteristics that reveal membership in a negatively valenced reference group. Goffman (1967) labeled these strategies as "impression management." Impression management strategies often encompass a range of behaviors through which an individual attempts to impact others' perceptions of their identity by tailoring his or her image and communication to a situation. Stigmatized individuals may engage in impression management to achieve higher-level social status or access. Major and O'Brien (2005) noted that social access is dependent upon acceptance or denial of presented identities. Goffman (1967) posited that individuals who can hide a stigmatized characteristic may learn over time to be more adept at impression management due to: (a) desire for social access, (b) greater opportunities for practice, and (c) prior experience with the social consequences of stigma. Although stigma avoidance strategies may benefit the stigmatized individual in the short term, impression management strategies reinforce negative group assessments by the dominant group and maintain a status quo that denies the minority group respect and power (Link & Phelan, 2001). Therefore, the stigmatized individual who engages in stigma avoidance and impression management perpetuates hegemony, stigma, and the continued necessity of impression management strategies in future communication interactions for his or her group.

Passing is one specific type of impression management that has been recognized as a stigma avoidance strategy (Goffman, 1963). According to Goffman (1963), passing is a specific set of communicative behaviors employed by stigmatized individuals in an effort to hide a stigmatized characteristic and construct a normative identity. Smart and Wegener (2000) explained that engaging in passing behaviors by subordinate group members can confer benefits and privileges accorded to members of the dominant group, yet can also come at the cost of extra psychological effort and denial of one's "authentic" self, which can lead to psychological distress.

Specific acts of passing can include deliberate manifestations of verbal and nonverbal behaviors to reflect membership in the dominant group (Bolin, 1992; Brown, 1991; Corbett, 1994; Corbin & Strauss, 1985 Edwards, 1996; Jackson & Mohr, 2016; Yep & Pietri, 1999). For example, passing can be accomplished through intentional alteration of adornment (i.e., clothing, hairstyle, jewelry), posture (i.e., legs crossed, back reclined or erect), proxemics (i.e., physical space between communicative partners, amount of contact), kinesics (i.e., gestures, walking patterns), and vocalics (i.e., vocal pitch, speech patterns). Over time, negative reference group members may develop such communicative skill at enacting passing behaviors that these become second nature. Brown (1991) defined *unaware passing* as acts that occur without explicit planning. Goffman (1963) argued that unintentional passing consists of a series of passing behaviors that creates an unaware "natural cycle" of passing (p. 79). An individual who engages in the act of passing is, perhaps without awareness, supporting the dominant group's superior position and power, which can contribute to further disempowerment of their stigmatized identity and group.

PASSING BY LGBTQ INDIVIDUALS

LGBTQ individuals are one stigmatized group that may engage in heteronormative passing behaviors as a means to appear heterosexual and avoid stigma within social contexts. Heteronormative passing may help LGBTQ persons appear communicatively competent and achieve their personal goals in situations, yet it is important to understand the contexts and ramifications that may accompany such actions. Engaging in heteronormative passing requires increased mental and emotional energy to *code switch* (Lumby, 1976), which contributes to higher levels of minority stress in LGBTQ individuals (Meyer, 1995, 2003; Smart & Wegener, 2000). Spradlin (1998) viewed passing not only as an act of stigma avoidance but also as a psychological coping strategy that entails flight from one's own personal identity, leading to self-denial and mental duress. Vargo (1998) addressed several negative outcomes that heteronormative passing may cultivate. He explained:

Remaining in the closet may create or intensify existing identity problems and generate feelings of anxiety, self-loathing, guilt, and depression as a predictable result, especially given the time and energy that one must expend to ensure that the mask does not slip off. (p. xvi)

In addition, Brown (1991) concluded that the decision to enact a LGBTQ identity is dependent not only upon the social environment, but also the individual's own feelings about being LGBTQ. Individuals who are LGBTQ may consider sexual orientation as a private personality characteristic that is not relevant in all social contexts. For instance, Eichberg (1990) explained:

We are brought up by heterosexuals, taught that it is best not to be homosexual (if homosexuality is mentioned at all), and grow up in communities and in a society in which there has been a very clear and pervasive message that being different is bad, and that *"queer"* is the worst kind of different one can be. (p. 12)

Also, Brown (1991) pointed out that LGBTQ individuals' attempts to pass for heterosexual can create an internal dilemma, and even self-loathing, stating:

One paradoxical consequence of passing is that individuals who do so are forced actively or tacitly to agree with expressions of mainstream attitudes toward themselves. This can create feelings of disloyalty and self-contempt which can exacerbate a sense of alienation. (p. 45)

In order to understand the social conditions that lead a LGBTQ individual to feel the need to employ passing behaviors, it is necessary to understand the social contexts in which passing occurs. For example, Spradlin (1998) and McNaught (1993) studied LGBTQ passing in the workplace and assessed several possible threats and perceived needs to pass as heterosexual. As of this writing, LGBTQ individuals can still be fired from their jobs in 28 US states. Among males, workplace threats may manifest in *overcompensating* passing acts that include homophobic or sexist comments, and extreme masculine behaviors that promote heterosexuality as "normal" male behavior (Jome & Tokar, 1998; Miller, 1998). For women, heteronormative passing may include denial of masculine traits and acquiescence to embrace femininity and female submissive roles (Brooks Gardner, 1995; Daley, 1998; Spradlin, 1998; Malinsky, 1997). Other contexts that may encourage heterosexual passing include: education (Malinsky, 1997; Woods & Harbeck, 1991), gender-specific social situations (Brooks Gardner, 1995; Jome & Tokar, 1998; Miller, 1998), and decisions to seek health care (Daley, 1998; McKee, Hayes, & Axiotis, 1994; O'Byrne, & Watts, 2014). In each context, there is both gained privilege from presenting as heterosexual and also personal loss of LGBTQ identity.

LGBTQ PASSING IN HEALTH CARE INTERACTIONS

Only a few studies have identified the phenomenon of passing by LGBTQ individuals within the health care context. For example, McKee, Hayes, and Axiotis (1994) recognized heterosexism in college health delivery; Edwards (1996) found that gay adolescent males expressed a need for heteronormative passing in health care settings; and O'Byrne and Watts (2014) found young gay males may avoid seeking health care because of fear of stigma from health care providers. Finally, Hatzenbuehler (2014) and colleagues highlight the negative health effects of LGBTQ structural stigma within the health care system, particularly mental health care (Hatzenbuehler, McLaughlin, Keyes, & Hasin, 2010).

The limited past research has focused on LGBTQ individuals in health care contexts, and more research is needed; however, studies have not explored the impact of being in a long-term same-sex romantic relationship and passing in health care settings, or how involved male partners are in each other's health and interactions in the health care setting. Research has found that being in a same-sex romantic relationship and being "out" strengthen both LGBTQ identity and a sense of social belonging (Clausell & Roisman, 2009; Haas & Stafford, 1998). Yet, more needs to be understood about health-related issues within same-sex couples. This gap leads to the following research questions:

RQ1: Are male same-sex partners "out" to their health care providers as gay and in a long-term same-sex relationship?

RQ2: How involved are male same-sex partners in each other's personal health and interactions with health care providers?

METHOD

To explore the research questions, an IRB-approved qualitative study was conducted using (a) open-ended surveys ($n = 30$), and (b) a series of nine focus groups ($n = 31$). Gay males in long-term committed romantic relationships ($M = 12.5$ years, $SD = 9.14$) ($R = 8$ months to 37 years) either engaged in a written open-ended survey or participated in a 90-minute focus group discussion about their experiences with health care providers and how involved partners are in each other's health and health care. Mean age was 39 ($R = 19–71$). Race/ethnicity was primarily Caucasian (82%), followed by Hispanic (10%), and African American (8%). All were educated: bachelor's degree (64%), master's degree (18%), or a professional degree (18%). A majority (84%) had combined household incomes of $75,000 or greater.

Data were analyzed for commonalities through a process consistent with constant comparison across the qualitative data (Glaser & Strauss,

1967). Focus group discussions were transcribed verbatim and were reviewed for audibility and accuracy against the recordings (Lincoln & Guba, 1985). All transcripts were evaluated to be of high quality. Next, open-ended survey responses and focus group transcripts were analyzed for *meaning units*. Meaning units capture a single concept or issue. A meaning unit could be a word, phrase, sentence, or several sentences. First, open coding was used to identify meaning units within the data. Then, coded meaning units were organized into subcategories based on concept similarity. Thus, the thematic findings were derived inductively from the data. Through a process of axial coding, subcategories and categories were combined into larger superordinate categories. As patterns emerged, appropriateness of fit of the thematic structure to explain the data was compared to deviant cases within the data (i.e., dissimilar category instances are either reconciled or become a new category) until no new categories arose and saturation had occurred (Strauss & Corbin, 1990). A written analysis explaining the themes and a discussion of study findings was then undertaken. Emergent themes were derived across participant responses, and exemplar quotes were presented as evidence of validity in representing the lived experiences. All participant names presented in this manuscript have been replaced with pseudonyms to ensure anonymity.

FINDINGS

In exploring RQ1, "Are male same-sex partners 'out' to their health care providers as gay and in a long-term same-sex relationship?," a range of experiences were reported regarding perceptions of stigma in interactions with health care providers when individuals were "out" as gay and in a same-sex relationship. Only one-third of the participants reported that they were "out" to their primary care physician–both as a gay male and in a same-sex relationship. These individuals described feeling low levels of stigma from their health care providers. One factor that affected many of these participants' experiences was that they had actively sought out a gay physician. These individuals explained that either through their social networks or through LGBTQ city guides that included health care providers, they found a primary care physician who is either gay or gay-friendly, which increased their openness to and comfort in "coming out" during their health care interactions.

The majority, however, sought health care from providers they assumed to be heterosexual, and these individuals reported a range of sexual orientation disclosures and reported experiencing stigma. Some were not "out" to their providers, and believed sexual orientation was their private information. Many reported reasons that impacted their decision not to disclose their sexual orientation and to engage in heteronormative passing with their health care providers. Three main themes emerged that capture these reasons and the range of behaviors described in enacting passing.

Reasons for Engaging in Heteronormative Passing Behaviors

Male partners from these long-term same-sex romantic relationships described three primary reasons for engaging in heteronormative passing communication behaviors: (a) a fear of stigma and receiving poor health care, (b) self-assessed relevance of sexual orientation to the health problem, and (c) perceptions of provider comfort level with LGBTQ people. The decision to self-disclose a gay male identity and whether one is in a same-sex relationship relied on a combination of these three influences. Exemplar quotes will be used to give participants voice in explaining these three domains.

Fear of stigma and receiving lesser care. The most common influence on decisions to engage in heteronormative passing was a fear of being stigmatized as LGBTQ and the potential for receiving lesser care. Two-thirds of the sample described perceptions that gay stigma could negatively impact their care, or they had actually experienced stigma and discrimination for being gay from health care providers. For example, when participants were asked if they had ever tried to "pass" as heterosexual with health care providers, Conner explained:

Definitely, out of fear of being discriminated against, or getting bad treatment. You never know about a doctor's personal feelings, let alone his or her ability to stay objective in the office, and it's a very dangerous position in which to put yourself . . . bad treatment, verbal abuse, or whatever.

Similarly, Adam described using passing as a communicative defense mechanism:

At the beginning, I always try to pass as heterosexual because of the social implications or possible bias that I can encounter. For me, it [passing] is a way to protect myself against any possible kind of bias and try to get good medical treatment.

Thomas asserted, "I was protecting myself from an uncomfortable situation or biased health care," and Jason states, "Well, there is a genuine fear often that one will receive bad health care [as a result of expressing a LGBTQ identity]. It is statistically proven that minorities receive worse health care." Also, Juan said, "I have to worry about how I'll be treated because of it [expression of a LGBTQ identity]." Robert described not self-disclosing his sexual orientation this way:

It keeps a wall up between you and the health care provider, it's sort of analogous to asthma and breathing–less air–less communication. The doctor, nurse, or whoever will remain a stranger in my mind. It's safer to assume that, if they assume you're straight. You don't know if they're open-minded enough as to tolerate you not being straight, so you stay in the closet, and sort of give up on any real conversation beyond the medical stuff.

Furthermore, some participants described attempts to change the topic or control the conversation to avoid self-disclosure of sexual orientation out of fear of receiving a lower standard of care. These sentiments of fear can accumulate over time, and as a result, passing for heterosexual can become a defensive communicative act in which hiding one's sexual orientation is accepted and the self is reconstructed in order to obtain the equal access to health care services as heterosexuals.

There also were some participants who expressed a fear of poor treatment because they had experienced past discrimination or inferior health care. Roughly half of the participants reported past experiences of discrimination and fear-inducing incidents. For example, as Mitch explained:

I went to my primary care physician and told him, "I've got poison ivy. I need something. It's pretty bad." He looked at it and said, "You're not into any funny business, are you?" That was his way of saying, "Do you have sex with men?" I obviously played dumb, like, "I don't know what you mean by 'funny business,'" and he goes, "Do you have sex with men?" I said, "Yeah, I'm gay." He said, "Well then, this is not poison ivy, this is – what's the chickenpox version – shingles. This is shingles. You have to have an HIV test immediately." He just completely lost his mind on what he normally would have done, and did something completely different. He sent me out of that office in a panic. I spent two weeks in despair thinking I was HIV positive and waiting for the test results. Turns out, it was poison ivy. I'm not HIV positive. I left that doctor's care after this.

Also, Blake described experiencing discrimination when his partner was hospitalized:

My partner was hospitalized with meningitis, which is very serious. The staff would not let me back to be with him, even though we've been together for 10 years. Eventually his mother came, and she told them to let me back. I don't know what I would have done if she lived in another city. It was extremely upsetting.

Larry, who disclosed his sexual orientation on a dental intake form, recalled, "A dental hygienist made negative comments and refused to work on my teeth. The dentist was very professional, asked her to leave, and took care of the cleaning himself." Another participant, Charles, described an incident when his partner had surgery. When asking how his partner was doing in the recovery room, he explained:

The surgical nurse says, "Let me talk to him." She says, "Are you related to him?" I said, "I'm his partner." She said, "I'm sorry, we can't release information to anyone but next of kin." I said, "Well, if you check your records, you'll find I'm his health care surrogate, and I think you should talk to me." . . . . I didn't find out until much later that she'd been running around ranting and raving in the recovery room after that, saying, "I think I've got an [HIV] exposure risk here." This was at a university medical center.

Because of perceived risk, or actual received acts of discrimination, fear of lesser care was the predominant reason reported for engaging in heteronormative passing behaviors with health care providers.

Relevance of sexual orientation to the health problem. A second reason participants provided to judge the necessity of engaging in heteronormative passing with health care providers was the perceived relevance of sexual orientation to their health problem. More than half of participants used terms such as "relevant," "pertinent," or "necessary" to describe their decision-making process regarding whether to conceal or reveal their sexual orientation in health care interactions. Health care settings were one context in which these same-sex relationship partners described making conscious decisions about whether or not to self-disclose being gay or in a same-sex relationship. For instance, Tony stated, "It depends what I am in for, if it's just a cold who cares … but my gastro-oncologist, he knows." Dexter said, "I'm not 'out' to my dentist. It's not relevant, and doesn't come up." Thus, male same-sex partners in this sample believed their sexual orientation and relationship may or may not be relevant to a health issue.

Sexual orientation was most often disclosed if HIV testing or sexually transmitted infection (STI) was the reason for seeking health care. Several participants who sought testing for HIV, hepatitis, or other STIs described expressing their sexual orientation with providers because they assessed it to be relevant. For example, Trevor stated, "I told my physician when I 'came out' and started to be sexually active. I've told them because of HIV." Also, Nick explained,

After a few years, I was like, 'I need to be honest with this man' ["come out" to the provider] because I'm not serving myself any good by holding this back. When I go get a physical, I get blood work, and now I always order up the full spectrum because I think the default blood work does not include HIV testing. You always have to specify that, and he always looks at me, but I don't care, I want a full report.

Overall, however, there was little acknowledgment of potential negative health implications from omitting one's sexual orientation in a health care interview, even though research indicates gay males are at higher risk for some health conditions such as depression, suicide, eating disorders, substance use/misuse, and STIs (IOM, 2011; Lee, 2000). Participants also did not discuss whether or not their physician would make a similar judgment regarding relevance of sexual orientation to their health problem. Regardless, these participants described feeling comfortable with their self-assessments of relevance and their decisions to withhold sexual orientation information. Some also talked about using different health clinics for gay-related issues. For instance, Matt explained, "I use two different places, my family clinic for regular things, and then a gay clinic for other things like STD worries, etc." This is an example of both a physical and ideological separation between "regular health care are" and "gay-related care." The very use of terms such as *regular* and *gay* by participants supports adoption of heteronormative stigma assumptions in viewing these as different types of health care themselves.

Comfort level of the provider. While partners in these same-sex relationships were perhaps not fully aware of the implications of passing on their health care, they were concerned with their provider's comfort level with LGBTQ individuals. The majority stated that a provider's comfort with LGBTQ patients was never explicitly discussed in a medical interview. Instead, participants made their own appraisals of their provider's comfort level based on verbal or nonverbal cues in deciding whether or not to broach the subject of sexual orientation. Some described experiences in which they disclosed their sexual orientation and were presented with provider discomfort. For example, Todd explained, "It's really impossible to gauge how even the closest people to you will react, parents, best friends, siblings, never mind a doctor you've never met before." Most focused on negative provider reactions that patients had received after expressing a LGBTQ identity. For instance, Jake stated, "I was treated for an STD. Upon identifying myself as homosexual, I felt as though the doctor disapproved, although he said he did not care. Needless to say, I never returned to that doctor." Dillon recalled, "Once, while I was getting a blood test, the doctor said, 'Don't worry, only gay people contract AIDS.'" The implicit heterosexist assumption by this provider was that this patient (and perhaps no patient of his) could be LGBTQ. As a result of this comment, Dillon opted to continue passing as heterosexual while under this physician's care. Another participant, Karl, who was "out" to his doctor, explained:

He's fine when it comes to issues like a cold or normal, small things. On the other hand, he seems almost irritated when the visit seems to be around a sexual orientation issue. This is all based on perception, but he is hard to figure out which is sometimes a pain when going to the doctor because that is not what you want to worry about.

Here, Karl highlights the extra effort that must be exerted to assess provider acceptance or discomfort with LGBTQ patients.

Some participants admitted not mentioning that they are in a same-sex romantic relationship to avoid discomfort with physicians. For example, Andrew explained, "I would leave any mention of a partner out [of the health care setting] in order to avoid being uncomfortable." Two-thirds of participants stated they engage in casual rapport building conversations with their provider, but those topics are superficial in nature (e.g., weather, sports), and they avoided mention of their same-sex relationship. A few mentioned engaging in heteronormative code switching by changing the pronouns used to refer to their male partner as a female. For instance, Earl employed pronoun changes when discussing his partner with health care providers, stating,

"If I have problems of a sexual nature, I have made references to a girlfriend so the doctor doesn't ask too many questions." And Todd stated, "If a question is asked about my girlfriend or sex life, I usually change the subject or make a joke, and then change the subject." Jake stated, "I have talked around [sexual orientation] issues." Also, Alex admitted, "When I see doctors, I've left out a lot of my [gay] life."

Several other participants reported making allusions to being single despite being in a long-term same-sex relationship. Still others described replying "no" if directly asked if one is gay, and marking "single" on insurance and intake forms. Some also mentioned altering their nonverbal behaviors in order to pass as heterosexual; for instance, Andrew explains:

An audible lowering of my voice, hands stay down at my side, I try not to show too much emotion in my voice and facial features. While I generally retain my usual wit and charm, I try to filter it a little for any excess flamboyance . . . You learn how to bend the truth a little . . . it's sort of awful sometimes, but in general it's tolerable.

Similarly, Collin described changing his nonverbal behavior to pass as heterosexual, stating, "I try to hide my mannerisms, hand movements." Here, the presentation of a heterosexual identity is linked to nonverbal presentation behaviors rather than verbal strategies. This forfeit of an open gay identity can create a false perception of intimacy between the provider and patient which may be communicatively competent in achieving the goal of good health services, but also perpetuates the stigma that a gay sexual orientation is "abnormal."

Involvement in Partners' Health

In exploring RQ2, "How involved are male same-sex partners in each other's personal health and interactions with health care providers?," male same-sex partners in this study were found to describe a continuum of partner health involvement within their relationships, ranging from autonomy over managing their health to high involvement in their partner's health (e.g., attending physician appointments together). Three-fourths reported high autonomy concerning their personal health management and interactions with health care providers. Most participants described partners as having independence related to their health. One factor that may impact high health autonomy within male same-sex relationships is the influence of *hegemonic masculinity* (Connell, 1995; Connell & Messerschmidt, 2005; Johansson & Ottemo, 2015). Hegemonic masculinity involves male gender socialization and patriarchal power structure reinforcement of predominant male heterosexual norms and stereotypes that promote males as psychologically and physically dominant, self-reliant, emotionally detached, aggressive or violent, and enacting machismo (Connell, 1995; Connell & Messerschmidt, 2005). Health self-care ideals are in line with these types of masculinity principles.

Presence of masculine ideals of autonomy and independence were expressed by many of the participants and were described as playing a role in how involved partners are in each other's health. Partners described making health suggestions and influencing each other's health behaviors, but the majority of participants reported principles of health independence dominating their relationships. For example, Eli explained, "For our relationship, mostly, each person gets to make their own health choices. I don't think either of us could tell the other what to do. We can offer suggestions." Charles stated, "I don't tell him what to do. He's basically in charge of his own workouts and I'm in charge of my own workouts." Drake said, "We try and remind each other about things, like staying hydrated, but we don't impose on each other. We just let each other do what they wanna do." Pierce described his relationship philosophy by saying, "'I want you to do what you wanna do. I'm gonna do what I wanna do, and hopefully, those things match up, and continue to match you over time' . . . He's not in a relationship with me for me to keep him controlled . . .. I just learned pretty quickly, just don't try to back him into anything. I don't wanna be backed into anything, either."

When participants were asked if there are health rules they impose on each other in their relationship, Colin stated, "Neither of us is the police, so we don't police each other. We have no accountability whatsoever, so they're kind of said, but they're never enforced by any means or anything." Sam asserted, "I think we influence each other, but we don't actively tell each other, 'No, you shouldn't be eating that.' Or, 'You shouldn't be doing that.'" And Rex stated, "I think it's equal as far as encouraging to go to the doctor – time for your annual appointment, go to the dermatologist, that kinda stuff. I think that feels equal between both of us." Andy also explained that separate health insurance (because they are not married) has an influence, "We kind of operate independently, I think. Maybe part of that is because, you know, he's on his insurance; he has his own dental insurance, that kind of stuff, and I have mine. I take care of myself. If I need a checkup, he may not even know that I went, or something like that. I mean, most of the time, I can't think of a time when he didn't know, but I mean, I wouldn't know if he went, necessarily, unless he told me so."

Male partners in this sample reported enacting masculine characteristics of self-reliance and personal control over their own health with little partner oversight, which may be influenced by masculine ideals. The only time partners did become temporarily more involved was if one partner had a health issue or crisis arise, such as an emergency room visit, surgery, or hospitalization. In other words, unless an acute health problem occurred, self-care and self-management of one's health was predominant. Only two individuals described being high monitors of their partner's health; for example, overseeing their partner's diet, exercise regimen, physician appointment scheduling, and the like. These individuals were in a minority in this sample. Most participants described relational dynamics based in health autonomy. The current findings provide initial evidence that the combination of masculinity, health autonomy, and self-care may be unique relational characteristics that impact male same-sex couples' involvement in their partner's health and health care.

DISCUSSION

For the majority, heteronormative passing was perceived as a necessary and effective communicative strategy to ensure positive health care experiences and adequate health care. Three predominant themes emerged as reasons for engaging in heteronormative passing behaviors in the health care setting: a) fear of lesser care, b) perceived relevance of sexual orientation to the health concern, and c) perceived physician discomfort with LGBTQ patients/health issues. Fear of lesser care was the most mentioned reason for engaging in heteronormative passing behaviors. Fears were grounded in perceptions of potential stigma or actual past discrimination experiences. These findings indicate that although LGBTQ issues have progressed (e.g., legal same-sex marriage; Gates, 2015), LGBTQ stigma persists in US society. All participants were concerned about the potential of receiving lesser health care, and took actions to either find a gay-friendly physician or enacted heteronormative passing.

Fear of lesser care due to a LGBTQ identity could be addressed through increased health care provider training. In general, participants in this study indicated that passing for heterosexual was taxing on their mental health, which has been found in prior studies (Denton, Rostosky, & Danner, 2014). In fact, passing can affect the mental health of those patients who employ it as a strategy (Meyer, 1995, 2003). The decision of whether or not to pass as heterosexual can induce high stress and anxiety, similar to the stress associated with concealing a secret (Smart & Wegener, 2000). If one does self-disclose a LGBTQ identity, additional situational monitoring and mental effort may be required in subsequent interactions with those health care providers to ensure good health care.

Fear of rejection and lesser care also was mentioned by a few participants as a reason to avoid seeking health care until a health problem has become very severe, as has been found in previous studies (Lee, 2000). Another possibility is that this fear can lead patients to believe that disclosing a LGBGTQ identity invalidates them as a person, and thus are knowingly conferring stigma on themselves. This is a difficult decision when LGBTQ individuals are seeking health care. Fear of stigma was prevalent for the majority. LGBTQ patients need to examine their identity and communication behaviors, and consider how interactions with providers may be impacting their health.

In general, heterosexuals often view homosexuality as the antithesis of masculinity (Dowsett, Williams, Ventunea, & Carballo-Diéguez, 2008). This creates a paradox for gay men who are socialized into the cultural norms of hegemonic masculinity (Kahn, Goddard, & Coy, 2013), and yet must reconcile their sexual attraction to males within these norms (Lanzieri & Hildebrandt, 2011). This creates the likelihood that male same-sex couples retain some aspects of hegemonic masculinity, and yet may alter others. For instance, in an investigation of same-sex versus different-sex couples' health relational roles, Liu, Reczek, and Brown (2013) found that females in opposite-sex couples tended to take on a role of "health expert" and oversaw the health of both partners, yet they found in male same-sex couples that neither partner was more dominant in overseeing health-related issues within their relationships. Lui et al. (2013) posited that norms of hypermasculinity may be operating, and the current study findings also support the presence of egalitarian, masculinity-based relational dynamics.

Finally, some participants did report having satisfying interactions with their providers and offered prescriptions for effective interactions. Overall, participants were looking for providers who are open and accepting. Several suggestions for how providers could improve interactions with LGBTQ patients were offered, such as: (a) expressing an open and accepting demeanor, (b) directly asking about sexual orientation and explaining the relevance to certain health conditions, and (c) informing patients about LGBTQ-specific health risks. Providers could increase their knowledge of LGBTQ health by creating opportunities for themselves to interact with LGBTQ individuals to learn how to tailor their patient care for LGBTQ patients. Physician efforts should invite dialogue. Other suggestions included placing an inclusive non-discrimination clause in a visible place in the waiting room, including more open-ended questions about sexual activity, gender identity, and relationship status on intake forms, and providing LGBTQ interest magazines in the waiting room as ways to suggest an open and accepting environment.

Limitations

This study has limitations. First, the sample was exclusively gay male, predominantly white, educated, and middle-to-upper class. Minority group recruitment is challenging, and subgroups more so (e.g., long-term same-sex couples; and subgroups within this subgroup such as lesbian, bisexual, transgender, and racial or economic differences). Still, future research should continue to attempt to access and recruit diverse representation within populations. Second, the findings from this study are exploratory and are not generalizable beyond this sample. The strength of qualitative research is its depth of insight into people's lived experiences. Validity is heightened as readers are exposed to participants' lives, concerns, and issues through representative quotes that capture common themes. Yet, same-sex couples remain understudied in the literature. Future studies are needed to continue to explore relational dynamics and issues in LGBTQ relationships.

CONCLUSION

The decision to self-disclose a LGBTQ identity and same-sex relationship can have an impact on health care interactions. Future research on fear of lesser care among LGBTQ patients, and perceiving the need to enact heteronormative passing behaviors to ensure quality health care are needed. Also, studies that explore the implementation of medical association suggestions for creating a LGBTQ-friendly medical practice (AMA, 2017) should be pursued. This study serves as a call to increase research on LGBTQ individuals' and same-sex couples' experiences within the health care setting.

REFERENCES

American Medical Association (AMA). (2017). Creating an LGBTQ-friendly practice. Retrieved from: https://www.ama-assn.org/delivering-care/creating-lgbtq-friendly -practice, May 25, 2017.

Bolin, A. (1992). Coming of age among transsexuals. In T. L. Whitehead & B. V. Reid (Eds.), *Gender constructs and social issues* (pp. 13–39). Urbana, IL: University of Illinois Press.

Brooks Gardner, C. (1995). *Passing by: Gender and public harassment.* Berkeley, CA: University of California Press.

Brown, P. (1991). Passing: Difference in our public and private self. *Journal of Multicultural Social Work, 1,* 33–50. doi: 10.1300/J285v01n02_3

Button, S. B. (2004). Identity management strategies used by lesbian and gay employees: A quantitative investigation. *Group & Organization Management, 29,* 470–494. doi: 10.1177/1059601103257417

Clark, W. M., & Serovich, J. M. (1997). Twenty years and still in the dark? Content analysis of articles pertaining to gay, lesbian, and bisexual issues in marriage and family therapy journals. *Journal of Marital and Family Therapy, 23,* 239–253. doi: 10.1111/j.1752–0606.1997.tb01034.x

Clausell, E., & Roisman, G. I. (2009). Outness, big five personality traits, and same-sex relationship quality. *Journal of Social and Personal Relationships, 26,* 211–226. doi: 10.1177/0265407509106711

Connell, R. W. (1995). *Masculinities.* Cambridge, MA: Polity Press.

Connell, R. W., & Messerschmidt, J. W. (2005). Hegemonic masculinity: Rethinking the concept. *Gender and Society, 19,* 829–859. doi: 10.1177/0891243205278639

Corbett, J. (1994). A proud label: Exploring the relationship between disability and gay pride. *Disability & Society, 9,* 343–357. doi: 10.1080/09687599466780381

Corbin, J., & Strauss, A. (1985). Managing chronic illness at home: Three lines of work. *Qualitative Sociology, 8,* 224–247. doi: 10.1007/BF00989485

Daley, A. (1998). Lesbian invisibility in health care services: Heterosexual hegemony and strategies for change. *Canadian Social Work Review, 15*, 57–71. Retrieved from: http://www.jstor.org/stable/41669660

Denton, F. N., Rostosky, S. S., & Danner, F. (2014). Stigma-related stressors, coping self-efficacy, and physical health in lesbian, gay, and bisexual individuals. *Journal of Counseling Psychology, 61*, 383–391. doi: 10.1037/a0036707

Dowsett, G. W., Williams, H., Ventunea, A., & Carballo-Diéguez, A. (2008). "Taking it like a man": Masculinity and barebacking online. *Sexualities, 1*, 121–141. doi: 10.1177/1363460707085467

Duck, S. W., & Wood, J. T. (1995). Off the beaten track: New shores for relationship research. In S. W. Duck & J. T. Wood (Eds.), *Understudied relationships: Off the beaten track* (pp. 1–21). Thousand Oaks, CA: Sage.

Edwards, W. J. (1996). A sociological analysis of an in/visible minority group: Male adolescent homosexuals. *Youth & Society, 27*, 334–355. doi: 10.1177/0044118X96027003004

Eichberg, R. (1990). *Coming out, an act of love: An inspiring call to action for gay men, lesbians, and those who care.* New York, NY: Plume.

Gates, G. J. (2015). Marriage and family: LGBT individuals and same-sex couples. *The Future of Children, 25*, 67–87. doi: 10.1353/foc.2015.0013

Glaser, B., & Strauss, A. (1967). *The discovery of grounded theory: Strategies for qualitative research.* Chicago, IL: Aldine.

Goffman, E. (1963). *Stigma: Notes on the management of spoiled identity.* Englewood Cliffs, NJ: Prentice Hall.

Goffman, E. (1967). *Interaction ritual: Essays on face-to-face behavior.* Garden City, NY: Anchor Books.

Gramsci, A. (1971). Selections from the prison notebooks. In Q. Hoare & G. N. Smith (Eds.), *Selections from the prison notebooks of Antonio Gramsci* (p. 328). New York, NY: International Publishers.

Greene, K. (2009). An integrated model of health disclosure decision-making. In W. A. Afifi & T. D. Afifi (Eds.), *Uncertainty, information management, and disclosure decisions* (pp. 226–253). New York, NY: Routledge.

Haas, S. M., & Stafford, L. (1998). An initial examination of maintenance behaviors in gay and lesbian relationships. *Journal of Social and Personal Relationships, 15*, 846–855. doi: 10.1177/0265407598156008

Haas, S. M., & Whitton, S. (2015). The significance of living together and importance of marriage in same-sex couples. *Journal of Homosexuality, 62*, 1241–1263. doi: 10.1080/00918369.2015.1037137

Hatzenbuehler, M. L., McLaughlin, K. A., Keyes, K. M., & Hasin, D. S. (2010). The impact of institutional discrimination on psychiatric disorders in lesbian, gay, and bisexual populations: A prospective study. *American Journal of Public Health, 100*, 452–459. doi: 10.2105/AJPH.2009.168815

Hatzenbuehler, M. L. (2014). Structural stigma and the health of lesbian, gay, and bisexual populations. *Current Directions in Psychological Science, 23*, 127–132. doi: 10.1177/0963721414523775

Institute of Medicine (IOM). (2011). *The health of lesbian, gay, bisexual, and transgender people: Building a foundation for better understanding.* Washington, DC: National Academies Press.

Jackson, S. D., & Mohr, J. J. (2016). Conceptualizing the closet: Differentiating stigma concealment and nondisclosure processes. *Psychology of Sexual Orientation and Gender Diversity, 3*, 80–92. doi: 10.1037/sgd0000147

Johansson, T., & Ottemo, A. (2015). Ruptures in hegemonic masculinity: The dialectic between ideology and utopia. *Journal of Gender Studies, 24,* 192–206. doi: 10.1080/09589236.2013.812514

Jome, L. M., & Tokar, D. M. (1998). Dimensions of masculinity and major choice traditionally. *Journal of Vocational Behavior, 52,* 120–134. doi: 10.1006/jvbe. 1996. 1571

Kahn, J. S., Goddard, L., & Coy, J. M. (2013). Gay men and drag: Dialogical resistance to hegemonic masculinity. *Culture & Psychology, 19,* 139–162. doi: 10.1177/1354067X12464984

Lanzieri, N., & Hildebrandt, T. (2011). Using hegemonic masculinity to explain gay male attraction to muscular and athletic men. *Journal of Homosexuality, 58,* 275–293. doi: 10.1080/00918369.2011.540184

Lee, R. (2000). Health care problems of lesbian, gay, bisexual, and transgender patients. *Western Journal of Medicine, 172,* 403–408. Retrieved from: https://www .ncbi.nlm.nih.gov/pmc/journals/183/

Lincoln, Y. S., & Guba, E. G. (1985). *Naturalistic inquiry.* Beverly Hills, CA: Sage.

Link, B. G., & Phelan, J. C. (2001). Conceptualizing stigma. *Annual Review of Sociology, 27,* 363–385. doi: 10.1146/annurev.soc.27.1.363rg/10.1146/annurev .soc.27.1.363

Liu, H., Reczek, C., & Brown, D. (2013). Same-sex cohabitors and health: The role of race-ethnicity, gender, and socioeconomic status. *Journal of Health and Social Behavior, 54,* 25–45. doi: 10.1177/0022146512468280

Lumby, M. E. (1976). Code switching and sexual orientation: A test of Bernstein's sociolinguistic theory. *Journal of Homosexuality, 1,* 383–399. doi: 10.1300/J082v01n04_03

Major, B., & Eccleston, C. P. (2005). Stigma and social exclusion. In D. Abrams, M. A. Hogg, & J. Marques (Eds.), *Social psychology of inclusion and exclusion* (pp. 63–88). New York, NY: Psychology Press.

Major, B., & O'Brien, L. T. (2005). The social psychology of stigma. *Annual Review of Psychology, 56,* 393–421. doi: 10.1146/annurev.psych.56.091103.070137

Malinsky, K. P. (1997). Learning to be invisible: Female sexual minority students in America's public high schools. *Journal of Gay & Lesbian Social Services, 7,* 35–50.

Martin, J. I., & Knox, J. (1997). Self-esteem instability and its implications for HIV prevention among gay men. *Health & Social Work, 22,* 264–273. doi: 10.1300/J041v07n04_03

McKee, M. B., Hayes, S. F., & Axiotis, R. A. (1994). Challenging heterosexism in college health service delivery. *Journal of American College Health, 42,* 211–216. doi: 10.1080/07448481.1994.993846

McNaught, B. (1993). *Gay issues in the workplace.* New York, NY: St. Martin's Press.

Meyer, I. H. (1995). Minority stress and mental health in gay men. *Journal of Health and Social Behavior, 36,* 38–56. http://www.jstor.org/stable/2137286

Meyer, I. H. (2003). Prejudice, social stress, and mental health in lesbian, gay, and bisexual populations: Conceptual issues and research evidence. *Psychological Bulletin, 129,* 674–697. doi: 10.1037/0033-2909.129.5.674

Miller, T. (1998). Commodifying the male body: Problematizing hegemonic masculinity? *Journal of Sport & Social Issues, 22,* 431–477. doi: 10.1177/019372398022004007

Nadal, K. L. (2013). *That's so gay! Microaggressions and the lesbian, gay, bisexual, transgender community.* Washington, DC; American Psychological Association.

O'Byrne, P., & Watts, J. (2014). Include, differentiate, manage: Gay male youth, stigma, and healthcare utilization. *Nursing Inquiry, 21*, 20–29. doi: 10.1111/nin.12014

Petronio, S. (2002). *Boundaries of privacy: Dialectics of disclosure*. New York, NY: State University of New York Press.

Rintamaki, L., & Brashers, D. E. (2010). Stigma and intergroup communication. In H. Giles, S. Reid, & J. Harwood (Eds.), *The dyamics of intergroup communication* (pp. 155–166). New York, NY: Peter Lang.

Rubin, R. B., Rubin, A. M., & Jordan, F. F. (1997). Effects of instruction on communication apprehension and communication competence. *Communication Education, 46*, 104–114. doi: 10.1080/03634529709379080

Smart, L., & Wegner, D. M. (2000). The hidden costs of hidden stigma. In T. F. Heatherton, R. E. Kleck, M. R. Hebl, & J. G. Hull (Eds.), *The social psychology of stigma* (pp. 220–242). New York, NY; Guliford Press.

Spradlin, A. L. (1998). The price of passing: A lesbian perspective on authenticity in organizations. *Management Communication Quarterly, 11*, 598–605. doi: 10.1177/0893318998114006

Strauss. A., & Corbin, J. (1990). *Basics of qualitative research: Grounded theory procedures and techniques*. Thousand Oaks, CA: Sage.

Vargo, M. E. (1998). *Acts of disclosure: The coming-out process of contemporary gay men*. Binghamton, NY: Haworth Press.

Woods, S. E., & Harbeck, K. M. (1991). Living in two worlds: The identity management strategies used by lesbian physical educators. *Journal of Homosexuality, 22*, 141–166. doi: 10.1300/J082v22n03_06

Yep, A., & Pietri, M. (1999). In their own words: Communication and the politics of HIV education for transgenders and transsexuals in Los Angeles. In W. N. Elwood (Ed.), *Power in blood: A handbook on AIDS, politics, and communication* (pp. 199–213). Mahwah, NJ: Lawrence Erlbaum Associates, Inc.

3

"Let's Take a Walk": Relationship Maintenance and Health Communication in Romantic Relationships

The expression "Let's take a walk" can mean many things. It could be an invitation to spend quality time together with one's partner. It could also reflect one's support-seeking communication in service of achieving health goals. Similarly, it could be meant to encourage one's partner to be healthy. All of these motives reflect the fact that people's health is inextricably linked to their involvement in relationships (House, Landis, & Umberson, 1988), particularly their romantic relationships (Kiecolt-Glaser & Newton, 2001). Moreover, these different motives illustrate the mutual influence that exists between partners in these relationships (Thibaut & Kelley, 1959).

Couples often try to capitalize on this inherent influence through their expression of health-related social control. That is, people in a relationship enact health-related social control to encourage their partner to adopt healthier behaviors (Lewis & Rook, 1999). This expression of influence is particularly salient in the context of diet and exercise, as these adaptable lifestyle factors are linked to being overweight or obese when poor choices are made (Miller, Koceja, & Hamilton, 1997). Given that approximately 69% of US adults are currently considered overweight or obese, and that obesity is related to conditions such as type 2 diabetes, hypertension, cardiovascular disease, and cancer (Poirier et al., 2006), it has become increasingly important to examine romantic partners as a potential point of intervention in healthy behavior change.

Research on couples' health communication includes social control and social support (Burke & Segrin, 2014), yet there is a limited focus on relationship maintenance as a form of relationship-sustaining communication. Just as health communication is ongoing in relationships (Butterfield & Lewis, 2002), relationship maintenance is an ongoing relational process enacted in the service of relational continuity (Canary & Zelley, 2000). Consequently, this study employed the relationship maintenance framework in conjunction with social control to examine the potential associations among relationship maintenance, diet- and exercise-related social control, and diet- and exercise-related social support in romantic relationships.

Relationship maintenance is a routine relational behavior that includes communicating positivity, openness, assurances, and sharing tasks and social networks in order to promote relationship quality and sustain relationships (Stafford & Canary, 1991). This study focused on positivity, openness, and assurances, specifically, as these behaviors are common in established relationships (Stafford & Canary, 1991; Guerrero, Eloy, & Wabnik, 1993) and are indicative of interactions in romantic relationships in particular (Canary et al., 1993). *Positivity* connotes optimism and courtesy on the part of partners; partners who engage in *openness* share their thoughts and feelings; and *assurances* signal partners' desire to continue the relationship in the future (Stafford & Canary, 1991). Given the relational focus of these forms of maintenance, they might be especially salient in the context of partners' health promotion, which was the focus of the current study.

Relationships are not self-sustaining; they require attention and continuous maintenance (Canary & Zelley, 2000). As relational partners become interdependent, their maintenance activities stabilize and become normative, prorelational expressions of their desire to continue the relationship (Dindia & Baxter, 1987). Thus, it is not surprising that relationship maintenance is a powerful predictor of proximal (Dainton, 2000) and longitudinal marital satisfaction (Weigel & Ballard-Reisch, 2001), as well as predicting other relationship characteristics, such as liking and commitment (Canary, Stafford, & Semic, 2002). Beyond these outcomes, relationship maintenance is also linked to relationship equity. Indeed, people in equitable relationships report a greater engagement with positive relationship maintenance behaviors (Messman, Canary, & Hause, 2000), as well as greater relationship satisfaction, than people in inequitable relationships (Stafford & Canary, 2006).

The cognitive calculus inherent within evaluating contributions to relationship maintenance illustrates the interactional nature of relationship maintenance, wherein both partners influence each other's relational perceptions and outcomes. Considering that individuals' enactment of prosocial relationship maintenance reflects their investment in and commitment to their partner and their desire to maintain their relationship (Canary & Stafford, 1992), it is possible that this effect carries over into the realm of relational health communication and influence as well. Although relationship maintenance has been examined in conjunction with a variety of topics including relationship equity (Canary & Stafford, 1992), interdependence (Stafford & Canary, 2006), relationship types (Canary et al., 1993), relational expectations and satisfaction (Dainton, 2000), and relational characteristics

(Canary et al., 2002), the potential overlap with health communication has largely been ignored in the literature.

RELATIONSHIP MAINTENANCE AND HEALTH COMMUNICATION

Similar to relationship maintenance, health-related communication and influence are ongoing in relationships (Lewis & Butterfield, 2007), demonstrating that they may co-occur when it comes to partners facing health issues in relationships. Indeed, one study on relationship maintenance in the context of weight loss surgery found that open communication was a crucial element of navigating the changes and relational issues associated with participants' weight loss intervention (Aramburu, Alegría, & Larsen, 2017). Other research suggests that relationship talk, which includes constructs akin to relationship maintenance (e.g., discussing relationship expectations, planning for the future), is beneficial to both cancer patients and their partner (Badr, Acitelli, & Taylor, 2008). Finally, relationship maintenance norms and bonds appear to drive friends' and family members' attempts to communicate with patients experiencing a communication-debilitating illness or injury (Bute, Donovan-Kicken, & Martins, 2007). These studies suggest that relationship maintenance is a salient factor in couples' health-related communication, as relational continuity is at least partly determined by partners' health. Accordingly, in the current study, relationship maintenance was examined alongside health promotion communication, such as social control and social support.

HEALTH-RELATED SOCIAL CONTROL

Research on social influence, diet, and exercise generally suggests that social influence can foster healthy behavior changes in diet and exercise. A meta-analysis of social influence and exercise indicates that exposure to social influence accounts for some of the variance in people's adherence to and compliance with exercise recommendations (Carron, Hausenblas, & Mack, 1996); however, this research does not consider the relational context in which these influence messages are delivered. Research indicates that the inherent interdependence among individuals in romantic relationships (Thibaut & Kelley, 1959) fuels an environment in which partners serve as a source of health-related influence and behavior change (Lewis & Butterfield, 2007; Lewis & Rook, 1999). With regard to communication about diet and exercise specifically, such social influence is associated with couples' diet and exercise habits (Markey, Markey, & Gray, 2007) and behaviors (Burke & Segrin, 2014), and with relationship quality (Burke & Segrin, 2016).

Health-related social control is often examined in terms of positive and negative social control messages. Whereas positive social control reflects partners' positive emotions, suggestions, and praise, negative social control might involve negative emotions, guilt, and withdrawal (Butterfield & Lewis, 2002). Positive social control should facilitate constructive and confirming communication that likely benefits the relationship (Laing, Phillipson, & Lee, 1966) and generate the desired change in partner behavior (Lewis & Butterfield, 2007). In contrast, a by-product of negative social control might include negative affect and disconfirming communication that could harm the relationship (Gottman, 1994) and limit healthy behavior change (Tucker & Anders, 2001). In the same vein, individuals' perceived positive social control from partners is associated with increased relationship satisfaction, but their perceived negative social control is unrelated to their relationship satisfaction (Burke & Segrin, 2016). Given the well-established links between relationship satisfaction and relationship maintenance (Dainton, 2000; Weigel & Ballard-Reisch, 2001), health-related social control could be associated with relationship maintenance, as well.

As mentioned previously, similar to relationship maintenance (Stafford & Canary, 2006), health promotion messages are communicated routinely in romantic relationships (Lewis & Rook, 1999). By communicating these health promotion messages, partners reinforce their desire to maintain each other's health and, consequently, their relationship. As a result, this study examined relationship maintenance in conjunction with social control communication to gain a more comprehensive understanding of the relational environment in which couples communicate diet- and exercise-related health promotion.

H1: Perceived partner relationship maintenance is positively associated with individuals' (a) *use of* positive social control, and (b) their *perceptions of* positive social control from the partner.

H2: Perceived partner relationship maintenance is negatively associated with individuals' (a) *use of* negative social control, and (b) their *perceptions of* negative social control from the partner.

HEALTH-RELATED SOCIAL SUPPORT

Research suggests that beyond social control communication, social support is a salient communication process when it comes to couples communicating about health (Burke & Segrin, 2014; Franks et al., 2006); therefore, this study also examined relationship maintenance in conjunction with perceived support from the partner. In general, research suggests that individuals' perceptions of available support from significant others is associated with well-being and physical health (House et al., 1988; Kiecolt-Glaser & Newton, 2001). When people have support available to them, it provides them with an extra resource on which they can depend when they face challenges. Adhering to healthy diet and exercise programs might be one of these challenges, particularly in romantic relationships, where dietary habits often converge (Bove, Sobal, & Rauschenbach, 2003). Couples often make dietary decisions and prepare meals together (Anderson, Marshall, & Lea, 2004); thus, an individual's perception that his or her partner is available to provide support might be especially salient in the context of diet- and exercise-related communication.

Indeed, results from a review of studies, including social support in weight management interventions, suggest that people's weight management is linked to support from significant others (Verheijden et al., 2005). Similarly, when partners participate in weight management programs together, they are more likely to report eating more reduced-fat foods, fruits, and vegetables (Burke et al., 1999). Supportive partners are also helpful when it comes to exercise behaviors. Partners who participated in a weight loss program together reported that partner support was helpful in changing their behaviors to incorporate light exercise into their daily activities (Burke et al., 1999). Although partner support might offer benefits in general (Lewis et al, 2004), less is known about health-related support in a relational health promotion context (Franks et al., 2006).

Similar to relationship maintenance, social support is a communicative phenomenon that reflects interdependence and coordination between significant others (Albrecht, Burleson, & Goldsmith, 1994). It is typically conveyed in the service of providing aid (MacGeorge, Feng, & Burleson, 2011), and can take various forms, ranging from nurturant to action-facilitating messages (Cutrona & Suhr, 1992). Support messages are closely aligned with relationship maintenance expressions of positivity, openness, and assurances, as they are communicated for the purpose of improving others' outcomes. Although diet and exercise communication has been examined in families and friendships (Sallis et al., 1987), it is pertinent to understand its salience within the context of relationship maintenance and relational health promotion.

H3: Perceived partner relationship maintenance is positively associated with individuals' perceived (a) diet-related and (b) exercise-related social support from the partner.

Given the significance of the relationship context in this study, it is also important to consider these interactions in conjunction with relationship quality. Beyond the obvious association between relationship maintenance and relationship quality (Dainton, 2000; Weigel & Ballard-Reisch, 2001), research indicates that social control (Burke & Segrin, 2016) and social support (Cramer, 2006; Cutrona, 1996) are both associated with relationship quality. Consequently, to elucidate further the relational dynamics that occur within the context of diet- and exercise-related communication in relationships, social control and social support were examined as potential moderators of the association between relationship maintenance and relationship satisfaction.

RQ1: Will individuals' (a) *use of* positive social control, or (b) *perceptions of* positive social control from the partner, moderate the association between their perceived partner relationship maintenance and relationship satisfaction?

RQ2: Will individuals' (a) *use of* negative social control, or (b) *perceptions of* negative social control from the partner, moderate the association between their perceived partner relationship maintenance and relationship satisfaction?

RQ3: Will individuals' perceived (a) diet- related partner support, or (b) exercise-related partner support, moderate the association between their perceived partner relationship maintenance and relationship satisfaction?

METHOD

Participants and Procedure

Participants were recruited through student referral at a large southwestern university. Students were offered extra credit toward their course grade in exchange for referring a couple (older than 18 years of age and in a relationship for at least 6 months, married or cohabiting) to complete an online questionnaire. Both partners in the couple were required to be willing to participate, and were recruited through emails sent to separate email addresses provided by the student. These emails included a link to the online questionnaire and a unique code number to enter at the end of the questionnaire. The code numbers matched partners' responses to each other and to the referring student without the provision of identifying information.

After completing the questionnaire, participants were directed to a separate webpage where they entered their mailing address in order to receive a $10 gift card in appreciation for their participation. The response rate was 90% among the 466 participants who were recruited (i.e., 418 individuals responded). However, data from 20 uncoupled participants, and data from seven couples including at least one partner who completed the questionnaire in less than ten minutes, were removed from analysis.

Of the 192 heterosexual couples (N = 384 individuals) whose data were retained, 91% reported being married (9% reported that they were unmarried but cohabiting). Participants had a mean age of 48 years (SD = 11.26, range = 22–86), and couples had a mean relationship length of 21.33 years (SD = 10.77, range = 1–44). A majority of the couples in the sample reported they had children (85%). The sample comprised primarily white individuals (85%), followed by 9% Latino/a, 2% African American, 3% Asian/Pacific Islander, and 1% other. Most participants in the sample were fairly well educated, with 25% reporting that they had a graduate/professional degree, 46% a bachelor's degree, 25% some college/associate's degree; 4% reported having completed only high school. In addition, the majority of participants reported being employed full time (68%), with 16% employed part-time, 8% unemployed, 3% students, and 5% retired.

Measures

Means, standard deviations, and correlations for study variables are presented in Table 3.1.

Relationship maintenance. The positivity, openness, and assurances sub-scales of Stafford and Canary's (1991) Relationship Maintenance Strategy Measure (RMSM) were used to assess relationship maintenance. The current study included 16 items, with eight items for positivity, five for openness, and three for assurances. Sample items included, "My partner attempts to make our interactions enjoyable" (positivity); "My partner seeks to discuss the quality of our relationship" (openness); and, "My partner stresses his/her commitment to me" (assurances). Participants responded to this measure on a 1 (*strongly disagree*) to 7 (*strongly agree*) scale. Cronbach's alpha indicated acceptable reliability ($\alpha = 0.91$) for both females and males.

Diet- and exercise-related social control. Individuals' *use of* social control, as well as their *perceptions of* social control from the partner, were measured with an adapted version of Butterfield and Lewis' (2002) Health-Related Social Influence Scale. Their original measure assessed health-related social influence in general, but was adapted for this study to measure 16 different influence tactics relative to diet- and exercise-related social control, specifically: asking, bargaining, invoking guilt, expressing negative emotions, showing persistence, attempting persuasion, expressing positive emotions, reasoning, stating importance, making suggestions, invoking obligation, telling, using withdrawal, changing behavior, modelling/hinting, and praising. Consistent with Tucker and Anders (2001), participants indicated how often in the last six months they (a) *used* each strategy to influence their partner to engage in healthier diet or exercise behaviors, and (b) *perceived* that their partners used each strategy to encourage them to engage in healthier diet and exercise behaviors. Participants responded on a 1 (*never*) to 7 (*daily*) scale.

A principal components analysis was conducted to determine how people's *use of* each of the social control tactics loaded onto factors; direct oblimin factor rotation was used to determine how the items loaded onto the factors. Two distinct factors emerged for individuals' reported social control strategy

TABLE 3.1 *Descriptive statistics and correlations among study variables*

	M(SD)	1	2	3	4	5	6	7	8
		4.89 (0.97)	2.84 (1.14)	3.11 (1.24)	0.13 (0.18)	0.16 (0.19)	4.74 (1.19)	4.19 (1.27)	5.93 (0.96)
1. Relationship Maintenance	4.90 (1.03)	**0.43*****	0.14†	0.29***	-0.13†	-0.06	0.38***	0.39***	0.60***
2. Positive Social Control Use	3.22 (1.29)	0.17*	**0.21****	0.69***	0.47***	0.26***	0.41***	0.33***	-0.01
3. Perceived Partner Positive Control	2.86 (1.31)	0.29***	0.57***	**0.24****	0.30***	0.39***	0.58***	0.51***	0.11
4. Negative Social Control Use	0.17 (0.19)	-0.07	0.53***	0.11	**0.25****	0.64***	0.05	0.02	-0.32***
5. Perceived Partner Negative Control	0.11 (0.17)	-0.04	0.37***	0.42***	0.57***	**0.28****	0.06	0.09	-0.27***
6. Diet Support	3.90 (1.27)	0.28***	0.24**	0.59***	0.04	0.33***	**0.13†**	0.53***	0.23**
7. Exercise Support	4.09 (1.31)	0.45***	0.20**	0.53***	-0.06	0.14*	0.61***	**0.32****	0.37***
8. Relationship Satisfaction	5.85 (1.06)	0.66***	0.11	0.21**	-0.20**	-0.13	0.23**	0.37***	**0.47****

Note. Intraclass correlations are in bold along the diagonal descriptives and correlations for males are above the diagonal. Descriptives and correlations for females are to the left of/below the diagonal. ***$p < 0.001$, **$p < 0.01$, *$p < 0.05$, †$p < 0.10$.

use (i.e., how frequently people reported *using* these strategies to encourage their partner to be healthier): *positive* social control strategy use and *negative* social control strategy use. Both factors had an eigenvalue greater than 1 and were above the elbow of the Scree plot; together the factors accounted for 70% of the variance.

The *positive* social control strategy factor included the following items: asked, expressed positive emotion, stated importance, made suggestions, changed behavior, modelled/hinted, and praised. *Negative* actor social control strategy use included the following items: bargained, guilt, expressed negative emotions, invoked obligation, told, and used withdrawal. The factor loadings for *positive* social control ranged from 0.58 to 0.89 and the factor loadings for *negative* social control ranged from 0.67 to 0.84. The following items did not load onto either dimension: persistence, persuasion, and reasoned. The results were identical for individuals' *perceived* social control from their partners, except that the two factors accounted for 61% of the variance. Reliability for positive social control strategy *use* was $\alpha = 0.88$ for females and $\alpha = 0.84$ for males and for negative social control strategy *use* it was $\alpha = 0.87$ for females and $\alpha = 0.88$ for males. Reliability for *perceived* positive social control from the partner was $\alpha = 0.87$ for females and $\alpha = 0.83$ for males, and for *perceived* negative social control from the partner it was $\alpha = .89$ for both sexes.

Diet- and exercise-related partner support. Diet- and exercise-related support from the partner was measured using items adapted from Sallis et al. (1987). Sample items from the 10-item diet- and exercise-related support measure included, "My partner reminds me not to eat unhealthy food" and, "My partner offers to exercise with me." Participants indicated their agreement with these items using a 1 (*strongly disagree*) to 7 (*strongly agree*) scale. The five diet support items were averaged into a diet support subscale and the five items for exercise support were averaged into an exercise support subscale. Reliability for diet support was $\alpha = 0.87$ for females and $\alpha = .87$ for males. Reliability for exercise support was $\alpha = 0.88$ for females and $\alpha = 0.86$ for males.

Relationship measures. Relationship measures included relationship type (e.g., married, cohabiting), relationship length, and relationship satisfaction. Relationship satisfaction was assessed using Hendrick's (1988) 7-item Relationship Assessment Scale (RAS). Sample items included, "How well does your partner meet your needs?" and "How good is your relationship compared to most?," where items were measured on a 1 (*negatively valenced*) to 7 scale (*positively valenced*). Reliablity was $\alpha = 0.90$ for females and $\alpha = 0.88$ for males.

Data Analysis

Analyses were conducted using actor–partner interdependence models (APIMs; Kenny, Kashy, & Cook, 2006) in SAS proc mixed. Following recommendations by Kenny et al. (2006), individuals were nested within dyads using repeated measures and compound symmetry functions to control for the interdependence among the couples in this sample. Including actor (the individual) and partner (the individual's partner) reports of predictor variables allows for estimation of the extent to which actors' outcomes are influenced by their scores on predictor variables while simultaneously controlling for the effect of their partner's scores on those variables. The hypotheses in this study were limited to actor effects; as such, partner effects were not interpreted, but were included as control variables in each model. Sex was also included as a control variable in each model.

The first six multilevel models examined H1 through H3, and included actors' and partners' perceived partner relationship maintenance as predictors of six health communication variables: (1) _use of_ positive social control, (2) _perceptions of_ positive social control from the partner, (3) _use of_ negative social control, (4) _perceptions of_ negative social control from the partner, and perceived (5) _diet_ support and (6) _exercise_ support from partners. The negative social control variables were positively skewed, so they were log transformed to obtain variables with more normal distributions. All analyses were conducted using the transformed variables.

To examine the interaction effects addressed in RQ1 through RQ3, six parallel multilevel models were run. All of these models included relationship satisfaction as the dependent variable and actors' and partners' relationship maintenance as predictor variables. Each of the aforementioned health communication variables were included as predictors in the six separate models, and interactions between each of the relationship maintenance variables and each of these six health communication variables were also included as predictor variables in the six separate models.

For example, the first model included the following predictors: (a) actor perceived relationship maintenance, (b) partner perceived relationship maintenance, (c) actor _use of_ positive social control, (d) actor perceived relationship maintenance*actor _use of_ positive social control, and (e) partner perceived relationship maintenance*actor _use of_ positive social control. The other models paralleled this example, but exchanged _use of_ positive social control for one of the other health communication variables. Significant interaction effects were decomposed following guidelines from Aiken and West (1991). Given that the guidelines permit authors to choose values "within the full range of _Z_" (p. 12) for plotting interactions, the conditional values were calculated at the 25th and 75th percentiles to illustrate the interaction effects in this study.

RESULTS

The first three hypotheses included individuals' perceptions of partner relationship maintenance as a predictor of their *use of* positive social control (H1a), *perceptions of* positive social control from the partner (H1b), *use of* negative social control (H2a), *perceptions of* negative social control from the partner (H2b), and perceived diet support (H3a) and exercise support (H3b) from the partner. As depicted in Table 3.2, the results indicated that perceived relationship maintenance from the partner positively predicted *use* of positive social control to encourage one's partner to be healthier ($b = 0.15$, $p < 0.05$; H1a), and *perceptions of* positive social control from one's partner ($b = 0.34$, $p < 0.001$; H2a). Thus, H1 was confirmed.

In contrast, perceived relationship maintenance from the partner was marginally negatively associated with *use of* negative social control to encourage one's partner to be healthier ($b = -0.02$, $p = 0.05$; H1b), and was unrelated to *perceptions of* negative social control from the partner ($b = -0.01$, *ns*; H2b). Finally, perceived relationship maintenance from one's partner positively predicted perceived *diet*-related support from the partner ($b = 0.40$, $p < 0.001$; H3a) and perceived *exercise*-related support from the partner ($b = 0.48$, $p < 0.001$; H3b). Although H2 was not confirmed, H3 was confirmed.

In terms of RQ1 through RQ3, four significant interaction effects emerged (see bolded lines in Table 3.3). First, *perceived* positive social control from one's partner moderated the association between perceived relationship maintenance from the partner and relationship satisfaction ($b = -0.11$, $p < 0.001$; RQ1b), such that individuals who perceived less relationship maintenance from their partner reported greater relationship satisfaction with greater perceived positive social control from the partner (see Fig. 3.1). A parallel pattern emerged for *perceived* negative social control from the partner ($b = -0.48$, $p < 0.05$; RQ2b). That is, people who perceived less relationship maintenance from the partner reported greater relationship satisfaction with greater perceived negative social control from the partner (see Fig. 3.2).

A similar pattern emerged for perceived diet-related support from the partner ($b = -0.11$, $p < 0.001$; RQ3a); individuals who perceived less relationship maintenance from their partner reported greater relationship satisfaction with greater perceived diet support from the partner (see Fig. 3.3). In contrast, as individuals perceived greater relationship maintenance and greater diet-related support from their partner, their relationship satisfaction decreased. Finally, perceived exercise-related support from the partner moderated the association between perceived relationship maintenance and relationship satisfaction ($b = -0.09$, $p < 0.01$; RQ3b), such that individuals who perceived less relationship maintenance from their partner reported greater relationship

TABLE 3.2 *Perceived partner relationship maintenance as a predictor of health communication*

Outcome Variables	b	SE	df	t	Outcome Variables	b	SE	df	t
Model 1: Pos. Social Control Use	0.15	0.07	358	2.31*	Model 2: Perceived Partner Pos. Control	0.34	0.07	362	5.14***
Model 3: Neg. Social Control Use	-0.02	0.01	370	-1.98†	Model 4: Perceived Partner Neg. Control	-0.01	0.01	376	-0.98
Model 5: Perceived Diet Support	0.40	0.06	343	6.16***	Model 6: Perceived Exercise Support	0.48	0.06	366	7.77***

Note.***p < 0.001, **p < 0.05, *p < 0.05 †*p* = 0.05. Perceived partner relationship maintenance is the predictor variable in each model. Partner reports of perceived relationship maintenance and sex were included as control variables.

TABLE 3.3 *Health communication variables as moderators of the association between perceived partner relationship maintenance and relationship satisfaction*

Predictor Variables	b	SE	df	t	Predictor Variables	b	SE	df	t
Model 1					**Model 2**				
Perceived Partner Rel. Maint.	0.65	0.11	339	5.95***	Perceived Partner Rel. Maint.	0.89	0.10	357	9.03***
Pos. Social Control Use	-0.10	0.19	377	-0.51	Perceived Partner Pos. Control	0.72	0.19	380	3.67***
Perceived Maint. × Pos. Use	-0.02	0.03	336	-0.60	**Perceived Maint. × Perceived Pos.**	**-0.11**	**0.03**	357	-3.57***
Model 3					**Model 4**				
Perceived Partner Rel. Maint.	0.54	0.05	362	10.23***	Perceived Partner Rel. Maint.	0.70	0.08	372	8.23***
Neg. Social Control Use	-2.20	1.33	372	-1.65	Perceived Partner Neg. Control	0.38	0.31	379	1.25
Perceived Maint. × Neg. Use	0.10	0.22	347	0.44	**Perceived Maint. × Perceived Neg.**	**-0.48**	**0.22**	**362**	-2.15*
Model 5					**Model 6**				
Perceived Partner Rel. Maint.	1.02	0.13	364	7.95***	Perceived Partner Rel. Maint.	0.91	0.13	343	6.88***
Perceived Diet Support	0.60	0.16	373	3.66***	Perceived Exercise Support	0.57	0.17	378	3.37***
Perceived Maint. ×Diet Support	**-0.11**	**0.03**	363	-3.77***	**Perceived Maint. × Exer. Support**	**-0.09**	**0.03**	336	-2.98**

Note. ***$p < 0.001$, **$p < 0.01$, *$p < 0.05$ †$p = 0.05$. Partner reports of perceived relationship maintenance and sex were included as control variables. Significant interactions are bolded (and visually depicted in Figs. 3.1–3.4).

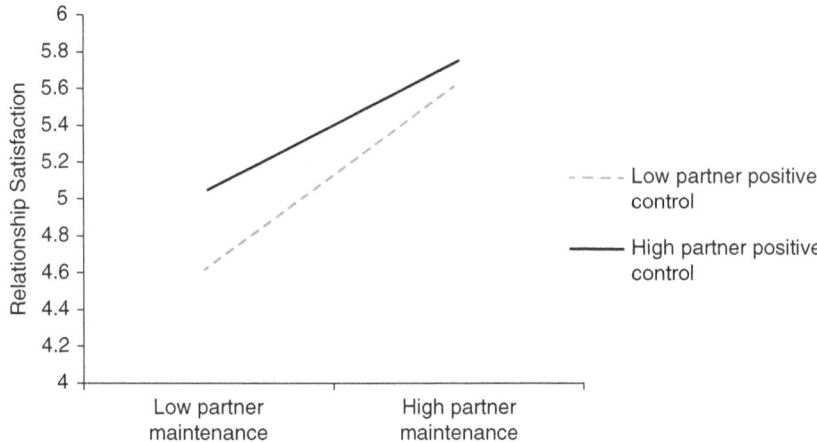

FIGURE 3.1   Perceived positive partner social control as a moderator of the association between perceived partner relationship maintenance and relationship satisfaction.

Note. Low perceived partner positive social control, $b = 0.67$, $SE = 0.05$, $p < 0.001$; high perceived partner positive social control, $b = 0.47$, $SE = 0.05$, $p < 0.001$.

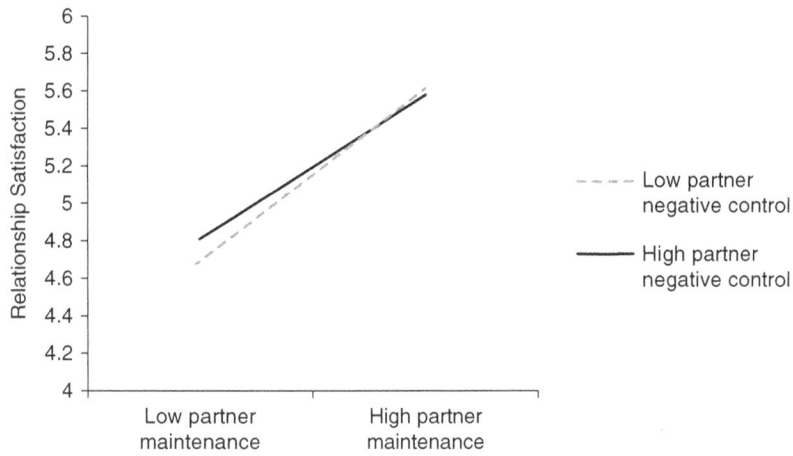

FIGURE 3.2   Perceived negative partner social control as a moderator of the association between perceived partner relationship maintenance and relationship satisfaction.

Note. Low perceived partner negative social control, $b = 0.63$, $SE = 0.04$, $p < 0.001$; high perceived partner negative social control, $b = 0.53$, $SE = 0.05$, $p < 0.001$.

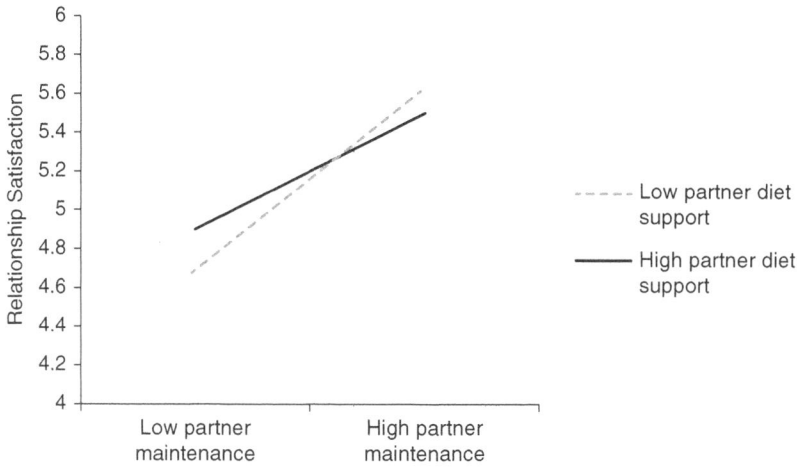

FIGURE 3.3 Perceived partner diet support as a moderator of the association between perceived partner relationship maintenance and relationship satisfaction.
Note. Low perceived partner diet support, $b = 0.60$, $SE = 0.04$, $p < 0.001$; high perceived partner diet support, $b = 0.40$, $SE = 0.05$, $p < 0.001$.

satisfaction as their perceived exercise support from the partner increased (see Fig. 3.4). Neither *use* of positive social control ($b = -0.02$, *ns*; RQ1a) or *use* of negative social control ($b = 0.10$, *ns*; RQ1b) moderated the association between perceived partner relationship maintenance and relationship satisfaction, however.

DISCUSSION

The purpose of this study was to investigate whether relationship maintenance was associated with diet- and exercise-related communication between relationship partners, as well as the potential role that diet- and exercise-related communication played in the association between relationship maintenance and relationship satisfaction. In this study, relationship maintenance was associated with health promoting communication in relationships, as evidenced by the positive associations with positive social control and diet- and exercise-related support from the partner. Moreover, individuals' *perceived* social control and social support influenced the association between relationship maintenance and relationship satisfaction.

This study fused two areas of study – relationship maintenance and health communication – in order to demonstrate that these interactional processes are intertwined in the context of relational communication. The results of this study illustrate that as people perceived greater relationship

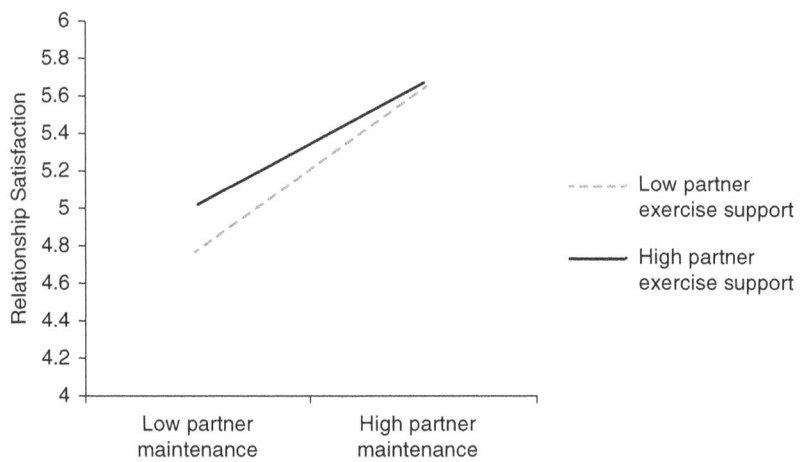

FIGURE 3.4 Perceived partner exercise support as a moderator of the association between perceived partner relationship maintenance and relationship satisfaction. *Note.* Low perceived partner exercise support, $b = 0.57$, $SE = 0.05$, $p < 0.001$; high perceived partner positive social control, $b = 0.43$, $SE = 0.05$, $p < 0.001$.

maintenance from their partner, they also reported using more positive social control to encourage their partner to be healthier (H1a). This finding demonstrates the interactional nature of relationships. That is, people were motivated to encourage their partner to be healthier when they also believed that their partner was contributing to the relationship through relationship maintenance. This finding suggests that people might have a relational motive for using social control to encourage their partner to be healthier. Prior research identified a similar relational effect, proposing that individuals' use of social influence is a function of both partners' experiences as agents and targets of social influence (Butterfield & Lewis, 2002).

Individuals' perceptions of their partner's relationship maintenance were also positively associated with their *perceptions of* greater positive social control (H1b) and diet- and exercise-related social support (H3a and H3b) from their partner. That is, when people perceived more relationship maintenance from a partner, they also perceived more communication of social control and social support from him or her. These couples appear to recognize that sustaining a partner's health is tantamount to sustaining a relationship; therefore, in addition to communicating maintenance to sustain their relationship (Canary & Stafford, 1992), they also understand the value of encouraging their partner to be healthier. These results are consistent with the idea that people tend to preference positive health-promoting communication (Markey et al., 2007) in service of fostering a healthy relational environment, given the limited findings for negative social control in this study. The lacking significant effects for negative social control are consistent with other research, which demonstrated mixed or limited effects of negative social control (Tucker & Anders, 2001).

Beyond these main effects, four significant interaction effects emerged in this study. At lower levels of perceived partner relationship maintenance, people reported greater relationship satisfaction when they perceived greater positive (RQ1b) and negative (RQ2b) social control from their partner, as well as greater diet (RQ3a) and exercise-related support (RQ3b) from their partner. It seems that when people feel that their partner is less attentive to routine relationship maintenance, they can still feel satisfied in their relationship to the extent that their partner is showing interest in their health. Perceived health influence (Markey et al., 2007) and social support are associated with relationship quality (Cramer, 2006; Cutrona, 1996), so it would follow that these types of health communication could promote relationship quality in the case of less perceived relationship maintenance.

Although these results might be expected for positive social control and social support, it is somewhat surprising that parallel results emerged for negative social control. Such disconfirming language is typically associated with adverse relational outcomes (Gottman, 1994). It is important to remember, however, that people have different ways of communicating their love and investment (Gottman & DeClaire, 2001). Thus, one possible explanation for these results is that individuals' perceptions of care from their partner trumped the negative connotation associated with these expressions of care. It is also important to note these participants' perceptions of social control and social support were not necessarily mutually exclusive. Individuals may have perceived a mix of positive social control, negative social control, and social support from their partner that, together, benefited their relationship quality, limiting the potential adverse effects of negative social control.

For the most part, people who perceived heightened relationship maintenance from their partner reported increased relationship satisfaction. There was one exception to this, however. Perceived partner relationship maintenance was more strongly associated with relationship satisfaction under conditions of *low* rather than high diet-related support from a partner. In other words, it seems as though relationship maintenance promotes relationship quality, unless a partner's maintenance behaviors become invasive or interfere with individuals' diet goals. This is consistent with the idea of reactance (Brehm, 1972), wherein people resist influence messages that they perceive to infringe on their freedom to make their own choices.

Relative to diet-related issues specifically, research suggests that mixed-weight partners report greater relational conflict when they eat together more frequently (Burke, Randall, Corkery, Young, & Butler, 2012). Similarly, individuals are less satisfied in relationships when they think their partner considers them to be overweight or unattractive (Markey & Markey, 2006).

Although partners in this study might have been well-intentioned in communicating diet-related support, this communication might be unwelcome if it makes people feel judged. It is important to keep in mind that these results are cross-sectional, and the direction of these effects cannot be determined. Nonetheless, it appears that couples need to be aware of each other's limits and preferences when it comes to discussing dietary habits and providing diet support.

Theoretical and Practical Implications

Relationship maintenance is a well-established relational communication process and plenty of evidence suggests that social control communication occurs in relationships, yet these frameworks were previously disparate in the literature. By combining these frameworks, it was possible to demonstrate that health communication might occur as a routine relationship maintenance process, akin to communicating positivity, openness, and assurances. Given research suggesting that couples' dietary habits converge (Bove et al., 2003) and that couples make dietary decisions and prepare meals together (Anderson et al., 2004) – a daily process – it is not surprising that this type of communication could demonstrate partners' commitment to and investment to each other's health, and ultimately to sustaining their relationship. Attention to diet and exercise continues to increase in the United States as the obesity epidemic continues to rise; thus, the results of this study illustrate that adding social control and social support to the relationship maintenance typology could be fruitful in terms of understanding the health communication that couples employ to fortify their committed relationships.

In addition to augmenting our understanding of relationship maintenance, the findings in this study highlight valuable information for practitioners who are trying to help couples navigate these potentially sensitive conversations. Individuals report engaging in health-enhancing behaviors in conjunction with their partner's reports of *positive* social influence strategy use (Lewis & Butterfield, 2007); therefore, it is important to educate partners on the value of enacting *positive* social influence to encourage healthy behavior adoption. This is especially true in light of the findings from this study, which suggest that positive social control and social support are generally constructive elements of people's relationship functioning. For instance, health practitioners could educate partners about how to effectively employ positive social control strategies, such as modeling healthy behaviors (e.g., eating a healthy meal together), to protect each other's health and relationship. In contrast, they could instruct partners to avoid using more negative strategies (e.g., inducing guilt), as they tend to be less reliably associated with healthy behavior change (Tucker & Anders, 2001) and, as evidenced in this study, with relationship maintenance. Given the results for diet support in this study, suggesting that there are times when support is less welcome, it would also be helpful to educate patients about how to communicate their preferences for supportive messages in order to preserve and sustain their relationships.

Limitations and Future Directions

Despite its contributions, this study could be improved in several ways. First, this study is limited by the cross-sectional nature of the data. That is, the directionality of the associations documented in this study cannot be reliably ascertained. Future research should study these variables longitudinally to parse out the direction of the effects among these variables. Second, the variables in this study were self-reported. Consequently, participants may have furnished socially desirable responses. There is some evidence of this occurring with the negative social control variable, given the positive skewness; however, the issue is somewhat mitigated by the fact that these variables were transformed to obtain a more normal distribution. This study is also limited by the relatively homogeneous sample; these participants were similar in terms of marital status, race/ethnicity, and education. It would be valuable to study the variables in this study across different populations to gain a more comprehensive understanding of health communication in a relational context. Finally, this study is limited in that it assessed both partners' perceptions of relationship maintenance from each other, but did not assess their enactment of relationship maintenance with each other. Understanding more about this behavior might provide more purposeful instruction about how to engage in effective health communication.

CONCLUSION

It is clear that significant effort is required to maintain committed relationships and to maintain healthy diet and exercise behaviors. This study combined these different areas of research to demonstrate that couples' health-promoting communication appears to correspond with their relationship maintenance. Specifically, people report using more positive social control, and perceiving more positive social control and diet- and exercise-related support from their partner in conjunction with greater perceived relationship maintenance from their partner. These findings reflect a relational environment in which partners work to sustain their relationship by communicating relationship maintenance (Canary & Stafford, 1992) as well as positive social control and social support to each other. These couples appear to understand that health is a crucial element of their relational continuity. As a result, it is possible that these relationship maintenance and health maintenance expressions will become normative

(Dindia & Baxter, 1987) in the service of promoting long-term relational and physical health.

REFERENCES

Aiken, L. S., & West, S. G. (1991). *Multiple regression: Testing and interpreting interactions.* Thousand Oaks, CA: SAGE.

Albrecht, T. L., Burleson, B., & Goldsmith, D. (1994). Supportive communication. In M. Knapp & G. Miller (Eds.), *The SAGE handbook of interpersonal communication* (pp. 419–459). Thousand Oaks, CA: SAGE.

Anderson, A. S., Marshall, D. W., & Lea, E. J. (2004). Shared lives-an opportunity for obesity prevention? *Appetite, 43,* 327–329. doi: 10.1016/j.appet.2004.07.007

Aramburu Alegría, C., & Larsen, B. (2017). Contextual care of the patient following weight-loss surgery: Relational views and maintenance activities of couples. *Journal of the American Association of Nurse Practitioners, 29,* 17–25. doi: 10.1002/2327-6924.12372

Badr, H., Acitelli, L. K., & Taylor, C. L. C. (2008). Does talking about their relationship affect couples' marital and psychological adjustment to lung cancer? *Journal of Cancer Survivorship, 2,* 53–64. doi: 10.1007/s11764-008-0044-3

Bove, C. F., Sobal, J., & Rauschenbach, B. S. (2003). Food choices among newly married couples: Convergence, conflict, individualism, and projects. *Appetite, 40,* 25–41. doi: 10.1016/S0195-6663(02)00147-2

Brehm, J. W. (1972). *Responses to loss of freedom: A theory of psychological reactance.* Washington, DC: General Learning Corporation.

Burke, T. J., Randall, A. K., Corkery, S. A., Young, V. J., & Butler, E. A. (2012). "You're going to eat *that?*" Relationship processes and conflict among mixed-weight couples. *Journal of Social and Personal Relationships, 29,* 1109–1130. doi: 10.1177/0265407512451199.

Burke, T. J., & Segrin, C. (2014). Examining diet- and exercise-related communication in romantic relationships: Associations with health behaviors. *Health Communication, 29,* 877–887. doi: 10.1080/10410236.2013.811625

Burke, T. J., & Segrin, C. (2016). Weight-related social control and relationship quality: Accuracy and bias effects. *Journal of Social and Personal Relationships, 33,* 999–1017. doi: 10.1177/0265407515615692

Burke, V., Giangiulio, N., Gillam, H. F., Beilin, L. J., Houghton, S., & Milligan, R. A. K. (1999). Health promotion in couples adapting to a shared lifestyle. *Health Education Research, 14,* 269–288. doi: 10.1093/her/14.2.269

Bute, J. J., Donovan-Kicken, E., & Martins, N. (2007). Effects of communication-debilitating illnesses and injuries on close relationships: A relational maintenance perspective. *Health Communication, 21,* 235–246. doi: 10.1080/10410230701307675

Butterfield, R. M., & Lewis, M. A. (2002). Health-related social influence: A social ecological perspective on tactic use. *Journal of Social and Personal Relationships, 19,* 505–526. doi: 10.1177/0265407502019004050

Canary, D. J., & Stafford, L. (1992). Relational maintenance strategies and equity in marriage. *Communication Monographs, 59,* 243–267. doi: 10.1080/03637759209376268

Canary, D. J., Stafford, L., Hause, K. S., & Wallace, L. A. (1993). An inductive analysis of relational maintenance strategies: Comparisons among lovers, relatives, friends, and others. *Communication Research Reports, 10,* 3–14. doi: 10.1080/08824099309359913

Canary, D. J., Stafford, L., & Semic, B. A. (2002). A panel study of the associations between maintenance strategies and relational characteristics. *Journal of Marriage and Family, 64*, 395–406. doi: 10.1111/j.1741-3737.2002.00395.x

Canary, D. J., & Zelley, E. D. (2000). Current research programs on relational maintenance behaviors. In M. E. Roloff (Ed.), *Communication yearbook 23* (pp. 305–339). Thousand Oaks, CA: SAGE.

Carron, A. V., Hausenblas, H. A., & Mack, D. (1996). Social influence and exercise: A meta-analysis. *Journal of Sport & Exercise Psychology, 18*, 1–16. Retrieved from: http://journals.humankinetics.com/journal/jsep

Cramer, D. (2006). How a supportive partner may increase relationship satisfaction. *British Journal of Guidance & Counseling, 34*, 117–131. doi: 10.1080/03069880500483141

Cutrona, C. E. (1996). Social support as a determinant of marital quality: The interplay of negative and supportive behaviors. In G. R. Pierce, B. R. Sarason, & I. G. Sarason (Eds.), *Handbook of social support and the family* (pp. 173–194). New York, NY: Plenum Press.

Cutrona, C. E., & Suhr, J. A. (1992). Controllability of stressful events and satisfaction with spouse support behaviors. *Communication Research, 19*, 154–174. doi: 10.1177/009365092019002002

Dainton, M. (2000). Maintenance behaviors, expectations for maintenance, and satisfaction: Linking comparison levels to relational maintenance strategies. *Journal of Social and Personal Relationships, 17*, 827–842. doi: 10.1177/0265407500176007

Dindia, K., & Baxter, L. A. (1987). Strategies for maintaining and repairing marital relationships. *Journal of Social and Personal Relationships, 4*, 143–158. doi: 10.1177/0265407587042003

Franks, M. M., Stephens, M. A. P., Rook, K. S., Franklin, B. A., Keteyian, S. J., & Artinian, N. T. (2006). Spouses' provision of health-related support and control to patients participating in cardiac rehabilitation. *Journal of Family Psychology, 20*, 311–318. doi: 10.1037/0893-3200.20.2.311

Gottman, J. M. (1994). *What predicts divorce? The relationship between marital process and marital outcomes.* Hillsdale, NJ: Lawrence Erlbaum.

Gottman, J. M., & DeClaire, J. (2001). *The relationship cure: A 5 step guide to strengthening your marriage, family, and relationships.* New York, NY: Three Rivers Press.

Guerrero, L. K., Eloy, S. V., & Wabnik, A. I. (1993). Linking maintenance strategies to relationship development and disengagement: A reconceptualization. *Journal of Social and Personal Relationships, 10*, 273–283. doi: 10.1177/026540759301000207

Hendrick, S. S. (1988). A generic measure of relationship satisfaction. *Journal of Marriage and the Family, 50*, 93–98. doi: 10.2307/352430

House, J. S., Landis, K. R., & Umberson, D. (1988). Social relationships and health. *Science, 241*, 540–545. doi: 10.1126/science.3399889

Kenny, D. A., Kashy, D. A., & Cook, W. L. (2006). *Dyadic data analysis.* New York, NY: Guilford Press.

Kiecolt-Glaser, J. K., & Newton, T. L. (2001). Marriage and health: His and hers. *Psychological Bulletin, 127*, 472–503. doi: 10.1037//0033-2909.127.4.472

Lewis, M. A., & Butterfield, R. M. (2007). Social control in marital relationships: Effect of one's partner on health behaviors. *Journal of Applied Social Psychology, 37*, 298–319. doi: 10.1111/j.0021-9029.2007.00161.x

Lewis, M. A., Butterfield, R. M., Darbes, L. A., & Johnston-Brooks, C. (2004). The conceptualization and assessment of health-related social control. *Journal of Social and Personal Relationships, 21*, 669–687. doi: 10.1177/0265407504045893

Lewis, M. A., & Rook, K. S. (1999). Social control in personal relationships: Impact on health behaviors and psychological distress. *Health Psychology, 18*, 63–71. doi: 10.1037//0278-6133.18.1.63

Laing, R. D., Phillipson, H., & Lee, A. R. (1966). *Interpersonal perception: A theory and a method of research*. London: Tavistock.

MacGeorge, E. L., Feng, B., & Burleson, B. R. (2011). Supportive communication. In M. Knapp & J. A. Daly (Eds.), *The SAGE handbook of interpersonal communication* (pp. 317–354). Los Angeles, CA: SAGE.

Markey, C. N., & Markey, P. M. (2006). Romantic relationships and body satisfaction among young women. *Journal of Youth and Adolescence, 35*, 271–279. doi: 10.1007/s10964-005-9013-6

Markey, C. N., Markey, P. M., & Gray, H. F. (2007). Romantic relationships and health: An examination of individuals' perceptions of their romantic partners' influences on their health. *Sex Roles, 57*, 435–445. doi: 10.1007/s11199-007-9266-5

Messman, S. J., Canary, D. J., & Hause, K. S. (2000). Motives to remain platonic, equity, and the use of maintenance strategies in opposite-sex friendships. *Journal of Social and Personal Relationships, 17*, 67–94. doi: 10.1177/0265407500171004

Miller, W. C., Koceja, D. M., & Hamilton, E. J. (1997). A meta-analysis of the past 25 years of weight loss research using diet, exercise or diet plus exercise intervention. *International Journal of Obesity, 21*, 941–947. doi: 10.1038/sj.ijo.0800499

Poirier, P., Giles, T. D., Bray, G. A., Hong, Y., Stern, J. S., Pi-Sunyer, F. X., & Eckel, R. H. (2006). Obesity and cardiovascular disease: Pathophysiology, evaluation, and effect of weight loss: An update of the 1997 American Heart Association Scientific Statement on Obesity and Heart Disease from the Obesity Committee of the Council on Nutrition, Physical Activity, and Metabolism. *Circulation, 113*, 898–918. doi: 10.1161/CIRCULATIONAHA.106.17101

Sallis, J. F., Grossman, R. M., Pinski, R. B., Patterson, T. L., & Nader, P. R. (1987). The development of scales to measure social support for diet and exercise behaviors. *Preventive Medicine, 16*, 825–836. doi: 10.1016/0091-7435(87)90022-3

Stafford, L., & Canary, D. J. (1991). Maintenance strategies and romantic relationship type, gender and relational characteristics. *Journal of Social and Personal Relationships, 8*, 217–242. doi: 10.1177/0265407591082004

Stafford, L., & Canary, D. J. (2006). Equity and interdependence as predictors of relational maintenance strategies. *The Journal of Family Communication, 6*, 227–254. doi: 10.1207/s15327698jfc0604_1

Thibaut, J. W., & Kelley, H. H. (1959). *The social psychology of groups*. New York, NY: John Wiley & Sons.

Tucker, J. S., & Anders, S. L. (2001). Social control of health behaviors in marriage. *Journal of Applied Social Psychology, 31*, 467–485. doi: 10.1111/j.1559-1816.2001.tb02051.x

Verheijden, M. W., Bakx, J. C., van Weel, C., Koelen, M. A., & van Staveren, W. A. (2005). Role of social support in lifestyle-focused weight management interventions. *European Journal of Clinical Nutrition, 59*, S179–S186. doi: 10.1038/sj.ejcn.1602194

Weigel, D. J., & Ballard-Reisch, D. S. (2001). The impact of relational maintenance behaviors on marital satisfaction: A longitudinal analysis. *The Journal of Family Communication, 1*, 265–279. doi: 10.1207/S15327698JFC0104_03

PART II

INFORMATION MANAGEMENT IN HEALTH AND
RELATIONSHIPS

4

Health-Related Issues That Individuals with Type 2 Diabetes Avoid Discussing with Their Romantic Partner

JOHN LEUSTEK AND JENNIFER A. THEISS

Type 2 diabetes is a chronic health condition that has approached near epidemic levels in the past decade (Centers for Disease Control and Prevention [CDC], 2014). As such, researchers and health care providers are becoming increasingly interested in the risk factors for type 2 diabetes and how patients manage this condition. Research has shown that, in addition to treatment, medication, and lifestyle changes, social and relational factors may also influence a patient's health outcomes and quality of life (Karlsen & Bru, 2014). Romantic relationships, in particular, provide vital support for individuals diagnosed with type 2 diabetes. Romantic partners can help to quell fears and uncertainty about the illness (Middleton, LaVoie, & Brown, 2012) and they may also facilitate healthy and adherent behaviors, such as improvements to diet and exercise (Theiss, Carpenter, & Leustek, 2016). One prerequisite for many of these positive health outcomes is a relationship in which partners can communicate openly about facets of their condition. Research on disclosure and topic avoidance suggests that managing a chronic health condition poses numerous threats to open communication about the illness (Goldsmith, Miller, & Caughlin, 2008). Individuals with a chronic illness are often motivated to avoid certain topics related to their health condition to mitigate the potential for face threats, embarrassment, or discomfort. Consequently, individuals with type 2 diabetes who avoid discussing their illness with a partner may miss opportunities to receive support, encouragement, or assistance in managing their treatment and achieving a healthier lifestyle. Thus, the goal of this study is to examine the topics that individuals with type 2 diabetes tend to avoid discussing openly with their romantic partner.

COPING WITH TYPE 2 DIABETES

According to the CDC (2014), 29.1 million Americans currently have diabetes, with about 95% of all cases classified as type 2 diabetes. Type 2 diabetes is classified as a self-management condition (Glasgow & Anderson, 1999), which suggests that techniques for managing the condition are performed primarily by the patient, usually outside of a medical setting (Rintala, Jaatinen, Paavilainen, & Astedt-Kurki, 2013). Individuals with type 2 diabetes may be required to change their eating habits, increase their exercise, manage their blood sugar, and take medication. Adhering to self-management treatments, as prescribed by a health care provider, can result in a reduction of comorbid conditions and can greatly improve a patient's quality of life and prognosis (Adam & Folds, 2014).

A number of issues can facilitate or interfere with patients' ability to self-manage their type 2 diabetes. Issues of finance, treatment duration, treatment complexity, and pain levels may all interfere with how adherent patients are toward their treatment regimen (Peyrot et al., 2005). In addition, the amount of social support patients receive from their close network may also impact adherence. For example, individuals who perceive high levels of social support from their network are more likely to remain adherent and to feel less stress about their condition (Osborn & Egede, 2012). In addition, close romantic relationships may also influence self-management. Patients with type 2 diabetes who reported higher levels of relational satisfaction and intimacy were more likely to also report higher quality of life concerning their condition (Trief, Himes, Orendorff, & Weinstock, 2001). Spouses are also a primary source of influence in common self-management techniques for people with type 2 diabetes, including controlling food in the home and making sure that the patient remains compliant with diet and exercise regimens (Beverly, Miller, & Wray, 2008).

Given the importance romantic relationships for effectively managing type 2 diabetes, researchers and health care providers would benefit from understanding the complexities of communicating about the condition between partners. The type of information an individual chooses to disclose about his or her symptoms and diet may also have implications for how much a romantic partner can be involved in lifestyle changes (Miller & DiMatteo, 2013). Avoiding topics about poor diet or mismanagement of medications may prevent individuals from being able to intervene and help their partner regain control of managing his or her condition. Similarly, individuals may choose to keep long-term or personal worries to themselves, such as worries that stem from the prognosis of the illness, quality of life, treatment, and stigma (Middleton et al., 2012). As such, partners may be less equipped to provide effective support related to the illness, particularly in instances where they lack contextual information about what their partner is feeling or experiencing.

TOPIC AVOIDANCE IN THE CONTEXT OF CHRONIC ILLNESS

Avoidance can occur in romantic relationships for a variety of reasons. Topic avoidance can function as a way for individuals to protect themselves from uncomfortable or embarrassing situations (Afifi & Guerrero, 2009), to forestall intense emotions (Turner, Kelly, Swanson, Allison, & Wetzig, 2005), or to limit relational transgressions and circumvent a partner's aggressive behaviors (Golish, 2000). People are also motivated to avoid certain conversational topics if they anticipate their partner will be unresponsive or might violate privacy boundaries (Caughlin, Afifi, Carpenter-Theune, & Miller, 2005). In some instances, repeated avoidance about a specific topic can also contribute to perceptions that the topic is taboo or off limits for conversation in the relationship (Roloff & Ifert, 2000). Although topic avoidance can sometimes be functional for protecting personal privacy or maintaining harmony in a relationship (e.g., Donovan-Kicken & Caughlin, 2010; Toller & McBride, 2013), studies typically point to detrimental outcomes of topic avoidance, such as decreased relationship satisfaction (Goldsmith et al., 2008) and increased mental health issues, physical distress, and destructive communication patterns (Afifi, Shahnazi, Coveleski, Davis, & Merrill, 2017).

Health contexts provide a unique backdrop for investigating people's motivations for topic avoidance. For example, individuals diagnosed with cancer tend to avoid discussing their illness with a spouse to protect their partner and preserve the relationship, to maintain a sense of hope and normalcy in their lives, and to avoid eliciting strong emotions (Goldsmith et al., 2008). Along these lines, breast cancer patients have reported avoiding conversations with their partner about their fears regarding the prognosis of their illness, the future, and death (Walsh, Manuel, & Avis, 2005). In addition, individuals with irritable bowel syndrome avoid discussing their illness because of the social stigma that surrounds the nature of the condition (Defenbaugh, 2013). Finally, individuals diagnosed with HIV often avoid disclosing their condition to others for a number of unique reasons, including maintaining privacy about their condition, fear of how others might react due to stigma, and a feeling of solidarity in managing their condition (Derlega, Winstead, Greene, Serovich, & Elwood, 2004). Together, these findings suggest that the characteristics and conditions of a health condition create unique circumstances that may discourage open communication about the illness.

There are a number of characteristics associated with the diagnosis and treatment of type 2 diabetes that can make individuals reluctant to discuss their condition with a romantic partner. Individuals with type 2 diabetes report heightened anxiety and uncertainty about the diagnosis and long-term prognosis of their condition (Karlsen & Bru, 2014; Middleton et al., 2012). Research also suggests that individuals with type 2 diabetes have diabetes-specific distress, or sources of anxiety, frustration, and demoralization that stem from often complicated treatment regimens (Fisher et al., 2009). Many of the sources of diabetes-specific stress may be threatening or embarrassing to discuss with a relational partner, which may encourage avoidance of conversation about the illness (Donovan-Kicken & Caughlin,

2010; Theiss & Estlein, 2014). Identifying and understanding the topics that individuals with type 2 diabetes are reluctant to discuss with a relationship partner can help patients and health care providers anticipate some of the potential barriers to managing the illness through communal coping and support. Thus, this exploratory study examines the issues and topics that individuals with type 2 diabetes are disinclined to discuss with their relationship partner. The following research question guides this investigation:

RQ1: What topics, if any, do individuals with type 2 diabetes avoid discussing with their romantic partner about their health condition?

METHOD

The data that were used for this inquiry were part of a larger study about the relationship dynamics and communication behaviors between individuals with type 2 diabetes and their romantic partner. This study recruited individuals through Amazon's Mechanical Turk (MTurk) for a study broadly described as being about health and relationships. MTurk is a crowdsourcing application designed and maintained by Amazon that asks workers to complete tasks given by requesters in exchange for compensation (Goodman, Cryder, & Cheema, 2013). MTurk was originally designed as a tool for private sector research and analysis, but has more recently become a powerful tool for social science sampling and data collection. Current research on samples collected from MTurk suggests that the validity of the data is comparable to that of other traditional survey sampling methods (Casler, Bickel, & Hackett, 2013).

As a first step, a prescreening survey asked participants to identify which health conditions they currently had from a list of common health conditions and to indicate their current relationship status. Individuals who indicated they were diagnosed with type 2 diabetes and had some degree of romantic involvement with a partner were invited to continue with the study. Individuals were excluded from the study if they indicated that they were diagnosed with more than five illnesses or selected contradictory health conditions (e.g., gestational diabetes as a male, high and low blood pressure). Qualified individuals were then given the primary survey, administered through Qualtrics, to complete. On successfully completing the survey, participants were awarded $5 through the Amazon MTurk payment system.

Sample

Our sample for the prescreening survey consisted of 23,234 individuals. Of those who completed the prescreening survey, 500 individuals who qualified as having type 2 diabetes and being in a romantic relationship successfully completed the survey. Of the 500 individuals who participated in the study, 236 were male and 264 were female. Participants ranged in age from 21 to 74 years (M = 42 years, SD = 11.82 years). A majority of participants reported their race as white (67.8%), with 15.2% identifying as Asian, 8.2% as African American, 7.8% as Indian, 4.8% as Native American, and 0.6% as other. A majority of participants were married (64.6%), and others were monogamously dating (23%), engaged to be married or to enter a civil union (9.8%), or in a civil union (2.6%).

The average time since type 2 diabetes diagnosis was 5.03 years (SD = 5.86 years). In addition, most participants (74.4%) reported that they were diagnosed with type 2 diabetes after they were already romantically involved with their partner. A majority of participants actively managed their type 2 diabetes (98.4%), which included daily blood glucose monitoring (58.2%), diet and exercise (78.2%), oral medication (71.8%), long-acting insulin treatment (21.2%), and rapid-acting insulin treatment before meals (14.8%). A majority of participants also experienced complications or comorbid conditions as a result of their type 2 diabetes condition (96.4%), with blood pressure changes (51%), high cholesterol (37.2%), and nerve disease (34.6%) being most frequently reported within the sample.

Measures and Analyses

The broader survey for this study included demographic questions and a variety of closed-ended, Likert-type scale items that have been analyzed and reported elsewhere (Leustek & Theiss, 2018). For this investigation, participants responded to an open-ended question asking them to describe their communication with a romantic partner about their illness. The open-ended question stated, "Information can sometimes be kept private from romantic partners for various reasons. In the space below, please describe the topics or information about your type 2 diabetes diagnosis that you keep private or avoid discussing with your romantic partner." Participants were given a text box to respond to this question, and were given unlimited time and space to complete their answer.

All 500 responses were analyzed using content analysis to explicate the emergent themes embedded within the data. Our analytical approach was based in grounded theory through the utilization of the constant comparative method (Glaser, 1978). A research team consisting of two independent coders carefully reviewed the open-ended responses. First, the research team read through the open-ended responses to familiarize themselves with the dataset. Next, open and axial coding processes were used to look for larger themes in the data (Corbin & Strauss, 2015). Open coding allowed the research team to explore the emergent and descriptive themes that were dominant within the data, and the axial coding process helped the research team organize the open codes into a hierarchical schema of more dominant themes. This analysis resulted in eight major themes regarding topic avoidance for individuals with type 2 diabetes in romantic relationships.

Using the eight major themes as a codebook, the research team went back through the responses and coded each response with a specific theme. Responses that included multiple answers or contained instances of more than one theme were unitized and separated as individual codes. A total of $N = 512$ units of analysis were observed in order to answer RQ1. We used Cohen's κ to calculate the intercoder reliability between the independent coders. The reliability between coders for each subset of data ranged from $\hat{k} = 0.82$ to $\hat{k} = 0.89$. After all of the coding was complete, disagreements between the coding team were resolved through discussion with the first author.

RESULTS

Our research question asked participants to describe the topics about their illness that they avoid discussing with their romantic partner (RQ1). A total of eight categories emerged from the data (see Table 4.1): (a) health and wellness, (b) symptoms/complications, (c) maintaining privacy boundaries, (d) uncertainty, (e) lack of partner support, (f) sexual intimacy, (g) financial risks, and (h) open communication. In addition, a miscellaneous category (11.9%) was used to account for thematic units that did not fit into any other category (e.g., "I would rather not say," "I can't think of anything we would avoid.").

Health and Wellness

The first theme described topic avoidance related to health, weight management, food consumption, sugar levels, and the overall guilt associated with not adhering to lifestyle changes necessary to manage the illness (14.9% of thematic units). For example, one participant (male, age 37) stated, "I'm sometimes not completely honest about how well I'm managing things. If I haven't been good about my diet or getting exercise I won't volunteer that information and sometimes actively hide it. I know I should do better; I feel like at that point it doesn't accomplish much to have another person disappointed in me." Partners also mentioned that issues relating to health and wellness might also influence their relationship in addition to health concerns, such as one participant (female, age 46) stating, "I always eat more when I'm eating alone than I do when I am with him. I snack way too much at night and to my knowledge, he doesn't know I do that when I'm not with him. I am around 30 pounds overweight and he was too, until he got ill around the beginning of this year. Because of his illness, he has dropped down to around his ideal weight. This makes me very insecure and I'm afraid he may start looking for someone 'closer to his size.'" Participants with responses in this theme described trying to hide or trivialize issues associated with their

TABLE 4.1 *Topic avoidance themes*

1. Health and wellness

"My husband doesn't have a very great understanding of nutrition, because he's never had a weight problem. I will occasionally eat something/more than I should, and he doesn't know the difference. He is very watchful of my condition, as he is of his own health, so I like to keep him a little in the dark about my food choices." (female, age 47)

"I do not like to share if I am feeling bad, due to my ingesting some clandestine food driving up my blood sugar. I sometimes cheat (on my diet) and do not want to be lectured by my wife." (male, age 66)

"I avoid telling him my daily glucose levels because they reflect when I've "cheated" my diet without him knowing. I get fast food sometimes in addition to my regular meals, or don't exercise when I should." (male, age 58)

2. Symptoms/complications

"I recently had a skin infection and it was extremely bad. I kept that fact from him because he had no idea how bad diabetes can cause damage in the body which can lead to severe blood infections or loss of limbs. I am constantly worried about infections on my body. I don't want him to worry." (female, age 49)

"On the whole, I discuss everything with my partner, as he is very understanding, caring etc. Some days, I may feel giddy and rest for some time which I will not tell my partner as I feel that he may think that I am sick. Some other days I feel like my vision is blurring which I will not convey to him." (female, age 33)

"There are some side effects of the medications that I do not talk about, such as the extremely dry skin and mouth (and resulting dental problems). I also don't generally discuss my blood glucose levels unless something is out of whack or doesn't seem right." (female, age 35)

3. Maintaining privacy boundaries

"As previously mentioned, I don't really involve my partner in my diabetes management. It is not due to wanting to hide anything about it from her, I simply don't need anything from her in regards to it." (male, age 40)

"I pretty much always try to avoid discussing the diabetes. I feel embarrassed about having it, especially at my age. It's just not something I want to be reminded about or that I want to remind him about. I'd rather us focus on our relationship and things we enjoy together rather than the mistakes I've made in my life that led to this diagnosis." (male, age 27)

"My symptoms seem to come and go with new ones and old ones. Some days I get tired of complaining and talking about medical issues I have, I can't even stand to hear my own voice anymore. I am certain that my partner has the same feelings towards me, as I do myself. I try my best to spare him, and tend to keep the pains and sensations of my diabetes inside." (female, age 31)

Continued

TABLE 4.1 *Cont.*

4. Uncertainty

"I avoid talking about the future, and how the condition might impair me a few more years down the road. Because my diabetes is compounded by many other health conditions, I view my future health concerns as very oppressive. The only thing I can really control is my attitude over my health. I constantly look for positive things that will help balance out the concerns." (male, age 38)

"I don't like to tell him that I am afraid my life will not be as long as I had hoped, because of this stupid diabetes. I try not to tell him how angry I am with myself for getting this in the first place." (female, age 40)

"Mostly, in those dark days when I am afraid, I will minimize or will not tell him my fears. We have discussed at one time or another those dark fears and at some level I do understand that it is an unreasonable fear. WE manage my disease as best as we can, and he is very supportive of anything I want to try." (female, age 39)

5. Lack of partner support

"He never asks anything about my condition. I've shared, but he's so disinterested. I don't share much anymore. Anytime I discuss feelings his response is always "I don't know what to say" or "This makes me uncomfortable." So, I just don't care much anymore." (female, age 33)

"He doesn't want to hear about any aspect of it, if I mention it he will tune me out or start an argument and tell me I am just fat and lazy. I tend to keep all of it to myself and I have to hide my medications and syringes as he sees those either as a danger to him or an opportunity to take them and sell them for booze." (female, age 47)

"I really don't discuss my diabetes very much with him, not because I want to keep it private – he is aware of my diagnosis & the treatment – I don't discuss it because he really is not interested." (female, age 67)

6. Sexual intimacy

"We don't discuss my lack of interest in sex very often, and I've tried to let him know that it's not how I feel about him, but how I feel in general that causes this." (female, age 47)

"I avoid telling him about the other side effects – I have PCOS as well – like masculinization, since he has not seen me balding and bearded." (female, age 35)

"I sometimes avoid the fact that I experience some sexual dysfunction as a result of my condition. We do avoid talking about it as it makes me uncomfortable." (male, age 55)

7. Financial risks

"My insurance only covers so much of the cost of my diabetes. I try not to tell her that my treatment is creating money problems. I go sometimes without medication or test strips when money is tight." (male, age 39)

Continued

TABLE 4.1 *Cont.*

"I keep money matters private. I don't discuss money I spend on medication with my partner because I don't like to argue about money." (female, age 48)

8. Open communication

"Nothing that I can think of. I am very open about my blood glucose levels. He talks with me nicely about them and encourages me without nagging. He asks if I am taking care of myself if we haven't talked about my numbers recently or if he sees me eating poorly more than once. I think we keep the communication open." (female, age 42)

"My partner and I have a good relationship. We are respectful, encouraging, and loving with one another. I am able to share with my partner everything about my diabetes diagnosis. It is difficult to share when I have not been as compliant as I should, because he is so supportive, but I do share that information with him and we work on it together. I am comfortable in asking him for love, understanding, and support with my diabetes." (female, age 57)

"There are no topics related to my diabetes that are off-limits in my relationship with my partner. My partner is intelligent and well-informed and understands the physiologic causes of diabetes as well as the long-term effects if the condition is not treated. The possibility that diabetes will shorten my life expectancy is understood. All aspects of diet, exercise, weight-loss and other diabetes-related topics are open for discussion at any time. In my relationship there is no need for secrets; there are no taboos." (male, age 59)

diet, conceal any cheating they do on their exercise or diet regimen, and avoid discussing their illness with their partner because they feel guilty about their health choices or fearful of what their partner might think. Another participant (male, age 42) stated that he often succumbed to his cravings for sweet foods, but avoided telling his partner because of the potential fallout in their relationship, stating, "I sometimes hide what I eat and do not tell her the carb ratio. I tend to do this behind her back from time to time, mostly when I get cravings for sweets and she is usually unaware. I make up for it by exercising more, but I do not share this info with her for the sake of not upsetting her."

Symptoms/Complications

The second theme described topic avoidance related to symptoms that are associated with complications arising from type 2 diabetes (13.6% of thematic units). In this theme, participants emphasized not wanting to talk about the specifics of their symptoms, such as nerve damage, body odor (i.e., bad breath, strong urine scent, etc.), loss of hearing, loss of eyesight, blood pressure changes, yeast infections, and overall pain. One participant (male, age 26) mentioned not wanting to discuss symptoms with his partner, stating that he did not want to her to know "how bad the pain I get in my liver and feet is. I don't want her to worry about me 24/7 or feel like I'm some kind of burden to her and think she has to treat me like my diagnosis." Participants indicated that discussing these symptoms could be embarrassing or an indicator that they were not properly managing their illness. Another participant (female, age 31) mentioned the day-to-day issues she faced related to her symptoms, and how she avoided certain topics to prevent her husband from worrying that her illness had progressed, stating, "I try not to discuss days when I have horrible fruity breath from my diabetes, and I don't mention my fears to him concerning whether or not that little nick from shaving my legs is healing too slow or not. My feet are often a little dry, so I wear socks a lot to hide them." Other participants said they avoided discussing symptoms with their partner because it could worry them or make them feel anxious about their prognosis, such as one participant (male, age 41) who stated, "I sometimes don't tell my wife when my hands and feet are tingling . . . I figure this is due to my blood-glucose becoming too high, and I don't want her to worry."

Maintaining Privacy Boundaries

The third theme described topic avoidance resulting from the desire to keep information about the illness private (11.6% of thematic units). Participants mentioned wanting to keep information private because disclosing it might upset or burden their partner. Discussing specifics of the illness could make communication awkward with their partner or shift some of the responsibility for controlling the illness onto their partner. For example, one participant (male, age 32) stated, "I try to avoid bringing stuff up in general, because I feel bad about the fact that I don't take care of myself enough. When I think 10 or 20 years down the line, if I go blind, and I need her help, she'd be upset with me because I didn't take care of myself the way I should have now. I feel like a burden towards her." In addition, some participants felt that keeping information private created a healthier relational environment, with few sources of stress and anxiety. One participant (female, age 52) described how she tries to mention only more serious issues pertaining to her illness, stating, "I generally don't tell him about any wounds I get on my lower legs. He is overly sensitive about this issue because an aunt of his lost both of her lower legs due to diabetes and he gets too obsessive and overbearing about this particular issue. I would tell him if I felt I had a wound or skin condition that needed emergency medical attention." Other participants with responses in this theme described feeling like their illness was "my problem, not my partner's," and wanted to keep some autonomy in the management of their illness, such as one participant (male, age 45) stating, "I keep it all private. It is my condition and not hers, thus my concern and not hers. I am a man and deal with my own problems as well as the problems of my loved ones."

Uncertainty

The fourth theme described topic avoidance related to the uncertainties surrounding the prognosis and severity of the illness (10.5% of thematic units). As one participant (female, age 47) stated, "I don't discuss how worried I am about my future health or about how much of a financial burden this will impose on our family in the future. I also don't tell him that I think I'm developing diabetic nerve damage." Specifically, participants mentioned avoiding topics about their own personal fears and uncertainty about the expected course of their illness, their quality of life in the future, and unforeseen complications arising later in life. One participant (female, age 59) discussed that she worried about the uncertainty surrounding her long-term prognosis, stating, "I am 22 years older than my fiancé. So, I'm not eager to share with him a couple of potential extreme outcomes of diabetes that could happen, in time, if I'm not careful: blindness or amputation of a limb. I don't want him to get the feeling that he could eventually have an invalid on his hands." In addition, another participant (female, age 37) felt uncertain about the implications for her illness in the context of her relationship with her husband, stating "My fear is that he will leave me because I'm not able to do as much as I used to, like cooking all the meals, do the laundry, etc. I'm also afraid to talk about losing my life and what to do about my son if that happened. I know he would care for him, but it would be so much harder, and I don't want to leave them." Participants also noted that if they were to become incapacitated or pass away due to their illness, they were uncertain as to whether their partner or family would be provided for, both financially and emotionally.

Lack of Partner Support

The fifth theme described topic avoidance with regard to requests for social support, as participants predicted a negative or poor outcome as a result of their request (8.1% of thematic units). For example, one participant (male, age 35) expressed his frustration when trying to seek support from his partner, stating, "It doesn't really matter, because she won't listen to anything I say anyway – and in the unlikely event that she does listen, she usually forgets about it quickly so I can tell her anything and it is as if I kept it private." Participants noted that they avoided seeking support when they felt their partner would be uninterested, not want to discuss the problem, or make disparaging remarks toward them. Another participant (female, age 45) mentioned that her partner seemed disingenuous when providing support, stating, "I don't share much about how my condition effects [sic] me with my partner – he is simply in his own world or gives me an 'I'm sorry' and has no memory of it later. So I just don't bother." In addition, participants with responses in this theme also felt as though their requests for support would be unheard, or that their partner would not be able to handle the request. For example, one participant (female, age 60) stated, "We don't really discuss anything having to do with my condition, because it typically turns into a one-sided conversation about what issues he has, and how I just don't understand, so I keep mostly everything to myself."

Sexual Intimacy

The sixth theme described topic avoidance surrounding sexual intimacy and sexual capabilities (5.7% of thematic units). Participants mentioned avoiding topics related to their sex drive, desirability, and sexual functioning. Participants described wanting to avoid discussion about sexual dysfunction issues, such as erectile dysfunction, and reproductive health issues, such as polycystic ovarian syndrome. In addition, partners also described avoiding topics related to changes in their sex drive and sexual desire. One participant (male, age 38) stated that he avoided topics about sex with his partner because he noticed a change in his sexual capabilities, stating, "I have kept the issue of intimacy very private – simply for the fact that it's far and few in between right now so I know she has not noticed the gradual decrease in performance and or quality of intimacy as it is related to my diabetes." Another participant (male, age 47) discussed his frustration about his partner conflating sexual dysfunction with relational interest and desire, stating, "It is difficult to discuss erectile dysfunction with my partner, because she tends to see things of that nature as me not loving her or desiring her enough." Topic avoidance in this category was often driven by participants' desire to avoid drawing attention to the loss of intimacy and eliciting concern from one's partner, such as one participant (female, age 59) who stated, "I avoid discussing my lack of sex drive. Because the diabetes limits my sleep, I am often not interested in sex, but I do not tell him for fear he will worry about our sex life."

Financial Risks

The seventh theme described topic avoidance about issues related to finance and cost of care for the illness (5.1% of thematic units). Participants mentioned not discussing the cost of medication or care because their partner was either unaware of the true cost, or they did not want to argue with their partner about money. For example, one participant (female, age 36) stated, "I did not inform him that I have developed lesions on the back of my eye because we do not have insurance for him to see his doctor for his eyes and he has needed new script for last three years! Also, my insurance only covers one visit to the eye doctor for me so telling would just add undue stress to our situation. Since it can't be helped, why bring it up?" Participants also mentioned that when they had to forgo treatment, medicine, and procedures due to a lack of funds, they avoided mentioning it to their partner to prevent any additional stress about the topic. Another participant (female, age 45) discussed having trouble being able to afford regular blood sugar testing, stating, "I avoid talking to him about testing my sugar because we don't have health insurance right now and he doesn't grasp how expensive the test strips are and just gets impatient with me. I pretty much keep to myself concerning this with my partner."

Open Communication

Notably, a relatively large number of participants indicated that they strive to remain open in communication with their partner rather than avoiding certain topics about their illness (19.6% of thematic units). Partners mentioned that open communication was important because their type 2 diabetes was a "team effort" to keep under control. Participants with responses in this theme specifically mentioned that they appreciated the deeper understanding their partner had as a result of their open communication. For example, one participant (female, age 53) stated, "I tell him pretty much everything. We've been doing this for a while now, he knows a lot about diabetes and isn't afraid of it or of learning more about it, whether from me or other sources. He knows where my numbers fall and where on the scale they fall. I'm not obsessed about it, although it is part of every choice it seems, he kind of follows my lead. I can't think of anything I don't tell him – except my weight of course." Often, participants mentioned that open communication was possible because their partner also had type 2 diabetes, or there was a close family member/friend who had type 2 diabetes. Another participant (male, age 62) mentioned that prior experiences from both partners regarding type 2 diabetes was a motivational factor for open communication, stating, "Oh gosh, we share everything . . . having witnessed the experience of diabetic members of both our families, we are quite motivated to beat this – as a team."

DISCUSSION

Managing chronic illness can be a complicated factor for romantic relationships, as partners often co-manage the treatment, symptoms, lifestyle changes, and progression of the condition. Considering that many of the maintenance tasks involved with patient adherence to treatment of type 2 diabetes take place at home (Glasgow & Anderson, 1999), understanding the ways that individuals involve or exclude their romantic partner in the management of their illness can have implications for health outcomes. Our study examined the health-related topics that individuals avoid discussing with a romantic partner and identified eight distinct themes of topic avoidance: (a) health and wellness, (b) symptoms/complications, (c) maintaining privacy boundaries, (d) uncertainty, (e) lack of partner support, (f) sexual intimacy, (g) financial risks, and (h) open communication. In the following sections, we highlight and discuss the relational, health, and communicative implications of our findings in this study. We also discuss the strengths and limitations of our study.

Implications for Relationships

The results of this study point to some notable implications for close relationships. One notable finding was that many of the reasons for topic avoidance that emerged in this study suggest that the potential for embarrassment and shame encourages avoidance of certain topics. A growing body of research has looked at the effects of stigma on communication in relationships and the motivations couples have for disclosing health information (Della, Ashlock, & Basta, 2016). Type 2 diabetes has a unique set of stigmatized stereotypes that characterize the condition, such as individuals with type 2 diabetes being perceived as lazy, careless, overindulgent, lacking self-control, and making poor lifestyle choices (Schabert, Browne, Mosely, & Speight, 2013), despite the fact that genetics and hereditary insulin resistance are important risk factors for the development of type 2 diabetes (Lyssenko et al., 2008). Thus, avoiding topics related to one's illness that are perceived as stigmatizing, such as failures to comply with treatment, undesirable symptoms and complications, or unexpected sexual dysfunction, can help an individual save face in the eyes of a romantic partner.

The results also point to uncertainty as a driving force for topic avoidance about type 2 diabetes in romantic relationships. Some participants mentioned that they were uncertain about facets of their illness, such as their ability to manage the illness, control symptoms, or foresee their long-term prognosis. Although these issues specifically reflect illness uncertainty (Johnson Wright, Afari, & Zautra, 2009; Mishel, 1990), ambiguity about one's health can reverberate into broader concerns about the well-being of one's self or a relationship. Not surprisingly, then, a number of the themes of topic avoidance in this study reflected an unwillingness to discuss one's health condition owing to uncertainty about how the illness might dampen a partner's attraction, or enthusiasm for the relationship. Studies show that relational uncertainty encourages topic avoidance about a variety of issues (Knobloch & Carpenter-Theune, 2004; Knobloch, Sharabi, Delaney, & Suranne, 2015; Theiss & Estlein, 2014; Theiss & Nagy, 2013) and our results suggest that managing chronic illness may exacerbate some of these uncertainties.

Finally, a unique finding in this study was that a notable number of participants specifically mentioned avoiding support requests relating to their type 2 diabetes. Many participants noted that they wanted to request support from their partner, but felt that their partner either could not provide adequate support or did not want to provide adequate support, so they chose to forgo the request. When attempts were made to request support, partners wound up making superficial attempts to provide support, and others used communication tactics to either avoid or reverse the support request. Prior research has shown that self-efficacy about one's ability to provide support can influence how an individual approaches a support request (Bodie, Burleson, & Jones, 2012). Given the nuanced and technical nature of type 2 diabetes maintenance and complications, it may be that relational partners feel as though they do not possess the knowledge or skill to effectively support their partner. When individuals anticipate that a partner lacks the motivation or skills required to enact effective support, they may side-step sensitive issues to avoid the disappointment of receiving poor support.

Implications for Communication

Surprisingly, a sizable percentage of participants specifically mentioned that they rarely avoided topics with their partner and strived to communicate openly about their illness. One explanation for this finding may be that open communication is an important quality in a relationship in which one partner has a chronic health condition (Goldsmith, 2009). Open, honest, and direct communication about one's illness can be beneficial for clarifying expectations between partners, coordinating actions and routines for a healthier lifestyle, and managing complicated treatments (Goldsmith et al., 2008). If topics such as symptoms, worries, lifestyle changes, and financial issues are openly discussed between partners rather than avoided, then the relationship can provide an important source of support and facilitation for managing type 2 diabetes. An alternative explanation for this finding is that participants failed to recognize the various issues that they avoid discussing with their partner out of an ideology of openness. Cultural expectations about relationships tend to favor open and honest communication between partners over secrecy or dishonesty. Thus, individuals in this study may have been motivated to characterize their relationship in such a way that reflected cultural norms equating openness with intimacy without considering the true complexities of their relational communication.

Although open communication is often idealized in representations of close relationships, there are certain conditions in which constant openness can be detrimental to establishing intimacy and connection between partners. Along these lines, many participants also noted that privacy boundaries were an important part of choosing whether to disclose certain information to their partner. Taken together, these findings point to a core dialectical tension for individuals with type 2 diabetes, such that they desire open communication with their partner about the illness, but also want to protect their privacy to prevent embarrassment and stigma. These competing desires can create quite a quandary. For example, individuals may want the privacy and autonomy that comes with managing their condition by themselves, but they may also feel as though they want their partner's support and help in self-managing at home. Individuals may also feel as though they do not want to burden their partner with their self-care and worries about their condition, but may also feel overwhelmed and distressed trying to manage it alone. Thus, coping with chronic illness in the context of a close relationship requires that partners find an acceptable balance between openness and privacy.

Implications for Health

As previously mentioned, our results suggest that individuals with type 2 diabetes may be reluctant to request support from their romantic partner, despite the fact that social support can be an important component of managing chronic illness. Given that social support is a factor that has consistently been shown to have a positive association with wellness and self-management (Gallant, 2003), future research should look at the mechanisms of support efficacy in the context of type 2 diabetes. Whereas individuals with type 2 diabetes may feel comfortable seeking informational or tangible support to cope with their illness, such as researching treatment options or adhering to a healthy diet, requesting emotional and esteem support, such as reassurance from their partner or recognition for making difficult lifestyle changes, can be much more face-threatening. Thus, romantic partners can be most effective in providing support when they offer multifaceted messages that address both relational and health-based needs.

In addition, health care providers should be aware of the potential topics that individuals with type 2 diabetes might avoid discussing outside of a medical context. Communication about adherence to treatments and lifestyle changes may function differently between health care providers and romantic partners. Topics that patients may feel comfortable discussing and communicating about with their health care provider, such as health and wellness, symptoms/complications, sexual intimacy, or uncertainty, may be uncomfortable to discuss with romantic partners. As such, health care providers should be proactive in addressing the importance of involving romantic partners or family members in the management of their condition.

Limitations and Future Directions

This study was not without its share of limitations. First, given that participants responded to an open-ended survey question about topic avoidance, we were unable to probe their responses to achieve the level of detail that would be possible in an interview setting. A more interactive method of data collection would have provided for more depth in the responses. Next, our study only looked at sources of topic avoidance for type 2 diabetics in romantic relationships. As such, our findings were limited in highlighting any of the antecedents and consequences of topic avoidance in these relationships. In addition, given the cross-sectional nature of this study, we were unable to observe how prolonged avoidance of communication about health-related issues may have long-term implications for people's health and well-being Future research may wish to consider how topic avoidance exists during certain stages of chronic illness (e.g., immediately after diagnosis, during management, after symptoms manifest) and how topic avoidance influences romantic relationships over time.

REFERENCES

Adam, J., & Folds, L. (2014). Depression, self-efficacy, and adherence in patients with type 2 diabetes. *The Journal for Nurse Practitioners, 10*, 646–652. doi: 10.1016/j.nurpra.2014.07.033

Afifi, T. D., Shahnazi, A. F., Coveleski, S., Davis, S., & Merrill, A. (2017). Testing the ideology of openness: The comparative effects of talking, writing, and avoiding a stressor on rumination and health. *Human Communication Research, 43*, 76–101. doi: 10.1111/hcre.12096

Afifi, W. A., & Guerrero, L. K. (2009). Some things are better left unsaid II: Topic avoidance in friendships. *Communication Quarterly, 46*, 231–249. doi: 10.1080/01463379809370099

Beverly, E. A., Miller, C. K., & Wray, L. A. (2008). Spousal support and food-related behavior change in middle-aged and older adults living with type 2 diabetes. *Health Education & Behavior, 35*, 707–720. doi: 10.1177/1090198107299787

Bodie, G. D., Burleson, B. R., & Jones, S. M. (2012). Explaining the relationships among supportive message quality, evaluations, and outcomes: A dual-process approach. *Communication Monographs, 79*, 1–22. doi: 10.1080/03637751.2011.646491

Casler, K., Bickel, L., & Hackett, E. (2013). Separate but equal? A comparison of participants and data gathered via Amazon's MTurk, social media, and face-to-face behavioral testing. *Computers in Human Behavior, 29*, 2156–2160. doi: 10.1016/j.chb.2013.05.009

Caughlin, J. P., Afifi, W. A., Carpenter-Theune, K. E., & Miller, L. E. (2005). Reasons for, and consequences of, revealing personal secrets in close relationships: A longitudinal study. *Personal Relationships, 12*, 43–59. doi: 10.1111/j.1350-4126.2005.00101.x

Centers for Disease Control and Prevention (CDC). (2014). National Diabetes Statistics Report: Estimates of Diabetes and Its Burden in the United States, 2014. Atlanta, GA: U.S. Department of Health and Human Services. http://www.cdc.gov/diabetes/pubs/statsreport14/national-diabetes-report-web.pdf

Corbin, J., & Strauss, A. (2015). *Basics of qualitative research: Techniques and procedures for developing grounded theory* (4th ed.). Thousand Oaks, CA: SAGE.

Defenbaugh, N. L. (2013). Revealing and concealing ill identity: A performance narrative of IBD disclosure. *Health Communication, 28,* 159–169. doi: 10.1080/10410236.2012.666712

Della, L. J., Ashlock, M. Z., & Basta, T. B. (2016). Social constructions of stigmatizing discourse around type 2 diabetes diagnoses in Appalachian Kentucky. *Health Communication, 31,* 806–814. doi: 10.1080/10410236.2015.1007547

Derlega, V. J., Winstead, B. A., Greene, K., Serovich, J., & Elwood, W. N. (2004). Reasons for HIV disclosure/nondisclosure in close relationships: Testing a model of HIV-disclosure decision making. *Journal of Social and Clinical Psychology, 23,* 747–767. doi: 10.1521/jscp.23.6.747.54804

Donovan-Kicken, E., & Caughlin, J. P. (2010). A multiple goals perspective on topic avoidance and relationship satisfaction in the context of breast cancer. *Communication Monographs, 77,* 231–256. doi: 10.1080/03637751003758219

Fisher, L., Mullan, J. T., Skaff, M. M., Glasgow, R. E., Arean, P., & Hessler, D. (2009). Predicting diabetes distress in patients with type 2 diabetes: A longitudinal study. *Diabetic Medicine: A Journal of the British Diabetic Association, 26,* 622–627. doi: 10.1111/j.1464-5491.2009.02730.x

Gallant, M. P. (2003). The influence of social support on chronic illness self-management: A review and directions for research. *Health Education & Behavior, 30,* 170–195. doi: 10.1177/1090198102251030

Glaser, B. G. (1978). *Theoretical sensitivity: Advances in the methodology of grounded theory.* Mill Valley, CA: Sociology Press.

Glasgow, R. E., & Anderson, R. M. (1999). In diabetes care, moving from compliance to adherence is not enough: Something entirely different is needed. *Diabetes Care, 22,* 2090–2092. doi: 10.2337/diacare.22.12.2090

Goldsmith, D. J. (2009). Uncertainty and communication in couples coping with serious illness. In T. D. Afifi & W. A. Afifi (Eds.), *Uncertainty, information management, and disclosure decisions* (pp. 203–225). New York, NY: Routledge.

Goldsmith, D. J., Miller L. E., & Caughlin, J. P. (2008). Openness and avoidance in couples communicating about cancer. In C. Beck (Ed.), *Communication yearbook 31* (pp. 62–115). Malden, MA: Blackwell.

Golish, T. D. (2000). Is openness always better? Exploring the role of topic avoidance, satisfaction, and parenting styles of stepparents. *Communication Quarterly, 48,* 137–158. doi: 10.1080/01463370009385587

Goodman, J. K., Cryder, C. E., & Cheema, A. (2013). Data collection in a flat world: The strengths and weaknesses of Mechanical Turk samples. *Journal of Behavioral Decision Making, 26,* 213–224. doi: 10.1002/bdm.1753

Johnson Wright, L., Afari, N., & Zautra, A. (2009). The illness uncertainty concept: A review. *Current Pain and Headache Reports, 13,* 133–138. doi: 35400060180081.0007

Karlsen, B., & Bru, E. (2014). The relationship between diabetes-related distress and clinical variables and perceived support among adults with type 2 diabetes: A prospective study. *International Journal of Nursing Studies, 51,* 438–447. doi: 10.1016/j.ijnurstu.2013.06.016

Knobloch, L. K., & Carpenter-Theune, K. E. (2004). Topic avoidance in developing romantic relationships: Associations with intimacy and relational uncertainty. *Communication Research, 31,* 173–205. doi: 10.1177/0093650203261516

Knobloch, L. K., Sharabi, L. L., Delaney, A. L., & Suranne, S. M. (2015). The role of relational uncertainty in topic avoidance among couples with depression. *Communication Monographs, 83,* 25–48. doi: 10.1080/03637751.2014.998691

Leustek, J., & Theiss, J. A. (2018). Factors that shape cognitive and behavioral coping among individuals with type 2 diabetes: Features of illness versus features of romantic relationships. *Health Communication, 33,* 1549–1559. doi: 10.1080/10410236.2017.1384346

Lyssenko, V., Jonsson, A., Almgren, P., Pulizzi, N., Isomaa, B., Tuomi, T., . . . Groop, L. (2008). Clinical risk factors, DNA variants, and the development of type 2 diabetes. *The New England Journal of Medicine, 359,* 2220–2232. doi: 10.1056/NEJMoa0801869#t=article

Middleton, A. V., LaVoie, N. R., & Brown, L. E. (2012). Sources of uncertainty in type 2 diabetes: Explication and implications for health communication theory and clinical practice. *Health Communication, 27,* 591–601. doi: 10.1080/10410236.2011.618435

Miller, T. A., & DiMatteo, M. R. (2013). Importance of family/social support and impact on adherence to diabetic therapy. *Diabetes, Metabolic Syndrome and Obesity: Targets and Therapy, 6,* 421–426. doi: 10.2147/DMSO.S36368

Mishel, M. H. (1990). Reconceptualization of the uncertainty in illness theory. *Image: The Journal of Nursing Scholarship, 22,* 256–262. doi: 10.1111/j.1547-5069.1990.tb00225.x

Osborn, C. Y., & Egede, L. E. (2012). The relationship between depressive symptoms and medication nonadherence in type 2 diabetes: The role of social support. *General Hospital Psychiatry, 34,* 249–253. doi: 10.1016/j.genhosppsych.2012.01.015

Peyrot, M., Rubin, R. R., Lauritzen, T., Snoek, F. J., Matthews, D. R., & Skovlund, S. E. (2005). Psychosocial problems and barriers to improved diabetes management: Results of the Cross-National Diabetes Attitudes, Wishes and Needs (DAWN) Study. *Diabetic Medicine, 22,* 1379–1385. doi: 10.1111/j.1464-5491.2005.01644.x

Rintala, T. M., Jaatinen, P., Paavilainen, E., & Astedt-Kurki, P. (2013). Interrelation between adult persons with diabetes and their family: A systematic review of the literature. *Journal of Family Nursing, 19,* 3–28. doi: 10.1177/1074840712471899

Roloff, M. E., & Ifert, D. E. (2000). Conflict management through avoidance: Withholding complaints, suppressing arguments, and declaring topics taboo. In S. Petronio (Ed.), *Balancing the secrets of private disclosures* (pp. 151–163). Mahwah, NJ: Lawrence Erlbaum Associates.

Schabert, J., Browne, J. L., Mosely, K., & Speight, J. (2013). Social stigma in diabetes: A framework to understand a growing problem for an increasing epidemic. *The Patient, 6,* 1–10. doi: 10.1007/s40271-012-0001-0

Theiss, J. A., Carpenter, A. M., & Leustek, J. (2016). Partner facilitation and partner interference in individuals' weight loss goals. *Qualitative Health Research, 26,* 1318–1330. doi: 10.1177/1049732315583980

Theiss, J. A., & Estlein, R. (2014). Antecedents and consequences of the perceived threat of sexual communication: A test of the relational turbulence model. *Western Journal of Communication, 78,* 404–425. doi: 10.1080/10570314.2013.845794

Theiss, J. A., & Nagy, M. E. (2013). A relational turbulence model of partner responsiveness and relationship talk across cultures. *Western Journal of Communication, 77,* 186–209. doi: 10.1080/10570314.2012.720746

Toller, P. W., & McBride, M. C. (2013). Enacting privacy rules and protecting disclosure recipients: Parents' communication with children following the death of a family member. *Journal of Family Communication, 13,* 32–45. doi: 10.1080/15267431.2012.742091

Trief, P. M., Himes, C. L., Orendorff, R., & Weinstock, R. S. (2001). The marital relationship and psychosocial adaptation and glycemic control of individuals with diabetes. *Diabetes Care, 24,* 1384–1389. doi: 10.2337/diacare.24.8.1384

Turner, J., Kelly, B., Swanson, C., Allison, R., & Wetzig, N. (2005). Psychosocial impact of newly diagnosed advanced breast cancer. *Psycho-Oncology, 14,* 396–407. doi: 10.1002/pon.856

Walsh, S. R., Manuel, J. C., & Avis, N. E. (2005). The impact of breast cancer on younger women's relationships with their partner and children. *Families, Systems, & Health, 23,* 80–93. doi: 10.1037/1091-7527.23.1.80

5

Closeness, Recipient Response, and Interaction Effectiveness: An Application of the Actor–Partner Interdependence Model in Mental Health Disclosures

MARIA K. VENETIS, PATRICIA E. GETTINGS, AND
SKYE CHERNICHKY-KARCHER

Friends, including college-aged friends, often share important, personal information with each other (Mathews, Derlega, & Morrow, 2006). This information extends to health-related information such as mental illness diagnoses (Chaudoir & Quinn, 2010; Greene et al., 2012; Venetis, Chernichky-Karcher, & Gettings, 2018). Models predicting disclosure such as the disclosure decision-making model (DD-MM; Greene, 2009) and the revelation risk model (RRM; Afifi & Steuber, 2009) demonstrate that disclosure literature has largely focused on disclosers' cognitive processes and perceptions. However, disclosure is inherently a dyadic process that unfolds and is evaluated by the communicative behaviors of both interactants (i.e., discloser and recipient). Although disclosers may prepare for and script their disclosure (Bute, 2013), recipients may not have anticipated the disclosure and, therefore, simply react to information rather than preparing a response. Recipient response is an instrumental component of the disclosure interaction evaluation. Both disclosers and recipients will evaluate how disclosers shared the information (Williams & Mickelson, 2008) and how recipients responded, and they will make judgments concerning if the conversation went well. Interestingly, partners may experience the same event, such as shared conversation, yet report disparate recollections of that shared event. We seek to better understand how recipient responses influence interaction evaluation from both perspectives within the college-friend dyad. Specifically, this chapter aims to: (a) explicate the nature of interactions surrounding sharing mental illness within college-friend dyads, (b) review the role of the recipient and the complexities of recipient response in disclosure interactions, and (c) present results based on actor–partner interdependence model (APIM) analysis in a study of college-aged friend pairs.

MENTAL ILLNESS AND COLLEGE STUDENTS

Mental illness is a frequent diagnosis on college campuses, as each year more than one in four college students are diagnosed or treated by a professional for mental illness (American College Health Association, 2012). Mental illnesses are "health conditions involving changes in thinking, emotion or behavior (or a combination of these)" that are "associated with distress and/or problems functioning in social, work or family activities" (American Psychiatric Association, 2015). College students report a range of diagnoses; in a National Alliance on Mental Illness (NAMI, 2012) survey, for instance, participants reported the following primary diagnoses: depression (27%), bipolar disorder (24%), other (12%; e.g., borderline personality disorder, eating disorders, autism spectrum disorder), anxiety (11%), schizophrenia (6%), posttraumatic stress disorder (PTSD) (6%), and attention deficit and hyperactivity disorder (ADHD) (5%), among others. Although many students with mental illness have successful college careers, others report negative implications such as academic underperformance, difficulty establishing relationships, and possibly dropping out (Iarovici, 2014; NAMI, 2012). Beyond academic underachievement, mental illness might contribute to feelings of loneliness and isolation, which may impede social relationships (e.g., Kessler, Walters, & Forthofer, 1998).

College students may be motivated to disclose their mental illness status with friends for various reasons including catharsis, to strengthen a relationship, or because they feel the other has the right to know (e.g., Derlega, Winstead, Greene, Serovich, & Elwood, 2004). Furthermore, owing to the communal nature of college life in which students are likely to spend many hours with peers in close quarters, friends may notice behavioral markers of mental illness (e.g., difficulty concentrating, panic attacks). Such cues may motivate or oblige potential disclosers to share their mental illness. Despite disclosers' motivations for sharing, recipients' responses to mental illness disclosures can have serious implications for college student disclosers. Responses to mental illness disclosure can range from acceptance to rejection (Brohan et al., 2012). For example, positive disclosure experiences promote enhanced psychological benefits for the discloser, such as reduced fear of future disclosure and increased well-being (Chaudoir & Quinn, 2010). Conversely, negative responses may inhibit future disclosures (Chaudoir & Fisher, 2010). We now turn to a theoretical understanding of recipient response. Although research documents that how recipients respond is consequential to disclosers, less is known about the recipients' experiences of the disclosure process.

THE RECIPIENT EXPERIENCE AND DISCLOSURE RESPONSE

Disclosure research has thoroughly documented disclosers' predisclosure considerations. For example, Derlega et al. (2004) examined disclosure motivations and how recipient role influences the degree of information sharing. Similarly, Vangelisti, Caughlin, and Timmerman (2001) explored the criteria individuals use when determining whether to disclose family secrets (e.g., individuals who closely identified with their family secret tended to consider the nature of their relationship with a recipient before disclosing and were less likely to disclose simply because the information was contextually relevant). Several information management models position the intended recipient as an integral component of the disclosure decision. For example, the RRM (Afifi & Steuber, 2009) highlights how relational closeness to recipients influences both potential disclosers' evaluation of the risk in sharing the information (i.e., risk assessment), as well as their motivations for revealing (i.e., willingness to reveal conditions). Another example, the DD-MM (Greene, 2009), accounts for disclosers' sense of relational closeness with potential recipients as well as how others are expected to respond to the shared information. However, these models predict disclosure decisions, and the role of the recipient is logically limited to the extent to which disclosers can accurately anticipate their reactions.

Another framework, the model of disclosure decision-making in a single episode (Greene, Derlega, & Mathews, 2006), also describes the decision-making process. It explains that potential disclosers are influenced by their background (i.e., culture and personality), motivations for revealing, and conversational-level considerations (efficacy, flow of conversation, relational quality with other, and anticipated response). Should individuals decide to disclose, they then balance message design choices of whom to tell and how and where to share the information (see also the RRM and disclosure strategies, Afifi & Steuber, 2009). The Greene et al. (2006) model describes disclosure as a transactional process and posits that the disclosure elicits both discloser and recipient behavioral, emotional, and cognitive reactions. How the disclosure is managed and how the dyad interacts after the disclosure both have relational implications for the dyad. We examine the postdisclosure decision (i.e., after the discloser has decided to share the information) by dyadically exploring how relational closeness predicts perceptions of recipient response and the conversational implications and evaluations of those reactions.

The recipient perspective. Previous research gives us some idea about possible disclosure effects on recipients, albeit across a range of contexts (e.g., sexual orientation, chronic illness). A growing body of literature, for instance, documents the experiences of recipients of sexual assault or rape disclosures especially on college campuses. One study found that rape victims were most likely to disclose to informal (rather than formal) sources, such as friends, and the majority of recipients indicated they believe they were able to support the victim (e.g., by listening, comforting, or giving advice; Dunn, Vail-Smith & Knight, 1999). However, other studies found at least a third of recipients reported they were unsure how to appropriately respond to a disclosure of sexual assault or rape, and some reported less than optimal responses such as blaming the victim (Ahrens & Campbell, 2000; Dunn et al., 1999). Perhaps more germane to the current study, a proportion of disclosure recipients who felt they were supportive of the victim also indicated personal distress as a result of the interaction (Ahrens & Campbell, 2000; Banyard et al., 2010). Taken together, findings like these underscore the idea that receiving a disclosure and/or comforting the discloser can be mentally and emotionally taxing, even when the interaction could be considered successful.

The role of response. In the current study, we focus on perceived, post-disclosure recipient response. Rather than assessing anticipated response, we chose to collect data from individuals who had already disclosed (as described in Methods in more detail). Magsamen-Conrad (2014) reviewed how response has been operationalized across several information management theories and, in doing so, demonstrated the integral nature of recipient response within disclosure decisions and processes. Beyond positive or negative response, her examination identified four dimensions of recipient response: emotional reaction, support, reciprocity, and avoidance. Emotional reaction includes positive, negative, or neutral responses. Support is described as offering emotional, instrumental, or informational support. Reciprocity occurs when recipients match the disclosure by sharing information or openness. Finally, topic avoidance occurs when recipients avoid responding to the disclosure. Little research to date has examined how these four dimensions are associated with other disclosure variables. The current study extends Magsamen-Conrad's (2014) findings by exploring how these four response dimensions function in the context of mental health disclosures among college students.

Closeness and recipient response. As described earlier, theoretical consideration of recipients is often operationalized as relational quality, or closeness, with the other. In the context of anticipated disclosures, the degree of closeness influences disclosers' perceptions of recipient response (Greene, 2009) and, similarly, their perceived risk of disclosure (Afifi & Steuber, 2009). Greater closeness is associated with more positive anticipated response and reduced risk of sharing. This relationship also exists in postdisclosure examinations of how disclosure strategy influences response and interaction evaluations (Venetis, Chernichky, & Gettings, 2015). Because of this established relationship and because it connects with a feature of message choice in

Greene and colleagues' (2006) model, we examine how relational closeness predicts recipient reaction.

Recipient response and interaction effectiveness. Just as which information and how information is disclosed are consequential for self, other, and relational outcomes, the ways in which recipients respond to disclosures are important (Ahrens et al., 2007). For example, models of disclosure also explain that disclosers' perceptions of recipient response influence disclosers' future goals of revealing or concealing information (Chaudoir & Fisher, 2010; Greene, 2009), and negative responses often hinder future sharing. Among individuals disclosing mental illness information, research reports that some – although not all – recipients respond in ways that lead disclosers to feel stigmatized, resulting in feelings of embarrassment, anxiety, and isolation (Dinos, Stevens, Serfaty, Weich, & King, 2004). We argue that how disclosers and recipients recall recipient response (as supportive and open or negative and avoidant) will influence how both partners evaluate the interaction. We recently examined discloser perceptions of interaction effectiveness and found that among disclosers, support positively predicts interaction effectiveness (Venetis, Chernichky, et al., 2015). However, we are interested in dyadically examining the relationships between recipient support and interaction effectiveness, recognizing that the role of discloser or recipient may influence how interactions are recalled and evaluated.

To preview, the current study applies the APIM (Cook & Kenny, 2005) to data that include reports from 51 dyads in which one individual disclosed his or her mental illness diagnosis to a friend. Both members of the friend dyad separately completed an online questionnaire about their experiences following the disclosure of a mental illness diagnosis, including measures of relational closeness, recipient response, and interaction effectiveness.

METHOD

Participants

Participants were 51 dyads (N = 102) that were college-aged friends in which one friend shared his or her mental illness information with the other. Disclosers identified as female (n = 32, 62.7%), male (n = 18, 35.3%), and one did not report sex; recipients identified as female (n = 32, 62.7%), male (n = 18, 35.3%), and one did not report sex. Discloser age ranged from 18 to 27 years (M = 20.68, SD = 1.76); recipient age ranged from 18 to 27 years (M = 20.68, SD = 1.76). Disclosers self-identified as white/Caucasian (n = 35, 68.6%), Asian (n = 12, 23.5%), Hispanic or Latino/a (n = 2, 3.9%), American Indian (n = 1, 2%), or black/African American (n = 1, 2%). Similarly, recipients self-identified as white/Caucasian (n = 35, 68.6%),

Asian (n = 12, 23.5%), Hispanic or Latino/a (n = 2, 3.9%), American Indian (n = 1, 2%), or black/African American (n = 1, 2%). Disclosers were college students identifying as freshmen (n = 8, 15.7%), sophomores (n = 13, 25.5%), juniors (n = 9, 17.6%), seniors (n = 18, 35.3%), graduate level (n = 2, 3.9%), or other (n = 1, 2%). Recipients were college students identifying as freshmen (n = 8, 15.7%), sophomores (n = 13, 25.5%), juniors (n = 9, 17.6%), seniors (n = 18, 35.3%), graduate level (n = 2, 3.9%), or other (n = 1, 2%). Disclosers described that at the time of disclosure, recipients were friends (n = 46, 90.2%) or significant others (n = 4, 7.8%). Disclosers reported that they had known the recipient for varying lengths of time, including less than 1 year (n = 13; 25.5%), 1 year (n = 5; 9.8%), 2 years (n = 7, 13.7%), 3 years (n = 7, 13.7%), 4 years (n = 4, 7.8%), or more than 4 years (n = 14, 27.5%). Although the majority of pairs had been in the relationship for one year or less (n = 3, 62.8%) when disclosers shared their mental illness information, some pairs had been in the relationship for more than 4 years at the time of disclosure (n = 8, 15.7%).

Disclosers reported the following mental illness diagnoses: anxiety disorders (n = 15, 29%), depression (n = 14, 27%), attention deficit disorder (ADD) and/or ADHD) (n − 11, 22%), obsessive–compulsive disorder (n = 5, 10%), other (e.g., body dysmorphic disorder, epilepsy) (n = 6, 11%), bipolar disorder (n = 3, 6%), and borderline personality disorder (n = 3, 6%). Participants provided the details of their mental illness in an open-ended fashion and could report more than one illness. Because of this, percentages total greater than 100%. Category designations were made using the NAMI (2012) groupings for mental illness.

Procedure

On receiving university Institutional Review Board (IRB) approval, we recruited dyads for the study. Dyads were considered eligible if one member had a mental illness (i.e., discloser) and had disclosed his or her mental illness to the other member (i.e., recipient) within the past five years, if both members of the dyad were at least 18 years of age and college students, and if both members of the dyad considered the other to be a friend. For the purpose of this research, the term "friend" was used in the broadest sense, and participants themselves determined whether or not the recipient was classified as a "friend."

One member of each dyad enrolled in the study through a university online research participation system. Once enrolled, participants received an email describing the study in greater detail; participants were asked to provide both their own and their partner's email address, and their role as discloser or recipient. No details about specific mental health-related information were exchanged via email. After participants replied with contact information for both members of the dyad, researchers sent individual emails to disclosers and recipients with a web link to online surveys and unique identification codes. Once participants completed the survey online, participants received course credit (if applicable) and were entered into a drawing for a gift card.

Measures

Variables measured for both disclosers and recipients included closeness, recipient response (support, emotional reaction, reciprocity, topic avoidance), and interaction effectiveness (see Table 5.1 for correlations among study variables). We used SPSS 23 to generate descriptive statistics, create variables, and establish reliability. Composite scores were created by averaging responses of individual items, and variables were screened for normality and multicollinearity.

Closeness. College friends were asked to consider everyday interactions with the study participant and to rate their relational intimacy (Buchanan, Maccoby, & Dornsbusch, 1991). Eight of the nine scale items were retained; items included, "How well does your friend know what you are really like?" and "How satisfied are you with the relationship you have with your friend?" Responses ranged from 1 (*Not at All*) to 5 (*A Lot*). Higher scores indicated greater relational closeness ($M = 4.33$, $SD = 0.57$, $\alpha = 0.81$, disclosers; $M = 4.38$, $SD = 0.68$, $\alpha = 0.94$, recipients).

Recipient response. Discloser perception of recipient response and recipient perceptions of their own response were measured with a 16-item, 4-factor scale which included support, emotional reaction, reciprocity, and topic avoidance (Magsamen-Conrad, 2014). For disclosers, the items' stem asked participants to consider "how your friend responded when you talked about your mental illness." For recipients, the items' stem asked participants to consider "how did you respond at the time when your friend told you about his/her mental illness?" All responses ranged from 1 (*Strongly Disagree*) to 7 (*Strongly Agree*). Because we could not achieve acceptable reliability for the recipient support factor ($\alpha = 0.63$) and because the support and emotional reaction subfactors were highly correlated ($r = 0.78$, disclosers; $r = 0.74$, recipients), we performed a principal component exploratory factor analysis with varimax rotation that included the support and emotional reaction items, resulting in a one-factor solution called support. *Support* (eight items) assessed social support and positive response; higher scores indicate greater received support ($M = 5.65$, $SD = 1.36$, $\alpha = 0.91$, disclosers; $M = 5.80$, $SD = 0.70$, $\alpha = 0.87$, recipients). Items included, "My friend/I listened sympathetically." *Reciprocity* (three items) assessed reciprocated sharing; higher scores indicate greater reciprocity ($M = 5.05$, $SD = 1.49$, $\alpha = 0.81$, disclosers; $M = 3.97$, $SD = 0.80$, $\alpha = 0.76$, recipients). Items included, "My friend/I shared personal/

TABLE 5.1 *Zero-order correlation matrix of closeness, recipient response, and interaction effectiveness*

Scale Variable	1	2	3	4	5	6	7	8	9	10
1. Discloser Closeness	1.00	—	—	—	—	—	—	—	—	—
2. Discloser Interaction Effectiveness	0.51***	1.00	—	—	—	—	—	—	—	—
3. Discloser Support	0.49***	0.47***	1.00	—	—	—	—	—	—	—
4. Discloser Reciprocity	0.28*	0.01	0.42***	1.00	—	—	—	—	—	—
5. Disclosure Topic Avoidance	−0.59***	−0.52***	−0.68***	−0.17	1.00	—	—	—	—	—
6. Recipient Closeness	0.66***	0.43***	0.49***	0.30*	−0.41***	1.00	—	—	—	—
7. Recipient Interaction Effectiveness	0.42***	0.40***	0.38***	0.01	−0.25	0.36**	1.00	—	—	—
8. Recipient Support	0.52***	0.33**	0.64***	0.15	−0.62***	0.52***	0.49***	1.00	—	—
9. Recipient Reciprocity	0.29*	0.12	0.20	0.42***	−0.22	0.20	0.21	0.43***	1.00	—
10. Recipient Topic Avoidance	−0.46***	−0.37**	−0.68***	−0.15	0.62***	−0.48***	−0.50***	−0.83***	−0.34**	1.00

Note. N ranges from 48 to 51.
***Correlation is significant at the 0.001 level (2-tailed).
**Correlation is significant at the 0.01 level (2-tailed).
*Correlation is significant at the 0.05 level (2-tailed).

private thoughts and/or emotions." *Topic avoidance* (three items) assessed recipients' rejection to engage in the conversation; higher scores reflect more avoidance (M = 2.13, SD = 0.1.47, α = 0.90, disclosers; M = 1.65, SD = 0.88, α = 0.90, recipients). One item included, "My friend/I changed the subject or somehow avoided talking about my/my friend's mental illness."

Interaction effectiveness. Friends were asked to reflect on the mental illness disclosure and to evaluate the overall message effectiveness (Goldsmith & MacGeorge, 2000). Participants used four 7-point semantic differentials to rate the degree that the disclosure was *inappropriate* to *appropriate, insensitive* to *sensitive, ineffective* to *effective*, and *incompetent* to *competent*. All items were retained, and higher scores indicated a higher evaluation of the conversation (M = 5.91, SD = 1.03, α = 0.84, disclosers; M = 5.80, SD = 1.12, α = 0.86, recipients).

RESULTS

Preliminary Analyses

We initially conducted paired-sample t-tests to evaluate differences in discloser and recipient perspectives for study variables (see Table 5.2). Results revealed significant differences for college-friend disclosers and recipients in evaluations of topic avoidance and reciprocity. Disclosers (M = 5.06, SD = 1.50) reported that recipients provided greater reciprocity than did recipients (M = 3.97, SD = 0.79), t (48) = 5.63, p < 0.001. Disclosers (M = 2.08, SD = 1.45) reported that recipients were less avoidant and were more responsive than did recipients (M = 1.64, SD = 0.88), t (48) = 2.71, p < 0.01.

Substantive Analyses

Using path analysis in StataIC 14, analyses were conducted to examine relationships among both disclosers' and recipients' reports of (a) relational closeness, (b) recipient response, and (c) interaction effectiveness. More specifically, the data were analyzed using the APIM (Cook & Kenny, 2005). The APIM is "a model of dyadic relationships that integrates a conceptual view of interdependence in two-person relationships with the appropriate statistical techniques for measuring and testing it" (p. 101). By applying the APIM, researchers can calculate if a discloser's reports of relational closeness have an effect on his or her own reports of interaction effectiveness (i.e., an actor effect), as well as on his or her friend's (the recipient) reports of interaction effectiveness (i.e., a partner effect). Furthermore, we explored whether these effects are mediated by each individual's perceptions of the recipient's response (see Figure 5.1). Owing to small sample size (N = 48), three

TABLE 5.2 *Preliminary analyses: Summary table of paired-sample t-tests between disclosers and recipients*

Study Variables	Paired-Sample t-Test (2-Tailed)	Discloser *M, SD*	Recipient *M, SD*
Closeness	$t = -0.25$	$M = 4.36, SD = 0.57$	$M = 4.38, SD = 0.68$
Support	$t = 0.65$	$M = 5.71, SD = 1.32$	$M = 5.80, SD = 0.70$
Reciprocity	$t = 5.63^{**}$	$M = 5.06, SD = 1.50$	$M = 2.46, SD = 1.07$
Topic Avoidance	$t = 2.71^{*}$	$M = 2.09, SD = 1.46$	$M = 3.97, SD = 0.80$
Interaction Effectiveness	$t = 0.71$	$M = 5.89, SD = 1.03$	$M = 5.77, SD = 1.11$

$^{*}p < 0.01,^{**}p < 0.001.$

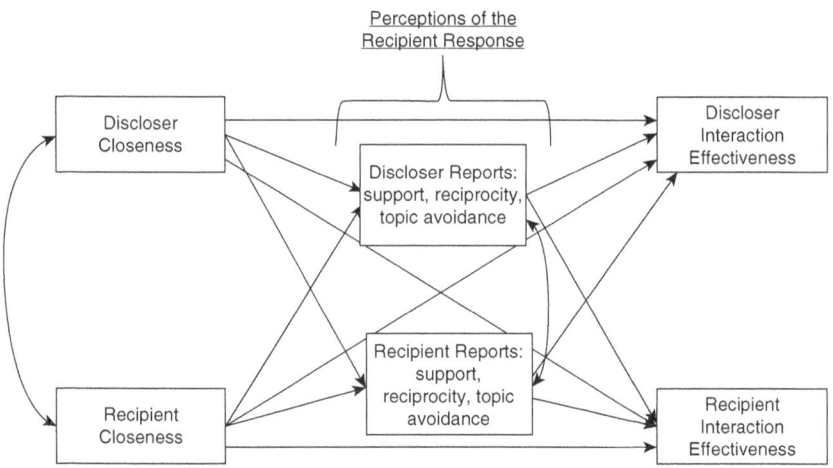

FIGURE 5.1   Proposed APIM of dyadic mental health disclosure interactions.

separate models were run, such that each model included only one recipient response variable (e.g., support, reciprocity, or topic avoidance).

Models were estimated using maximum likelihood. When appropriate, indirect effects were evaluated using the product of coefficients method, such that the path coefficient for the effect of the independent variable to the mediator is multiplied by the path coefficient for the effect of the mediator to the outcome (MacKinnon, Lockwood, Hoffman, West, & Sheets, 2002). The standard error of the product was calculated using the delta method (Oehlert, 1992). Significance of the indirect effect was used as evidence for mediation (i.e., the confidence interval must not contain zero). Model fit was assessed using the obtained chi-square (χ^2), Confirmatory Fit Index (CFI), and root mean square error of approximation (RMSEA). Good model fit was determined when the χ^2 value was nonsignificant, CFI was above 0.90 (i.e., Bentler & Bonett, 1980; Hu & Bentler, 1999), and RMSEA values were below 0.10 (Browne & Cudeck, 1993). If model fit was originally poor, items with nonsignificant path loadings were removed until acceptable model fit was achieved. All models are represented in Figure 5.2.

Recipient support response. Results for the model testing the relationships among relational closeness, recipient support, and interaction effectiveness are represented in Figure 5.2. The hypothesized model did not originally demonstrate good fit; thus, the nonsignificant direct path between recipient closeness and discloser interaction effectiveness was removed. This adjusted model demonstrated good fit to the data, χ^2 (2, $N = 48$) = 2.49, $p = 0.29$; CFI = 0.99, RMSEA = 0.07. Relational closeness and recipient support accounted for 33% of variance in discloser reports of interaction effectiveness and 28% of variance in recipient reports of interaction effectiveness.

As can be seen in the support model, several actor effects were significant. First, discloser reports of relational closeness were positively associated with their own reports of interaction effectiveness, and were marginally associated with their own reports of recipients' supportive responses. Additionally, discloser reports of recipients' supportive responses were positively associated

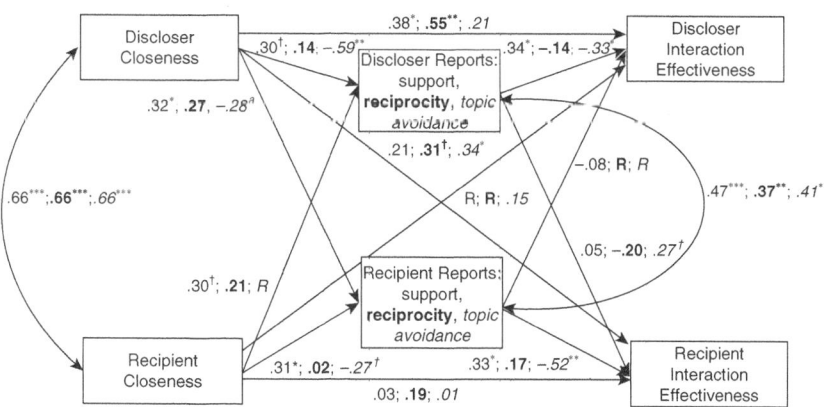

FIGURE 5.2 Model testing actor, partner, and indirect effects for closeness, recipient response variables, and interaction effectiveness.
Note. $N = 48$; $\dagger p < 0.10$, $^*p < 0.05$, $^{**}p < 0.01$, $^{***}p < 0.001$. For each set of results, the first result reflects support. Results for reciprocity are in bold. Results for topic avoidance are in italics. Results including R represent paths that were removed to improve model fit for the represented recipient response variable.

with their own reports of interaction effectiveness. For recipients, relational closeness was directly, positively associated with their own reports of support, which in turn were positively associated with their reports on interaction effectiveness.

This model revealed only one significant partner effect, such that discloser reports of relational closeness were positively associated with recipient reports of their own supportive response. The reverse relationship between recipient reports of closeness and discloser reports of support was only marginally significant, but was in the same positive direction. Finally, there were no significant indirect effects in this model. The lack of significant indirect effects in this model suggests that recipient support response does not mediate the relationships between relational closeness and interaction effectiveness.

Recipient reciprocity response. Results for the reciprocity model testing the relationships among relational closeness, recipient reciprocity, and interaction effectiveness are represented in Figure 5.2 and are bolded. The hypothesized model did not originally demonstrate good fit; thus, the nonsignificant direct paths between recipient closeness and discloser interaction effectiveness and between discloser reciprocity and recipient interaction effectiveness were removed. This adjusted model demonstrated good fit to the data, $\chi^2(3, N = 48) = 3.38$, $p = 0.34$; CFI = 0.99, RMSEA = 0.05. Relational closeness and recipient reciprocity accounted for 28% of variance in discloser reports of interaction effectiveness, and 23% of variance in recipient reports of interaction effectiveness.

The results for reciprocity are not robust. In this model, there was one actor effect: a positive relationship between discloser reports of relational closeness and their reports of interaction effectiveness. Additionally, a positive partner effect between discloser closeness and recipient interaction effectiveness approached significance. Owing to the lack of significant actor effects in the reciprocity model, indirect effects were not directly tested. Overall, these results demonstrate that compared to recipient support, recipient reports of relational closeness and both individuals' reports of recipient reciprocity did not predict their ratings of interaction effectiveness.

Recipient topic avoidance. Finally, results for the topic avoidance model testing the relationships between relational closeness, recipient topic avoidance, and interaction effectiveness are represented in Figure 5.2 and are italicized. The hypothesized model did not originally demonstrate good fit; thus, the nonsignificant direct paths between recipient closeness and discloser topic avoidance and between recipient topic avoidance and discloser interaction effectiveness were removed. This adjusted model demonstrated good fit to the data, $\chi^2(3, N = 48) = 3.45$, $p = 0.33$; CFI = 0.99, RMSEA = 0.06. Relational closeness and recipient reciprocity accounted for 34% of variance in discloser reports of interaction effectiveness and 34% of variance in recipient reports of interaction effectiveness.

As can be seen in Figure 5.2, there is a negative relationship between disclosers' reports of relational closeness and their reports of recipients' topic avoidance during their mental health disclosure interaction. Additionally, disclosers' reports of recipients' topic avoidant responses during the disclosure were negatively related to their own reports of interaction effectiveness.

Thus, if disclosers perceived the relationship with their friend to be close, they reported lower levels of recipient topic avoidance, which in turn predicted increased ratings of interaction effectiveness. Furthermore, this indirect path between discloser reports of closeness, topic avoidance and interaction effectiveness was significant, $\beta = 0.20$, $p < 0.05$, 95% CI [0.02, 0.38]. This relationship suggests that discloser reports of recipients' topic avoidance behaviors mediated the direct relationship between relational closeness and interaction effectiveness.

For recipients' reports, the actor effect between closeness and topic avoidance was in a negative direction but only marginally significant. Additionally, the relationship between recipient reports of topic avoidance and their reports of interaction effectiveness was negative, indicating that when recipients report engaging in higher levels of topic avoidance, they reported the interaction as less effective. Unlike discloser reports, the indirect path between recipient reports of closeness, topic avoidance, and interaction effectiveness was not significant, $\beta = 0.14$, $p = 0.10$, 95% CI [−0.03, 0.31].

Partner effects were also present in the topic avoidance model. First, there was a positive relationship between discloser reports of relational closeness and recipients' reports of interaction effectiveness. Additionally, the partner effect between discloser closeness and recipient topic avoidance approached significance.

DISCUSSION

This study of mental illness disclosures between college-student friends aimed to better understand the dyadic nature of mental illness disclosures and, in particular, the recipient experience. We examined the extent to which closeness predicts recipient response (support, reciprocity, and topic avoidance), and whether response contributed to discloser and recipient perceptions of interaction effectiveness. Our findings from a sample of close friends demonstrate that both disclosers and recipients tend to recall these disclosures similarly, and when differences occur, disclosers evaluate recipient behavior more favorably than do recipients. We also found evidence that one partner's evaluation of closeness predicts the other's evaluation of recipient support. That is, discloser evaluation of closeness predicts recipient evaluations of support, and recipient evaluation of closeness predicts discloser perceptions of recipient support. Finally, this investigation finds that within the context of college friends disclosing mental illness, three dimensions of response are supported. We discuss implications of each of these findings in the text that follows.

Discloser and Recipient Disclosure Evaluation

Examination of dyadic data allows for the comparison of how both dyadic partners contribute to an overall assessment. We first discuss similarities and then differences in how close college-student friends recall mental illness disclosure with special attention to interaction effectiveness and closeness.

Interaction effectiveness. We had anticipated that college friend disclosers and recipients could offer very different evaluations of the overall interaction effectiveness. We speculated that for the discloser, the interaction potentially involved an elaborate sequence including steps of predisclosure contemplation (see the DD-MM, Greene, 2009), disclosure strategy selection (Afifi & Steuber, 2009), possible angst in disclosure preparation, the disclosure interaction itself, recipient response, and the evaluation of the process. However, because recipients may lack a parallel experience of preparing for the interaction and anticipating the exchange, their recollection of the disclosure interaction may be somewhat abridged (i.e., they may recall the disclosure, their response, and the overall conversation but not have engaged in preplanning, strategy selection, or the like). Furthermore, we anticipated that unlike recipients, disclosers may have had greater emotional investment in the interaction, and positive recipient response may have further heightened the discloser's evaluation of the interaction. Despite this reasoning, findings from the present study suggest that friends evaluated the interaction similarly. Both disclosers and recipients were asked to evaluate the overall disclosure interaction in terms of appropriateness, sensitivity, effectiveness, and competence. Both parties rated the disclosure as relatively successful and effective (M = 5.89, disclosers and M = 5.77, recipients, range = 1–7). Although beyond the scope of this investigation, closer inspection of mean comparisons demonstrated that disclosers and recipients significantly differed in evaluations of interaction sensitivity, in which disclosers reported that the interaction was more sensitive (M = 6.20) than did recipients (M = 5.65). Disclosers provided a higher evaluation that the information was bad (M = 5.12) and negative (M = 4.92) than did recipients (M = 3.24 for evaluation as bad, M = 3.53 for evaluation as negative). The difference of sensitivity evaluation may reflect the concept of information ownership and its salience to identity (Petronio, 2002). Communication privacy management theory (Petronio, 2002) describes that individuals claim ownership of their information. Furthermore, disclosers tend to anticipate negative recipient response; post disclosure, they often report that responses were not as negative as anticipated (Caughlin, Afifi, Carpenter-Theune, & Miller, 2005). Finally, consequences of revealing such information are likely to be more severely evaluated by the information owner than co-owner and, taken together, these reasons offer rationale for why disclosers may perceive greater sensitivity than would recipients when disclosing. One practical implication of this finding is that despite recipients' and disclosers' differing evaluations of information as sensitive or problematic, recipients recognize that the information is important to disclosers, and recipients carefully manage their responses.

APIM also demonstrates similarity in how college friends conceptualize antecedents of interaction effectiveness. For example, both disclosers and recipients report that when recipients offer supportive responses, the interaction is more effective, and when recipients provide avoidant responses, the interaction is less effective. This summary seems to reflect an inherent expectation of close friendship: when a close other shares personal and private information, "competent" friends should be supportive and allow the discloser to dialogue about the matter rather than avoiding or changing topics. Recent research about mental illness and relationships (Henderson, Evans-Lacko, & Thornicroft, 2013) also supports this expectation regarding how those in relationships respond to mental illness disclosures. They found that although individuals may turn down a date with a person with mental illness, if the other is already an established friend, participants reported they would offer support and would be pleased that the other felt comfortable enough to disclose his or her mental illness.

Closeness. College friend disclosers and recipients reported similarly high degrees of relational closeness, and their evaluations were correlated. This is consistent with other research in which relational partners participated in dyadic investigations and reported high and similar degrees of closeness (e.g., Checton, Magsamen-Conrad, Venetis, & Greene, 2015; Magsamen-Conrad, Checton, Venetis, & Greene, 2015). In what follows, we discuss unique patterns between closeness and recipient responses of support, reciprocity, and topic avoidance.

Closeness and support. Models reflect complementary patterns of the effect of closeness and recipient response for friends. Consistent with dyadic reports of closeness and support among couples managing chronic illness (Checton et al., 2015), both discloser and recipient reports of closeness positively predict (or trend toward) respective discloser and recipient evaluations that the recipient was supportive. That is, discloser reports of closeness trend toward significance that they perceived recipients as supportive, and recipient reports of closeness predict recipient supportive responses. Furthermore, discloser evaluations of closeness significantly predict recipient reports of being supportive, and recipient evaluations of closeness trend toward discloser reports of recipient supportive responses. It appears that these close friends, in part, understand their relational quality by the degree of support offered when managing sensitive disclosures. Both disclosers and recipients recognize that close others are supportive during vulnerable times such as sharing a mental illness disclosure.

Closeness, support, and reciprocity.   One difference between discloser and recipient evaluations occurs in the support and reciprocity models. Within these two models, there is a direct effect between discloser closeness and discloser interaction effectiveness that is not mirrored in the recipient models. For disclosers, when recipients responded with what was perceived as positive intent, such as being supportive and communicating openly or sharing their own thoughts and feelings (i.e., reciprocating), closeness uniquely predicted support and reciprocity, and support and reciprocity uniquely predicted interaction effectiveness. However, closeness also directly predicted interaction effectiveness, suggesting that there is something intrinsic to being close that leads one to perceive that the interaction went well. For recipients, closeness separately predicted support and reciprocity, and support and reciprocity separately predicted interaction effectiveness, but the direct relationship between closeness and interaction effectiveness was not significant. This suggests that for recipients, perceiving their own behavior as supportive is necessary to evaluate that the interaction went well.

Closeness and topic avoidance. College friend participants reported that when the other was less close, there was a greater propensity for topic avoidance. For both dyad members, topic avoidance was significantly associated with reduced interaction effectiveness, demonstrating that it is dissatisfying for both friends. The relationship between topic avoidance and interaction effectiveness was stronger for recipients. The relationship between discloser perceptions of recipient topic avoidance and recipient interaction effectiveness trends toward significance. These two findings, taken together with the finding that disclosers reported that recipients engaged in less topic avoidance than did recipients, suggest that disclosers are less aware than are recipients of when topic avoidance is occurring. Recipients' greater awareness of their own topic avoidance may contribute to reduced recipient evaluations of an effective interaction. Furthermore, when recipients know that disclosers perceived that they were avoidant, interaction evaluation was reduced.

Dimensions of Response

Magsamen-Conrad's (2014) dimensions of recipient response were designed to evaluate how individuals contemplating disclosure may anticipate others' reactions. Other research has examined the relationship between these dimensions and disclosure outcomes such as disclosure intention, disclosure depth and breadth, and topic avoidance (Shields, 2017; Venetis, Magsamen-Conrad, Checton, & Greene, 2017). Within the ongoing cancer communication contexts (Venetis, Greene, Checton, & Magsamen-Conrad, 2015), reciprocity more strongly influenced cancer patient and partner decisions to disclose. Among women contemplating disclosure of their eating disorder, all four anticipated response dimensions were correlated with disclosure intention, but when examined holistically within the DD-MM (Greene, 2009), only reciprocity predicted disclosure intention. Interestingly, within this study context of mental illness disclosure, supportive responses, rather than returned openness and reciprocated sharing, predicted interaction effectiveness. Future research may examine how each of the four dimensions contributes to disclosure intention and retrospective disclosure evaluations.

Rather than four separate dimensions, this research supported three dimensions, given that support and emotional reaction loaded as a single factor. This may have occurred due to our limited sample size, the specific content, or the retrospective nature of recalling an event that had already occurred (i.e., Magsamen-Conrad's framework is prospective). Perhaps what is most salient to college-student friends is that when sharing personal and potentially stigmatizing information with another, friends provide positive support. Furthermore, that support can be enacted in the form of listening, demonstrating concern, withholding judgment, and affective behaviors such as offering a hug. Future research should continue to explore these dimensions of recipient support.

Limitations and Future Research

As in all research, this investigation presents limitations. One includes the limited sample size. On a practical level, we were challenged to recruit friends in which one had shared their mental illness information with the other and both were willing to participate. This speaks to the nature of dyadic data and motivating two individuals to complete surveys, particularly as our participants are college students and not all were necessarily eligible for extra course credit. The reduced sample size encumbered the number of variables we could entertain in our models. We recognize that variables beyond relational closeness are likely to influence recipient response and could be investigated in future research. However, owing to our sample size, closeness provided a succinct, one-factor variable that has been theoretically supported as predicting how individuals disclose and react in disclosure (Afifi & Steuber, 2009; Greene et al., 2012). Despite this limitation, we are pleased with our findings that demonstrate the value of closeness in predicting various recipient responses and how those responses contribute to discloser and recipient evaluations of interaction effectiveness.

A second limitation includes recruiting individuals who consider each other to be friends. Although this approach served the purposes of the current investigation allowing for exploration of disclosure as a dyadic process, there is value in investigating how the relationships between closeness, response, and interaction effectiveness differ among relational partners, friends, and others who are less close. For instance, given the close quarters and frequent interaction of many college students (e.g., dorm life), individuals with mental illness may feel compelled to disclose before they are ready to do so and/or to individuals with whom they are not particularly close. Extensions to the current research could look to incorporate a range of relational types in examinations of dyadic disclosure processes (perhaps even individuals who are no longer friends). Further, disclosure and recipient expectations of recipient response (e.g., degree of support) may differ based on closeness, and these expectations of response may influence perceptions of interaction effectiveness.

A third limitation is the lack of diversity within the sample. Our decision to recruit on a single Midwestern university campus may have constrained the age range and racial diversity of our participants (primarily white/Caucasian), which limits generalizability. Although we did not ask participants for their hometown/country of origin, it is likely that most participants were from the Midwest, which may reflect a unique, regional perspective on mental illness. Attitudes toward and beliefs about mental illness differ across ethnicities, cultures, and countries (e.g., Abdullah & Brown, 2011). Future research could replicate this study in a different US region and/or alter the study design so as to capture the role of cultural perspectives on mental illness.

Conclusion

The current research utilized APIM analyses to examine disclosers' and recipients' perceptions of the role of closeness, recipient response, and interaction effectiveness during disclosure interactions about mental illness. In terms of theory, results represent initial steps in how we might extend the boundaries of our current conceptualization of disclosure by incorporating both the discloser and the recipient. For instance, several disclosure models, including the DD-MM (Greene, 2009) and RRM (Afifi & Steuber, 2009), situate closeness in disclosure processes. The suggestion that closeness functions somewhat differently for disclosers compared to recipients (even though partners in this study evaluated their level of closeness with the other in similar ways) underscores the need to perhaps develop a complementary model that explains the disclosure process from the unique perspective of the recipient.

Practically speaking, results point to the importance of continuing to support college students with mental illness diagnoses in terms of how to manage health-related information. However, university administrators, mental health services, and other support initiatives should consider also supporting or providing information about mental health issues to the general student population. More specifically, the average college student is likely to receive a health-related disclosure, and current findings indicate that recipients who felt they were supportive evaluate the interaction as more effective. Educating college students about how best to be supportive may enhance their feelings of efficacy and, in turn, their evaluations of disclosure interactions. Ultimately, improving the disclosure experience so that both disclosers and recipients report satisfying experiences benefits both dyadic partners but likely has greater implications for the discloser. Supportive responses may reduce feelings of isolation, improve efficacy in further disclosures, and serve to strengthen dyadic closeness.

REFERENCES

Abdullah, T., & Brown, T. L. (2011). Mental illness stigma and ethnocultural beliefs, values, and norms: An integrative review. *Clinical Psychology Review, 31*, 934–948. doi: 10.1016/j.cpr.2011.05.003

Afifi, T., & Steuber, K. (2009). The revelation risk model (RRM): Factors that predict the revelation of secrets and the strategies used to reveal them. *Communication Monographs, 76*, 144–176. doi: 10.1080/03637750902828412

Ahrens, C. E., & Campbell, R. (2000). Assisting rape victims as they recover from rape: The impact on friends. *Journal of Interpersonal Violence, 15*, 959–986. doi: 10.1177/088626000015009004

Ahrens, C. E., Campbell, R., Ternier-Thames, N. K., Wasco, S. M., & Sefl, T. (2007). Deciding whom to tell: Expectations and outcomes of rape survivors' first disclosures. *Psychology of Women Quarterly, 31*, 38–49. doi: 10.1111/j.1471–6402.2007.00329.x

American College Health Association. (2012). *American college health association national college health assessment II: Reference group executive summary Spring 2012.* Retrieved from: www.acha-ncha.org/docs/ACHA-NCHA-II_UNDE RGRAD_ReferenceGroup_ExecutiveSummary_Spring2012

American Psychiatric Association. (2015). *What is mental illness?* Retrieved from: www.psychiatry.org/patients-families/what-is-mental-illness

Banyard, V. L., Moynihan, M. M., Walsh, W. A., Cohn, E. S., & Ward, S. (2010). Friends of survivors: The community impact of unwanted sexual experiences. *Journal of Interpersonal Violence, 25*, 242–256. doi: 10.1177/0886260509334407

Bentler, P. M., & Bonett, D. G. (1980). Significance tests and goodness of fit in the analysis of covariance structures. *Psychological Bulletin, 88*, 588–606. doi: doi.org/10.1037/0033-2909.88.3.588

Brohan, E., Henderson, C., Wheat, K., Malcolm, E., Clement, S., Barley, E. A., ... Thronicroft, G. (2012). Systematic review of beliefs, behaviours and influencing factors associated with disclosure of a mental health problem in the workplace. *BMC Psychiatry, 2*, 11–24. doi: 10.1186/1471-244X-12-11

Browne, M. W., & Cudeck, R. (1993). Alternative ways of assessing model fit. In K. A. Bollen & J. S. Long (Eds.), *Testing structural equation models* (pp. 136–162). Newbury Park, CA: SAGE.

Buchanan, C. M., Maccoby, E. E., & Dornbusch, S. M. (1991). Caught between parents: Adolescents' experience in divorced homes. *Child Development, 62*, 1008–1029. doi: 10.1111/j.1467-8624.1991.tb01586.x

Bute, J. J. (2013). The discursive dynamics of disclosure and avoidance: Evidence from a study of infertility. *Western Journal of Communication, 77*, 164–185. doi: 10.1080/10570314.2012.695425

Caughlin, J. P., Afifi, W. A., Carpenter-Theune, K. E., & Miller, L. E. (2005). Reasons for, and consequences of, revealing personal secrets in close relationships: A longitudinal study. *Personal Relationships, 12*, 43–59. doi: 10.1111/j.1350-4126.2005.00101.x

Chaudoir, S. R., & Fisher, J. D. (2010). The disclosure processes model: Understanding disclosure decision-making and post-disclosure outcomes among people living with a concealable stigmatized identity. *Psychological Bulletin, 136*, 236–256. doi: 10.1037/a0018193

Chaudoir, S. R., & Quinn, D. M. (2010). Revealing concealable stigmatized identities: The impact of disclosure motivations and positive first-disclosure experiences on fear of disclosure and well-being. *Journal of Social Issues, 66*, 570–584. doi: 10.1111/j.1540-4560.2010.01663.x

Checton, M. G., Magsamen-Conrad, K., Venetis, M. K., & Greene, K. (2015). A dyadic approach: Applying the developmental-conceptual model to couples coping with chronic illness. *Health Education & Behavior, 42*, 257–267. doi: 10.1177/1090198114557121

Cook, W. L., & Kenny, D. A. (2005). The actor–partner interdependence model: A model of bidirectional effects in developmental studies. *International Journal of Behavioral Development, 29*, 101–109. doi: 10.1080/01650250444000405

Derlega, V. J., Winstead, B. A., Greene, K., Serovich, J., & Elwood, W. N. (2004). Reasons for HIV disclosure/nondisclosure in close relationships: Testing a model of HIV-disclosure decision making. *Journal of Social & Clinical Psychology, 23*, 747–767. doi: 10.1521/jscp.23.6.747.54804

Dinos, S., Stevens, S., Serfaty, M., Weich, S., & King, M. (2004). Stigma: The feelings and experiences of 46 people with mental illness. *The British Journal of Psychiatry, 184*, 176–181. doi: 10.1192/bjp.184.2.176

Dunn, P. C., Vail-Smith, K., & Knight, S. M. (1999). What date/acquaintance rape victims tell others: A study of college student recipients of disclosure. *Journal of American College Health, 47*, 213–219. doi: 10.1080/07448489909595650

Goldsmith, D. J., & MacGeorge, E. L. (2000). The impact of politeness and relationship on perceived quality of advice about a problem. *Health Communication Research, 26*, 234–263. doi: 10.1111/j.1468-2958.2000.tb00757.x

Greene, K. (2009). An integrated model of health disclosure decision-making. In T. D. Afifi & W. A. Afifi (Eds.), *Uncertainty and information regulation in interpersonal contexts: Theories and applications* (pp. 226–253). New York, NY: Routledge.

Greene, K., Derlega, V. L., & Mathews, A. (2006). Self-disclosure in personal relationships. In A. Vangelisti & D. Perlman (Eds.), *The Cambridge handbook of personal relationships* (pp. 409–428). New York, NY: Cambridge University Press.

Greene, K., Magsamen-Conrad, K., Venetis, M. K., Checton, M. G., Bagdasarov, Z., & Banerjee, S. C. (2012). Assessing health diagnosis disclosure decisions in relationships: Testing the disclosure decision-making model. *Health Communication*, *27*, 356–368. doi: 10.1080/10410236.2011.586988

Henderson, C., Evans-Lacko, S., & Thornicroft, G. (2013). Mental illness stigma, help seeking, and public health programs. *American Journal of Public Health*, *103*, 777–780. doi: 10.2105/AJPH.2012.301056

Hu, L. T., & Bentler, P. M. (1999). Cutoff criteria for fit indexes in covariance structure analysis: Conventional criteria versus new alternatives. *Structural Equation Modeling: A Multidisciplinary Journal*, *6*, 1–55. doi: 10.1080/10705519909540118

Iarovici, D. (2014). *Mental health issues and the university student*. Baltimore, MD: Johns Hopkins University Press.

Kessler, R. C., Walters, E. E., & Forthofer, M. S. (1998). The social consequences of psychiatric disorders, III: Probability of marital stability. *American Journal of Psychiatry*, *155*, 1092–1096. doi: 10.1176/ajp.155.8.1092

MacKinnon, D. P., Lockwood, C. M., Hoffman, J. M., West, S. G., & Sheets, V. (2002). A comparison of methods to test mediation and other intervening variable effects. *Psychological Methods*, *7*, 83–104. doi: org/10.1037/1082-989X.7.1.83

Magsamen-Conrad, K. (2014). Dimensions of anticipated reaction in information management: Anticipating responses and outcomes. *Review of Communication*, *14*, 314–333. doi: 10.1080/15358593.2014.986514

Magsamen-Conrad, K., Checton, M. G., Venetis, M. K., & Greene, K. (2015). Communication efficacy and couples' cancer management: Applying a dyadic appraisal model. *Communication Monographs*, *82*, 179–200. doi: 10.1080/03637751.2014.971415

Mathews, A., Derlega, V. J., & Morrow, J. (2006). What is highly personal information and how is it related to self-disclosure decision-making? The perspective of college students. *Communication Research Reports*, *23*, 85–92. doi: 10.1080/08824090600668915

National Alliance on Mental Illness. (2012). *College students speak: Survey report on mental health*. Retrieved from: www.nami.org/collegereport.

Oehlert, G. W. (1992). A note on the delta method. *The American Statistician*, *46*, 27–29. doi: 10.1080/00031305.1992.10475842

Petronio, S. (2002). *Boundaries of privacy: Dialectics of disclosure*. Albany, NY: State University of New York Press

Shields, A. (2017). *Eating disorder disclosure/nondisclosure in close relationships: Applying the Disclosure Decision-Making Model. Unpublished master's thesis*, Purdue University, West Lafayette, IN.

Vangelisti, A., Caughlin, J., & Timmerman, L. (2001). Criteria for revealing family secrets. *Communication Monographs*, *68*, 1–27. doi: 10.1080/03637750128052

Venetis, M. K., Chernichky, S., & Gettings, P. (2015, November). Predicting mental health disclosure strategies. Paper presented at the annual meeting of the National Communication Association, Las Vegas, NV.

Venetis, M. K., Chernichky-Karcher, S., & Gettings, P. E. (2018). Disclosing mental illness information to a friend: Exploring how the Disclosure Decision-Making Model informs strategy selection. *Health Communication*, *33*, 653–663. doi: 10.1080/10410236.2017.1294231

Venetis, M. K., Greene, K., Checton, M. G., & Magsamen-Conrad, K. (2015). Decision making in cancer-related topic avoidance. *Journal of Health Communication*, *3*, 306–313. doi: 10.1080/10810730.2014.965364

Venetis, M. K., Magsamen-Conrad, K., Checton, M. G., & Greene, K. (2017, May). *Ongoing disclosure in cancer communication: The role of perceived response*. Paper presented at the annual meeting of the International Communication Association, San Diego, CA.

Williams, S. L., & Mickelson, K. D. (2008). A paradox of support seeking and rejection among the stigmatized. *Personal Relationships*, *15*, 493–509. doi: 10.1111/j. 1475–6811.2008.00212.x

6

From the Drawing Board to the Kitchen Table: An Analysis of Parental Messages Concerning Nutrition, Physical Activity, and Weight

EMILY SCHEINFELD, ERIN NELSON, AND BRITTANI CROOK

The rates of childhood obesity in the United States remain high (Olds et al., 2011), with one in three children classified as overweight or obese, three times the rate of thirty years ago (Ogden, Carroll, Kit, & Flegal, 2014). Childhood obesity is linked to several negative health consequences (Daniels, 2006), such as hypertension and type 2 diabetes (Kahn, Hull, & Utzschneider, 2006), and negative psychological outcomes including negative body image and low self-esteem (Williams, Wake, Hesketh, Maher, & Waters, 2005). With recognition that obesity is a serious issue for preventive public health care (National Preventative Taskforce, 2010; Ogden et al., 2014), various public health initiatives have been introduced to promote dialogue about health. Those health campaigns, which aim to target childhood obesity, suggest the family is a key site for intervention (Ristovski-Slijepcevic et al., 2010a).

The parent–child relationship is an important context for the study of health, particularly when examining conversations about nutrition, exercise, and weight. Parents are often the primary source of health-related information for their children (Shonkoff & Phillips, 2000), and are likely an important influence in shaping the child's nutrition and activity habits. Further, lifestyle behaviors are often influenced within the home environment (Neumark-Sztainer et al., 2010), and parents have influence over the information their children are exposed to about health and weight (Neumark-Sztainer et al., 2010).

Owing to the high prevalence and negative consequences associated with obesity in childhood and adolescence (Daniels, 2006; Ogden et al., 2012), it is critical for parents to understand how to share information about healthy living with their children. Engaging parents, however, requires an understanding of parents' health schemas and of how parents are accessing information on weight, diet, and physical activity and subsequently communicating it to their children. Thus, this study examines parental information seeking and family communication about exercise and nutrition.

PARENTAL INFORMATION SEEKING AND EVALUATION

Individuals seek health-related information from several sources, including the internet, television, medical professionals, friends and family, and news outlets. More specifically, parents rank health professionals and the internet as the top two sources of health-related information for their children (Bernhardt & Felter, 2004; Khoo, Bolt, Babl, Jury, & Goldman, 2008). Similarly, studies (Bernhardt & Felter, 2004; Khoo et al., 2008) demonstrate that parents of young children predominantly use the internet or a Google search as sources of information, but express concerns about reliability. Regardless of reliability, respondents prefer websites promoted by a clinical professional or by other parents (Bernhardt & Felter, 2004). Given the fact that we are submerged in the digital age, it is no surprise that parents turn to the internet. However, trust is an important factor in evaluating the specific sources and information obtained online. Relatively little is known about where parents seek information pertaining to their children's health, and how they evaluate that information. The sources that parents turn to for health information and the perceived credibility of those sources likely inform their perception of what healthy behaviors would be most appropriate for themselves and their family. To investigate the sources that parents rely on for health information and how those sources inform their thinking about health behavior, the following research questions are posited:

RQ1: Where do parents find information about health, nutrition, and exercise?
RQ2: How do various sources of health information inform parents' thinking about health, diet, and exercise, both for themselves and for their children?

FAMILY HEALTH

The family social environment is identified as a primary predictor of various health outcomes within childhood and adulthood, including weight, eating habits, and exercise preferences (Crossman et al., 2006). Parenting practices such as modeling (e.g., Hamilton & White, 2010), monitoring (e.g., Aalsma, Liu, & Wiele, 2011), and engagement in activities with children (e.g., Ornelas et al., 2007) play a significant role within the family social environment and influence child health behaviors. Empirical evidence suggests that parental control (e.g., Barber, 1996) and parent–child communication have a significant impact on child development; thus, these parenting behaviors are of specific interest in this study.

Parent–child communication is influential in the development of childhood health behavior (e.g., Barnes, Reifman, Farrell, & Dintcheff, 2000; Kaplan, Kiernan, & James, 2006). Specifically, Kaplan et al. (2006) observed families' use of communication about food as a successful mode of establishing healthy eating behaviors. Notably, not all talk about food is necessarily positive. That is, it is not simply talking about food that results in healthier eating habits. Despite empirical evidence demonstrating that open, frequent conversations can shape youth attitude toward health behaviors (Barnes et al., 2000), past research has some limitations in developing a more complex conceptualization of parent–child communication and examining its role in health behavior enactment (see Miller-Day & Kam, 2010). For example, many studies investigating health behavior related to communication (e.g., alcohol and drug use, healthy eating behaviors) focus on singular dimensions and, therefore, have offered a limited conceptualization of communication. Research conceptualizes parent–child communication as open conversation orientations (Ritchie & Fitzpatrick, 1990), or assesses the amount of talk between parent and child without discerning the strategies or approaches parents take within the conversations (Wills, Gibbons, Gerrard, Murray, & Brody, 2003). However, we argue that rather than rely on a singular trait of communication, it is necessary to understand the messages, communicative strategies, and processes within parent–child communication about health. Although an association between nonverbal modes of parent support, such as modeling, and children's diet and physical activity behaviors is well supported (Dave, Evans, Condrasky, & Williams, 2012; McMinn, Griffin, Jones, & van Sluijs, 2012), less is known about how parents verbally communicate information regarding weight, diet, and physical activity to their children. Thus, we pose a third research question:

RQ3: How do parents communicate about health information, nutrition, and exercise with their children?

METHODOLOGY

Participants and Procedures

Participants included 88 adults, ages 22–58 (M = 44.7; SD = 8.47) from a large Southwestern city. To participate, parents needed to speak English and have a child between the ages of 4 and 15 years. The majority of the participants were female (N = 80), and more than half of the sample identified as non-Hispanic and white (n = 58; 65.9%), followed by Hispanic or Latino/a (n = 11; 12.5%). About 50% (n = 43) of the participants indicated they felt the need to lose weight and/or were actively doing something to achieve that goal. Based on our recruitment efforts, which included advertising through a university-wide email, child development centers, preschools, and schools, it is not surprising that 22% of the participants reported having a graduate degree, and another 55% reportedly attended and/or graduated from a four-year institution. More than half (*n* = 57, 64.8%) fell within a normal body mass index (BMI) range (18.5–25). About 2% were underweight, 16 participants (18.2%) were overweight, and another eight participants (9.1%) were classified as obese.

Participants signed up online or by phone to participate in a one-on-one interview conducted by one of the researchers. Interviews were conducted in a private and quiet space to elicit honest and thorough responses. Each interview took about 45 minutes and was audio recorded and transcribed for analysis. Following the interview, participants completed an online questionnaire pertaining to their own health, their children's health, and closed-ended items about perceived communication behaviors.

Plan of Analysis

Data analysis began with a constant comparative technique (Strauss & Corbin, 1990) that was used to identify themes across the interviews and fine-tune the definition of each category (Glaser & Strauss, 1967). A subsample of the transcripts (20%) was coded by the authors, and Cohen's kappa was calculated for intercoder reliability (Stroud & Higgins, 2011). After intercoder reliability was achieved, the entire set of transcripts was analyzed by one coder to explore the presence of the themes and to identify exemplar quotations. The interview protocol focused on where parents received health and weight management information, what they may perceive as healthy behaviors, how they communicate this information to their children, and difficulties or barriers they perceive in communicating and implementing these healthy behaviors for their children.

RESULTS

This study sought to determine how parents of children ages 5–14 years perceive the health of their children but, moreover, how they perceive their communication pertaining to weight management practices to their children. Several themes emerged through the data analysis (see Table 6.1). Messages are presented verbatim as exemplars of each theme.

Overall Health Schema

When specifically prompted about health behaviors for themselves or for their children, asking, "What do you perceive to be physical activity?" or "What is nutrition?," parents often provided *traits* of health. Traits refer to the way parents characterized health to themselves and their families, and included concepts such as importance, definitions of health, and features of health. *Traits* of health were mentioned 69 times by parents. Many mentions of traits

TABLE 6.1 *Thematic analysis results*

Theme	Example	Occurrences
Health Schema		
Traits	Because health is paramount to life and happiness, I continually keep that in mind. Health is everything!	68
Recommendations	Fish, fish, fish! Vegetables – especially dark green ones, lean white meat (little to no red meat), lots of water, egg whites, legumes, garlic, peanut butter, yogurt (at least one a day), basil, and parsley	73
Other (strategies, family)	My child participates on different sorts of teams for little kids. I also think that playing outside with neighborhood kids is good physical activity.	153
Sources		
Unintentional	Usually I just run across information on the internet when I'm on various sites that have nothing to do with health or have a small health section.	32
Intentional	I do research about a sport or activity before letting my child participate in it.	
Mediated Formal	I would Google and then I would like to look specifically for sources that have medical doctors perhaps backing it. But then I'd have to figure out.	20
Mediated Informal	I was scanning Facebook and I see an article; depending on what the article is and what the title of the article is, may determine whether I click on it.	32
Face-to-Face Formal	I ask people at my gym who seem knowledgeable about physical activities. I also ask my doctor for health and nutrition information.	44
Face-to-Face Informal	We also have many discussions at work about dieting and nutrition (women always are talking about food and dieting).	26
Own Experience	I would also add, just from my education, my personal college education, I've taken classes that ... different classes that would address that as well. So just a personal knowledge of it.	14

Continued

TABLE 6.1 *Cont.*

Theme	Example	Occurrences
Information Assessment		
Trustworthiness/ Credibility	I find the doctors most trustworthy because it is their job and they have done plenty of research that makes them reliable. I don't like to use the internet because I feel that it makes things worse, but it is easier to find quick info.	24
Usefulness	I like posts from Skinny taste, organize yourself skinny, real food, *Fitness* magazine. I like these sources because they share recipes and exercise tips that I can really use.	10
Communication		
Direct Communication	Sometimes, I show my daughters nutrition labels. I educate them about added hormones to milk, eggs, and poultry.	31
Indirect Verbal Communication	It isn't something that we ever formally talked about. It was more about, "I need to lose weight so we are going to eat healthier." Or during sports training, making sure to lay off unhealthy foods.	14
Indirect Nonverbal Communication	I try to show them this by example, through lunches and dinners prepared in the house. I try to remind them of this daily, and allow sweets and other unhealthy snacks on a limited basis, but I do not deprive them of this.	Modeling – 45
	We do a lot of activities as a family to model a healthy lifestyle. I do pack my child's lunch; I do allow junk food – just not all the time.	Engaging – 39 Accessibility – 48
Barriers		
Accessibility	Eating junk food because it is convenient.	38
	I don't think that they have vending machines [at school] but I don't know if she has access to soda . . . I [would] despise that.	
Time	Also because of school work, if he doesn't finish homework before it	76

Continued

TABLE 6.1 *Cont.*

Theme	Example	Occurrences
	gets dark outside that limits his ability to go outside and exercise.	
Money	Healthy meal option restaurants can get very expensive. Also shopping for all organic foods can put a dent in the family budget.	30

included the notion that health is important. For example, "I think good health is important and everyone should strive for it." For some, parents simply defined what health is to them and their families: "I believe that health is about balance. It's important what we eat, think, exercise, stress, and reducing toxins in our environment and food. I believe living green is an important step in being healthy."

Another example of how parents characterized health by providing definitions and features of health included the outcomes of health: "Without good to excellent health, anyone's life will not be optimal and life expectancy will be reduced." Many parents also spoke of food as fuel, that food has a purpose and allows you to feel good. Similarly, parents wanted to teach their children that exercise and food are not punishments or rewards. This became especially true when there was a fear that later in life, their children may not choose a healthy lifestyle or may view exercise and activity as a chore. Parents mentioned their ability to influence choices, and therefore do so by expressing the notion that exercise can be fun, that choosing the apple over cake is a good choice. For example:

I'll give you an example, . . . I have the opposite relationship with food, where I spent my whole life dieting so I haven't really had these good and bad foods . . . That's part of the reason why I don't completely restrict any kind of junk food or snacks because I feel like it's important to learn to eat them and not binge eat them and not feel like I gotta eat the whole bag because I'll never get this again . . . Really, what I want them to do is learn to like foods that are good for you and be exposed to a lot of different foods.

Although some parents spoke generally of health definitions and features, others spoke specifically to their children and the goal they have for them:

I believe that teaching children to eat right at an early age will extend out to when they become autonomous and move out. I believe that it's important for me as a parent to use my influence as I have the time in their life because my influence will change and it already has. They only care about what their friends think. And I have become a moron.

At the same time, many parents freely provided *recommendations* for good health. Many parents noted they were "very conscious about just reviewing the food I am taking and kind of assessing whether it is a good choice or bad choice" when it came to their own health. When it came to how to help shape their children's health and to what physical activity and nutrition are, parents provided numerous recommendations. Many of them kept to their version of the USDA recommendations, including portion sizes, types of food to eat, time to exercise, and so on. As mentioned previously, health was often spoken about as balance and, therefore, some parents indicated that in addition to the guidelines, it is acceptable to treat yourself, or for a child to be a child now and then: "And I was just going to say it's always a balance because I wanted to have childhood food and things that taste good to them, but I want to also make sure they are getting what they need." In addition to recommendations based on USDA standards, many parents also believed that where the food came from was more important than the composition of food consumption. For example, they focused primarily on eating organic foods, and spoke less on the ratio of fruits and vegetables to meats and starches. This included foods with no genetically modified organisms (GMOs) or chemicals and no processed foods, only foods with organic and pronounceable ingredients.

Last, there was a difference in how parents spoke about *strategies* for health behaviors for themselves and how they spoke about health behaviors for their children. Parents often seemed to perceive there was an obligation to work out, to go to the gym, or to go for a run. In other words, they framed it as "working out" ($N = 79$ compared to $N = 27$ for mentioning the gym or runs for children). However, for their children, activity and food were about fun and enjoyment ($N = 51$). That is, children played sports, took dance classes, or went on walks with the family. Children were brought along on grocery shopping trips and helped make dinner as a form of entertainment. Parents reported on the children's extracurricular activities as forms of exercise, and made the activities fun for their children rather than a chore.

Sources of Health Information

The second theme that emerged revolved around characteristics of health information sources. Parents mentioned intentionally finding sources ($N = 85$), such as searching online or consulting family and friends, or mentioned unintentionally coming across health information sources ($N = 42$), such as on social media. Within the theme of intentional sources, parents mentioned signing up for listservs or actively collecting information on social media outlets. For example, one parent commented, "I have Pinterest boards, I'll save recipes on there. I'll find something that I think would be applicable for their lunch later. I don't know if I go and look for it, but I am actively collecting it." Similarly, parents mentioned intentionally picking up pamphlets or articles from medical offices or the children's school. For example, "I read the school hand outs of what activities my child does at school and complement this with outside activities to ensure he is getting enough exercise." Another parent mentioned the various information sources sought, as well as intentionally picking up a pamphlet, "News, talk shows, internet, reading magazines, podcasts. Anywhere really. When I see a brochure or pamphlet in a medical office, I usually take it and read it immediately."

The second way parents mentioned sources of information are through unintentional sources such as those shared on social media, or when media outlets posted announcements. Facebook, Instagram, and Pinterest were often mentioned as social media outlets on which friends, family, or professionals they "follow" share health information that participants happen to see while on these outlets. For example, "Most recently, I've really gotten interested in getting exercise tips and nutrition/food tips through Pinterest, as there is a greater variety of ideas on this website. However, seeing results from my friends who are using specific workouts or making special recipes are much more reliable sources than online resources." Another parent mentioned, "I usually just find information on the internet, a lot of times I like to look at news my friends post on Facebook."

The sources parents reported were also distinguishable by whether they were mediated by technology. Of those who mentioned any form of mediated sources, 20 participants identified a formal mediated source, while 32 mentioned an informal mediated source. Formal mediated sources included government sponsored websites, such as the Centers for Disease Control and Prevention (CDC), or large corporations that publish health information, such as WebMD. Informal mediated sources included social media and blogs. For example, one participant said, "I like fitness blogs because these women are moms just like me so I enjoy reading their advice and about their experience." In addition to general blogs, participants turned to blogs written specifically by other parents or moms. However, participants seemed to have different opinions about blogs, with some believing blogs are more valid accounts of information because these fellow mothers have similar experiences, while others "take it with a grain of salt."

There were 44 mentions of formal face-to-face, or nonmediated, sources, such as doctors, and 22 mentions of informal face-to-face sources, such as friends and family. For example, "Of course we read information in the newspaper about the healthy diets and what kids will eat and are continually working toward a healthier lifestyle. Mostly we just visit with other parents and friends about new ideas for cooking, snacking, and rewarding our children without totally indulging all of the time."

The last source parents mentioned is unique, as the source was themselves. Participants often commented on the fact that they mostly rely on their own experiences, such as their education, health background, and familial upbringing. For example, one mother said, "I don't search for most nutritional advice until there is a serious medical problem, I trust what I have tried myself and what is time-tested to be healthy but taste great or feel great." Similarly, another parent mentioned her education and that she thinks diet and exercise information should be personal, "I personally feel like . . . I'm well educated about it I don't really feel like I need anybody to tell me. It's just kind of being a person when you should just exercise and eat right. But really, I don't feel like I need an outside source to come in to tell me what my child should or should not be doing."

Information Assessment

Whether the information was sought out intentionally or it was stumbled upon unintentionally, parents assessed information on many dimensions. When deciding whether or not to accept the information, parents examined the source based on credibility or trustworthiness, their own common sense, whether it aligned with their own beliefs and ideas of truth, the usefulness, and the topic. The most often cited rationale for paying attention to information was the topic at hand, and therefore the usefulness of the material ($N = 10$). Parents mentioned information surrounding weight loss, nutrition, and physical activity as the primary topics they pay attention to. This was likely influenced by the prompt of the study and preceding questions in the interview. For example, one mother spoke about weight loss: "Weight loss as I'm like most other women, and always looking to lose a pound or two."

The most cited rationale for embracing information either intentionally or unintentionally sought out was credibility and overall trustworthiness ($N = 24$). One participant indicated, "I am most likely to pay attention to messages that come from those that I trust. For example, my doctor, trainer, or friends who have a high interest in health." Others indicated that information based on scholarly or scientific research was the only type of information they trusted, "[I trust] positive and scientific information in messages because they relay the information that I know to be true, but also imply the science behind what it supports to provide evidence." Parents also paid attention to social media and news sources when presented with information about health. They indicated that the pure frequency of the information, or even the amount of "likes" something has on Facebook, would warrant the information as credible and a worthwhile read.

Despite being exposed to the same information, and frequently, by way of the news or social media, some parents remained steadfast in their distrust:

Well I think I don't like blogs at all. Just because I feel that they are just opinions. And they have no validity, scientifically, unless some doctor writes blogs, usually but,

I think that would be my least sought out source. Probably lower than that would be something of a source that would be considered entertainment. Like a Yahoo news. Usually I think those tend to be more sensational just to get people to look at it.

Communicating to Children

When asked how they communicated these schemas and perspectives of what they considered good or healthy nutrition and physical activity, parents gave a variety of responses. We were able to separate the majority of responses into two main forms of communication: *indirect* and *direct*. Direct communication, outright conversations about nutrition and physical activity, was mentioned only 31 times by parents. These were concerted efforts by parents to talk to their children about physical activity and nutrition, and though they may not have sat down with their children to have a conversation, they did talk directly. The overall tones of conversations were reportedly more casual or conversational: "I just stay conversational. I don't sit them down and have a talk about it. It's just part of our lifestyle . . . . I verbally reinforce, just calling attention to what we're eating. Not in a way that is obnoxious. Just part of our normal conversation." Many of the conversations occurred while doing something else, or while partaking in the behavior together (e.g., dinner time, grocery shopping), using it as an opportunity. For example, one parent commented that her strategies depend on the situation:

I don't sit down and say okay, we're gonna now talk about health and fitness, because I think they would just completely turn off. It's more like piecemeal in connection to things, like my daughter, it'll be four in the afternoon, and she'll be like, "I'm hungry," and I'll be like well you can have an apple or you can have grapes and the reason is because we are going to eat dinner in two hours and that's a healthier option if you're still hungry. We will talk about it like that, sort of piecemeal, case-by-case kind of thing. I don't want it to come across as a lecture.

The direct verbal communication also took the form of education about physical activity and nutrition. For example, parents felt that while eating dinner, they could talk about food choice and portion size:

Just addressing when it is appropriate to have certain snacks. Trying to talk about timing of food. For instance you don't eat cookies in the morning for breakfast. Those types of things. And just calling attention to portion sizes.

Another mother discussed the idea of balance and moderation when discussing eating habits, and encouraged her daughter to collaborate in the cooking process in order to instill positive behaviors for the future:

I stress the importance of balance and not depriving yourself. I do talk to her about moderation. She also helps me cook and enjoys cooking herself when she has time. We have an open conversation that comes up more spontaneously not a sit down type of format. Maybe if we see something on TV or see a very unhealthy person out at a restaurant eating the wrong thing, or about bad choices we see celebrities or media people make that puts them in the hospital or leads to their death.

Similarly, parents used direct communication to encourage or suggest to their children to be physically active. For example, "Well, if we are at home, I just suggest that they go outside and play for a while." Others specifically engaged in physical activity with their children, and used the opportunity to talk about what activity can do for the body or why people should be active.

More often, parents indicated they use indirect communication with their children. Indirect verbal communication was the least used form ($N = 14$), as once parents started talking about certain behaviors, they began to talk about them in more detail, which then fell into the direct communication category. For example: "I make it a part of meal conversations. If I've cooked pasta, for example, and he asks for simple pasta with butter, I will suggest a tomato sauce. Or if we go out for sushi, I suggest that he eat a few edamame." Nonverbally, we saw indirect communication in the form of modeling behaviors and accessibility of resources. Modeling behaviors have been found to be amongthe most effective ways to encourage healthy behaviors in children (Hamilton & White, 2010); however, the literature often does not pay attention to whether these behaviors are intentional or occur by happenstance. The results here show that many parents purposely modeled healthy behaviors for their children ($N = 45$). For example, one parent commented on the importance of modeling: "It is important to model healthy behaviors otherwise my child gets mixed messages and is less likely to follow healthy habits if I don't." Another example of this involved the importance of both parents modeling healthy behaviors:

I try to model that. They know I get up at five in the morning and go running. They know I do that because I think it's a healthy thing to do. Their dad is a really competitive volleyball player and he plays like three nights a week. He's not with us right here, but he's always played. So they see that too and they sometimes come with him to the game. It plants in their mind that it's something fun to do. They go and sometimes they play with him, but also, they watch his games. I have also done races with the kids. We will all sign up for the five k together, then we all run it together. It's not super competitive, but it's a way to do it together as a family.

Other parents purposefully engaged in healthy behaviors with their children, partaking in the activity, or involving their children in their own activity (e.g., making dinner). For example, "For exercising, my daughter and I like to be active all the time. We dance around when we're getting dressed and making food in the kitchen, we take walks to nearby parks where we can play." More often than not, parents engaged in multiple forms of indirect communication, including modeling and talking indirectly about the behavior they were engaging in. For example, the parent in the following vignette mentions going grocery shopping together, planning out meals, and encouraging better choices of food via outcome, without directly saying why healthier options are a better choice (e.g., protein makes you stronger).

I like to take my children grocery shopping with me and we talk about what we would like to eat for the week and plan out lunch and dinners together. When they want something unhealthy I try to trade it out for something healthier and encourage them to pick that choice more than the unhealthy one. I also encourage him to eat everything if he wants to be able to play football or soccer and be big and good like all the professionals.

We also saw indirect nonverbal communication in the form of *controlled accessibility* ($N = 48$). Controlled accessibility was often portrayed in the form of packing lunches, not having certain foods in the house, or enrolling children in schools where healthy eating is required (e.g., schools that have a set list of food parents can pack for their child). For example:

And just to reinforce that, just making it available. So for instance we keep the apples, bananas, and oranges on the counter. So that they can visually see them as a choice in addition to knowing that they can go into the pantry and get a granola bar. I think that sometimes if things are out of sight, they're out of mind. So putting everything in the refrigerator may not be the best place for my kids to see it.

Concerning exercise, controlled accessibility took the form of making sports, classes, and exercise (often labeled as "play time") readily available. This included parents providing the funds to put their children through these activities, having equipment at home, and driving/showing up to practices, games, and recitals.

Barriers to Healthy Behaviors

Despite the desire to communicate positive weight management practices to their children, parents experienced a number of perceived barriers to both their own and their children's healthy eating and physical activity. Barriers are the reasons why parents reported they did not implement, or believed it was difficult to encourage, the behaviors they perceive to be healthy. Some parents also reported perceiving these barriers as related to their ability to communicate the need for these behaviors. Many parents mentioned *time, accessibility,* and *money* as the primary reasons why they and their family members have trouble eating healthy or meeting the recommended physical activity requirement during the week.

First, *time* was the most frequently mentioned perceived barrier for both physical activity and healthy eating behaviors. In fact, it was mentioned 76 times throughout the interviews, even when the interviewers did not prompt parents to think about barriers. Parents talked about full schedules, random changes in schedules, and exhaustion. For example, one parent wrote, "Random conflicts popping up keep me from exercising sometimes.

Exhaustion from our busy lifestyles can also be a barrier." These specific examples of barriers often surfaced in the context of physical activity, which was often discussed as a time commitment that required changing clothes, going somewhere to exercise, coming back, showering, and then changing clothes again. For example, "I feel my time is limited. Or not even so limited, but the free time I have is not conducive to getting on by. So maybe my free time is at nine o'clock at night, my kids are in bed, and I can't leave the house. So I can't go walk the dogs then, so I've missed that window." Time restrictions also overlap into their children's lives. Although many parents mentioned their children engaging in sports or dance rather than "working out," they continued to speak about time as a barrier, especially because many children need to be driven to these activities and parents wanted to show support.

Although time was mentioned frequently in the context of physical activity, it was also a perceived barrier for parents concerning healthy eating. Time was a major issue for parents, as balancing a family and the schedule of each person is difficult; Therefore, in that experience, the time it takes to grocery shop, cook, and clean dishes was perceived as difficult to fit in on a daily basis. One parent mentioned, "It is hard because sometimes we have very busy days where it is just easier to stop and get Whataburger on the way home." Additionally, when parents did manage to include physical activity into the schedule, adopting healthy eating, also, became a time issue. For example:

Barriers are definitely time constraints. For me it is working and family demands. For my daughter it is school, extracurricular activities and studies that sometimes cause her not to have time to get all her meals in. Going straight from school to cheer practice to a game may not allow the time to sit down and eat a meal and just grab something on the go.

One parent mentioned she does not perceive any barriers, because healthy living is a priority in their house: "None really, there are many options to choose from for sports and physical activity you just have to make it a priority." We therefore considered parents' making these behaviors a priority and their motivation to do so as a component of time. This subtheme was mentioned an additional 32 times by parents both in the sense that barriers were not perceived because parents made healthy behaviors a priority, and in the context of parents who did not necessarily make these behaviors a priority and chose an alternative. One parent mentioned her biggest fear was that her family just does not prioritize these healthy behaviors: "It requires time and energy and I worry my family does not prioritize working out."

Second, parents mentioned the *accessibility* of healthy foods and physical activity as a perceived barrier to engaging in weight management practices.

This theme is defined by the inability of parents to find the foods they believe to be healthy. Often, parents characterized accessibility as the inability to easily find or consume non-GMO, organic, or natural foods. Accessibility of nutritious food was also mentioned in relation to the ease of their families' accessibility to unhealthy food. For example, "Well my concern for her is school lunches. I know that she's not getting the healthiest things there because it's made for an army." This affected the entire family as well, especially when eating out: "Eating out is a concern because I don't know what they have back there. And things that I think may be scratch is actually a frozen or bagged product."

Accessibility also frequently referred to an individual's health. Health issues (e.g., chronic illnesses, diabetes, bad knees) are cited as rationales for why adopting a healthier diet or engaging in physical activity are limited for themselves or for their child. For example, "I have problems with my knee and foot that limits my ability to exercise. And there are no barriers that I can think of that would prevent my child from participating in sports. It is something that he thoroughly enjoys, and couldn't imagine taking him out of them." A few parents mentioned the development of health issues (e.g., eating disorders) as a rationale for allowing their children to behave in a particular manner. For example, "I have always been concerned about my children ever having eating disorders, as they are very present in today's society, especially at a young age. This is why I've always been open to them eating whatever they want, but also teaching them about the importance of healthy eating and exercise." Similarly, safety was cited as an accessibility issue. A family's neighborhood safety (e.g., crime that may be present) or daylight savings time (e.g., night taking away from the amount of time available to go outside) contribute to parents feeling uncertain about their children or themselves going outside to engage in activity. For example:

My concern about exercise is time management and neighborhood safety, community safety. Because I get home in the evening closer to nightfall and it's not safe for me and my daughter to be walking around in our own neighborhood. So that kind of takes away from our ability to always do it. So now in the winter it's getting dark at 6 o'clock. So by the time I get home there's no space to do it. So I need to find an alternative.

Last, and probably most consistent with previous family communication literature, money was the third most prevalent barrier mentioned by participants. Parents referenced the cost of healthy food, gym memberships, or organized sports as a barrier to their own and their children's regular diet and exercise habits. For example, one parent stated, "I would definitely say one of the biggest barriers about healthy eating is the cost. Food that is better for you is typically more expensive, and my family can't afford to make sure we're buying ONLY healthy food."

DISCUSSION

The purpose of this study was to examine how parents seek out health information for their children, process that information, and relay it to their children. Results suggest that parents retrieved information through several channels both intentionally and unintentionally. The majority sought out information from formal face-to-face channels, including doctors, nutritionists, and personal trainers. However, when parents retrieved information in a mediated setting, primarily online, they were consuming informal sources including blogs and posts on social media. Despite this information, parents perceived a number of barriers to keeping both themselves and their children engaging in weight management practices: these most frequently surfaced as time, accessibility, and money. Last, most parents used nonverbal and indirect methods of communicating what it means to engage in physical activity and adopt a healthy diet. This entailed modeling behaviors, controlling accessibility by making lunches, buying specific foods for the house, signing their children up for a sport, and engaging in behaviors such as inviting their children to cook or go grocery shopping with them.

It seemed as though parents knew "right/wrong" when discussing their definition of health. This remained a constant when they were prompted to talk about health generally and what it means to be physically active or eat healthy. For example, they frequently cited USDA recommendations, organic foods, and actual prescriptions or recommendations. However, when addressing where they sought information, the same parents expressed preference for information from other parents or nongovernment websites – which seems like it would contradict the "right" type of information source that they mentioned for the general health question.

Parents revealed a few types of strategies for talking with their children about health, diet, and exercise. Direct communication, or outright conversations about nutrition and physical activity, was mentioned only 31 times by parents. The reason was presumed to be the idea that talking about these behaviors can be a risky endeavor, as physical activity and nutrition are often associated with an individual's weight and body image. Research (Miller-Day & Kam, 2010; Ornelas, Perreira, & Ayala, 2007) argues that the best way to talk about challenging health behaviors is by having multiple conversations and remaining positive. Similarly, research demonstrates that direct efforts to influence another's health can undercut healthy behaviors and in fact have the reverse effect, primarily when this form of social control involves criticism (Rook, August, Stephens, & Franks, 2011). Therefore, the present study demonstrated that parents often use indirect methods as a form of social control over their children's health behaviors, which is a significantly understudied area. Most research focuses on modeling, which has mixed results for behavior promotion, and this study revealed a potential variation from modeling in which parents simply control the choices children (and parents) have in the home as a way of communicating healthy diet. Similarly, parents signed their children up for sports, or enrolled them in schools that also promote these healthy behaviors. These communicative efforts are a form of social control but are arguably a positive and indirect form in which parents model, restrict access, or narrate their own health and diet choices in order for their children to come to their own – albeit hopefully similar – conclusions and choices. This topic of positive forms of social control should be explored further to better understand their impact on behavior enactment for the long term.

Last, time was mentioned as a barrier to engaging in weight management practices. This mirrors recent research on understanding contemporary healthy living that demonstrated that time is an important factor that needs to be considered when evaluating family dynamics surrounding health, diet, and exercise (Chircop et al., 2015). More specifically, Chircop et al. (2015) found that time was a paradoxical idea in that families valued physical activity and healthy eating differently, with a higher value placed on physical activity than on healthy eating. Therefore, parents reported giving in to societal pressures of engaging their children in organized physical activity at the sacrifice of home-cooked family meals and consuming more fast food. Therefore, it is important to expand on the dimension of time and the important role it plays in family health behaviors as well as family communication surrounding health.

Practical Implications

This study provides insight into the way parents seek out and consequently communicate weight management practices, including nutrition and physical activity. The results of this study provide an opportunity to develop stronger, theory-based health interventions targeting parents and the healthy upbringing of their children that incorporate both direct and indirect communication strategies. Moreover, this study provided insight into the differences in how parents vary in their perspectives of health (e.g., fruits and vegetables are healthy, versus the need to be organic) and their ideas of how to communicate this to their children. Interventions targeting parents may help in streamlining what is healthy for children, dispelling myths, and explicating the pros and cons of organic food. The results of this exploration, along with that of future research, will allow us to understand fully what types of messages help promote healthy behaviors. Not only does this research help with parent–child communication, but it also provides guidance for health care providers in talking to their patients' parents about the best mode of communication to prevent children from being another statistic. Thus, the results of this study, in conjunction with past research, argue for more targeted health promotion tactics that also encourage talk, in conjunction with indirect tactics such as modeling, social control, and positive controlled accessibility.

Limitations and Future Research

Although this study aims to make unique contributions to communication and health scholarship, there are limitations. First, this study relied primarily on a university population. Therefore, many of our participants were of higher socioeconomic status, with 36% of them making more than $150,000 per household. Many of our participants (67%) identified as white or Caucasian and, on average, our parents were of normal weight range. By reaching out to a broader population, the data could be more generalizable, which could provide insight into the way different demographics vary in their communication. However, what does make our population more generalizable is that our population met the national average of overweight or obese children, at just over one third. Additionally, we had a broad range of parents, ages 22–58 years (M = 44.73), and children ranging the full 5–15 years (M = 11.23).

There is room to expand on this research in the future. For one, research should collect data from children about how they perceive the information that is being shared – what do they know? How do they make sense of it? How does it influence their decisions at lunch or at a friend's house? Exploring the other side of the communicative process will allow researchers to better understand not only how children perceive the communication and therefore act on it, but what motivates children in a positive way to partake in healthier behaviors. Understanding children's perceptions of communication can help us better shape messages from parents and health care providers without crossing the fine line that may push a child into unhealthy behaviors.

Furthermore, Li, Li, Guan, Ma, and Cui (2015) identified ten hotspots for research on health information seeking behavior, and three of the major areas are understanding adult health information seeking via mobile phone and its apps, attitudes and trust in online sources, and utilization of social media by parents. Future research should focus specifically on how parents obtain their health information "online" by specifying if it is through social media, applications, or traditional online research. This would be an interesting intersection for technology and health information seeking behaviors, to identify factors that influence credibility and retention of health information. For example, a few of the parents in our study mentioned the articles on social media that are titled with numbers, such as "10 Ways Blueberries Increase Health." One parent mentioned not trusting these sources, while another mentioned she liked the streamlined version of this health information.

Taking this a step further, it would be advantageous to investigate if preferential differences in health information influence parents' subsequent communication with their children. It is possible that parents may be more likely to discuss health information with children when it comes from a more simplistic source. As demonstrated in the present chapter, unintentional information seeking consisted of these types of articles on Facebook or Twitter, so this may be an avenue for future research.

Clearly, this project only begins to scratch the surface of our understanding of the parent–child dyad's communicative processes about weight management practices. Though the research on parent–child communication and health seems to be thorough, there are pieces missing. We aimed to start to fill that gap through a thorough examination of actual messages and communicative efforts. Future research connecting quantitative and qualitative data, as well as dyadic data, will continue to provide a more thorough understanding to help build stronger health promotion messages for parents through mass media and patient–parent–provider communication.

REFERENCES

Aalsma, M. C., Liu, G. C., & Wiehe, S. E. (2011). The role of perceived parent monitoring and support on urban child and adolescent problem behavior. *Community Mental Health Journal, 47*, 61–66. doi: 10.1007/s10597-009-9251-2aals

Barber, B. K. (1996). Parental psychological control: Revisiting a neglected construct. *Child Development, 67*, 3296–3319. doi: 10.2307/1131780

Barnes, G. M., Reifman, A. S., Farrell, M. P., & Dintcheff, B. A. (2000). The effects of parenting on the development of adolescent alcohol misuse: A six-wave latent growth model. *Journal of Marriage and the Family, 62*, 175–186. doi: 10.1111/j.1741-3737.2000.00175.x

Bernhardt, J. M., & Felter, E. M. (2004). Online pediatric information seeking among mothers of young children: Results from a qualitative study using focus groups. *Journal of Medical Internet Research, 6*, e7. doi: 10.2196/jmir.6.1.e7

Chircop, A., Shearer, C., Pitter, R., Sim, M., Rehman, L., Flannery, M., & Kirk, S. (2015). Privileging physical activity over healthy eating: "Time" to choose? *Health Promotion International, 30*, 418–426. doi: 10.1093/heapro/dat056

Crossman, A., Sullivan, D. A., & Benin, M. (2006). The family environment and American adolescents' risk of obesity as young adults. *Social Science & Medicine, 63*, 2255–2267. doi: 10.1016/j.socscimed.2006.05.027

Daniels, S. R. (2006). The consequences of childhood overweight and obesity. *Future Child, 16*, 47–67. doi: 10.1353/foc.2006.0004

Dave, J. M., Evans, A. E., Condrasky, M. D., & Williams, J. E. (2012). Parent-reported social support for child's fruit and vegetable intake: Validity of measures. *Journal of Nutrition Education and Behavior, 44*, 132–139. doi: 10.1016/j.jneb.2011.07.002

Glaser, B. G., & Strauss, A. L. (1967). *The discovery of grounded theory: Strategies for qualitative research.* Chicago, IL: Aldine Publishing.

Hamilton, K., & White, K. M. (2010). Identifying parents' perceptions about physical activity. *Journal of Health Psychology, 15*, 1157–1169. doi: 10.1177/1359105310364176.

Kahn, S. E., Hull, R. L., & Utzschneider, K. M. (2006). Mechanisms linking obesity to insulin resistance and type 2 diabetes. *Nature, 444,* 840–846. doi: 10.1038/nature05482

Kaplan, M., Kiernan, N., & James, L. (2006). Intergenerational family conversations and decision making about eating healthfully. *Journal of Nutrition Education & Behavior, 3,* 298–306. doi: 10.1016/j.jneb.2006.02.010

Khoo, K., Bolt, P., Babl, F. E., Jury, S., & Goldman, R. D. (2008). Health information seeking by parents in the Internet age. *Journal of Pediatrics and Child Health, 44,* 419–423. doi: 10.1111/j.1440-1754.2008.01322.x

Li, F., Li, M., Guan, P., Ma, S., & Cui, L. (2015). Mapping publication trends and identifying hot spots of research on internet health information seeking behavior: A quantitative and co-word biclustering analysis. *Journal of Medical Internet Research, 17,* e81. doi: 10.2196/jmir.3326

McMinn, A. M., Griffin, S. J., Jones, A. P., & van Sluijs, E. M. F. (2012). Family and home influences on children's after-school and weekend physical activity. *European Journal of Public Health, 23,* 805–810. doi: eurpub/cks160

Miller-Day, M., & Kam, J. (2010). More than just openness: Developing and validating a measure of targeted parent–child communication about alcohol health communication. *Health Communication, 25,* 293–302. doi: 10.1080/10410231003698952

Neumark-Sztainer, D., Bauer, K. W., Friend, S., Hannan, P. J., Story, M., & Berge, J. M. (2010). Family weight talk and dieting: How much do they matter for body dissatisfaction and disordered eating behaviors in adolescent girls? *Journal of Adolescent Health, 47,* 270–276. doi: 10.1016/j.jadohealth.2010.02.001

Ogden, C. L., Carroll, M. D., Kit, B. K., & Flegal, K. M. (2012). Prevalence of obesity and trends in body mass index among US children and adolescents, 1999–2010. *Journal of the American Medical Association, 307,* 483–490. doi: 10.1001/jama.2012.40

Ogden, C. L., Carroll, M. D., Kit, B. K., & Flegal, K. M. (2014). Prevalence of childhood and adult obesity in the United States, 2011–2012. *Journal of the American Medical Association, 311,* 806–814. doi: 10.1001/jama.2014.732

Olds, T., Maher, C., Zumin, S., Péneau, S., Lioret, S., Castetbon, K., . . . & Lissner, L. (2011). Evidence that the prevalence of childhood overweight is plateauing: Data from nine countries. *International Journal of Pediatric Obesity, 6,* 342–360. doi: 10.3109/17477166.2011.605895

Ornelas, I. J., Perreira, K. M., & Ayala, G. X. (2007). Parental influences on adolescent physical activity: A longitudinal study. *International Journal of Behavioral Nutrition and Physical Activity, 4,* 3. doi: 10.1186/1479-5868-4-3

Ristovski-Slijepcevic, S., Bell, Kg., Chapman, G. E., & Beagan, B. L. (2010). Being "thick" indicates you are eating, you are healthy and you have an attractive body shape: Perspectives on fatness and food choice amongst Black and White men and women in Canada. *Health Sociology Review, 19,* 317–329. doi: 10.5172/hesr.2010.19.3.317

Ritchie, L. D., & Fitzpatrick, M. A. (1990). Family communication patterns: Measuring intrapersonal perceptions of interpersonal relationships. *Communication Research, 17,* 523–544. doi: 10.1177/009365090017004007

Rook, K. S., August, K. J., Stephens, M. A. P., & Franks, M. M. (2011). When does spousal social control provoke negative reactions in the context of chronic illness? The pivotal role of patients' expectations. *Journal of Social and Personal Relationships, 28,* 772–789. doi: 10.1177/0265407510391335

Shonkoff, J. P., & Phillips, D. A. (Eds.). (2000). *From neurons to neighborhoods: The science of early childhood development.* Washington, DC: National Academies Press.

Strauss, A., & Corbin, J. (1990). *Basics of qualitative research* (Vol. 15). Newbury Park, CA: SAGE.

Stroud, N. J., & Higgins, V. (2011). Content analysis. In D. Sloan & S. Zhou (Eds.), *Research methods in communication* (2nd ed., pp. 123–143). Northport, AL: Vision Press.

US Preventive Services Task Force. (2010). Screening for obesity in children and adolescents: US Preventive Services Task Force recommendation statement. *Pediatrics,* peds-2009.

Williams, J., Wake, M., Hesketh, K., Maher, E., & Waters, E. (2005). Health-related quality of life of overweight and obese children. *Journal of the American Medical Association, 293,* 70–76. doi: 10.1001/jama.293.1.70

Wills, T. A., Gibbons, F. X., Gerrard, M., Murray, V. M., & Brody, G. H. (2003). Family communication and religiosity related substance use and sexual behavior in early adolescence: A test for pathways through self-control and prototype perceptions. *Psychology of Addictive Behaviors, 17,* 312–323. doi: 10.1037/0893-164X.17.4.312

PART III

UNCERTAINTY IN HEALTH AND RELATIONSHIPS

7

"We Have Been Robbed of the Life We Planned": Relational Turbulence and Experiences of Alzheimer's Disease

DANIELLE CATONA

The United States is an aging society. By 2030, the number of Americans aged 65 and older is expected to reach 71 million, or roughly 20% of the US population (Federal Interagency Forum on Aging-Related Statistics, 2008). One of the most significant health care issues facing an aging society is the prevalence of Alzheimer's disease (AD).

AD is a progressive disorder characterized by the onset of cognitive difficulties, ranging from minor confusion in its early stages to severe dementia in its later stages, and ultimately leading to death (Harwood, 2007). It is the most common form of dementia (it is estimated to account for more than half of all dementia cases) and affects an estimated 5 million people aged 65 and older (Hebert, Weuve, Scherr, & Evans, 2013). AD is the sixth leading cause of death in the United States (Alzheimer's Association, 2013). As the number of older Americans grows rapidly, so, too, will the numbers of new and existing cases of AD. By 2050, the number of people aged 65 and older with AD may nearly triple, from 5 million to a projected 13.8 million, without the development of medical breakthroughs to prevent, slow, or stop the disease (Hebert et al., 2013).

As the prevalence of AD increases, so, too, does the number of informal caregivers (Schulz & Martire, 2004). Informal caregiving refers to family members or friends attending to another individual's health needs. Informal caregiving often includes assistance with one or more activities of daily living, such as bathing and dressing (Gaugler, Kane, & Kane, 2002). In 2012, informal caregivers provided an estimated 17.5 billion hours of unpaid care for people with AD (Alzheimer's Association, 2013). The largest proportion of informal caregivers of people with AD are spouses, followed by children and children-in-law (Alzheimer's Association and National Alliance for Caregiving, 2004; Metlife Mature Marketing Institute, 2006). Because spouses are most likely to assume the role of informal caregiver, this study examines the diagnosis and progression of AD as significant transitions in older adult marriages.

Prior research has shown that AD can have both negative and positive effects on late-life marital relationships, depending on how couples view and communicate about the changes associated with the health condition. For example, Derksen, Vernooij-Dassen, Gillissen, Olde Rikkert, and Scheltens (2006) documented the effects of AD on 18 spousal caregiver–care recipient dyads. Caregivers felt burdened by the continuous care they provided for their partner and expressed a need for respite care. Care recipients were aware of the increasing burden on their partner, yet still wanted their relational partners to stay close to them. Care recipients put their trust in the strength of their long-term relationships and relied heavily on their partner's strength to cope with physical and cognitive declines. Caregivers also expressed the need to find ways to cope with changes in their marital relationships, such as focusing on the care recipient's remaining faculties instead of disabilities and preserving joint couple activities.

To further examine the effects of AD on late-life marital relationships, this study draws on the relational turbulence theory (RTT; Solomon, Knobloch, Theiss, & McLaren, 2016). The next section reviews claims advanced by the RTT, followed by a qualitative analysis of spousal caregiver blogs, and concludes with recommendations for how this study can facilitate future efforts to understand how older adult marital relationships are weakened or strengthened by the transition from care partner to caregiver and from partner interdependence to dependence.

THE RELATIONAL TURBULENCE THEORY

The RTT (Solomon et al., 2016) identifies relationship transitions as ripe for upheaval and turmoil, because they introduce changes to people's roles and routines and their goals for the relationship. The RTT has been applied to a number of relationship transitions that occur within marriages, such as adding children (Theiss, Estlein, & Weber, 2013), launching children (Nagy & Theiss, 2013), reintegrating after military deployment (Knobloch & Theiss, 2011), and the diagnosis of infertility (Steuber & Solomon, 2008) and breast cancer (Weber & Solomon, 2008). This study applies the RTT to identify and explain the relational issues faced by older adult married couples as they navigate the late-life, caregiving phase of their relationship. According to the RTT, the mechanisms that promote heightened reactivity to changes in the circumstances for the relationship are relational uncertainty and interference from a partner. Each mechanism is described in detail in the text that follows.

Relational Uncertainty

Relational uncertainty refers to the degree of confidence individuals have in their perceptions of involvement within interpersonal relationships (Knobloch & Solomon, 2002). Relational uncertainty consists of self, partner, and relationship uncertainty. *Self uncertainty* is defined as questions individuals have about their participation in a relationship, including their personal evaluation of the relationship's worth, or their goals within the relationship. *Partner uncertainty* refers to questions individuals have about their partner's participation in a relationship; it can include questions about the value the partner places on the relationship or about the goals that the partner has for the relationship. *Relationship uncertainty* is defined as questions about the viability of the relationship as a whole, including the behavioral norms for the relationship, the roles enacted within the relationship, the reciprocity of feelings between the partners, how the relationship is being defined, and where partners can expect the relationship to go in the future.

The RTT provides insight into both the causes and consequences of relational uncertainty within romantic relationships. For example, relational uncertainty could occur whenever changes in the circumstances for the relationship prompt people to revisit questions about their own involvement in the relationship, their partner's involvement, and the relationship itself. Tests of RTT have found that relational uncertainty is positively associated with negative appraisals of irritations (Solomon & Knobloch, 2004), perceptions of the difficulty of a conversation (Knobloch & Solomon, 2005), and threatening relationship talk (Knobloch & Theiss, 2011). Moreover, uncertain individuals are more likely to use indirect communication to address relational problems (Theiss & Solomon, 2006a), avoid talking about surprising relationship events (Knobloch & Solomon, 2002), enact less relationship talk (Knobloch & Theiss, 2011), and employ distancing behaviors (Knobloch & Carpenter-Theune, 2004; Knobloch & Theiss, 2011).

Interference from a Partner

Beyond questioning involvement in the relationship, other difficulties may emerge as partners coordinate daily routines and rely on one another to achieve daily goals. Partners can shape each other's daily activities in one of three ways: influence, interference, or facilitation (Solomon & Knobloch, 2001, 2004). *Influence* occurs when one partner is involved in the daily activities of the other partner. *Interference* refers to a situation in which one partner impedes or creates boundaries for the other partner to achieve his or her activities or goals. *Facilitation* is the extent to which an individual promotes or assists with the partner's daily activities.

The RTT predicts that experiences of interference from a partner increase when couples undergo changes in their patterns of interdependence. For example, during transitions, individuals may modify preexisting routines, which often leads to individuals being forced to adopt new/additional roles or to take on new/additional responsibilities. Empirical research suggests that partner interference is positively associated with perceived negativity of relational irritations (Solomon & Knobloch, 2004; Theiss & Solomon, 2006b), intensity of hurt, appraisal of the intentionality of hurt, and perceived damage to the relationship (Theiss, Knobloch, Checton, & Magsamen-Conrad, 2009). In addition, the directness of communication is positively associated with partner interference (Theiss & Solomon, 2006b), whereas communication positivity is negatively associated with interference from a partner.

A RELATIONAL TURBULENCE PERSPECTIVE OF ALZHEIMER'S DISEASE

Viewing AD through the RTT provides insight into how the progression from early- to mid- to late-stage AD sparks transitional periods in which spousal caregivers question or renegotiate aspects of their relationship. AD often comes as a surprise to older adult couples; it may upset retirement plans and growing old together (Alzheimer's Association, 2014). The following sections elaborate on the role of AD in relational uncertainty and the experience of interference from a partner.

Alzheimer's Disease and Relational Uncertainty

AD has an effect on both spouses and on the marital relationship (Hellstrom, Nolan, & Lundh, 2005, 2007). As the severity of AD increases, companionship and reciprocity decrease, which, in turn, transforms the marital relationship into more of a parent–child or caregiver–care recipient relationship (Sanders & Power, 2009). These changes have been found to prompt spousal caregivers to question the status of their marriage. Some may continue to feel married, while others may feel they no longer have a marriage (Evans & Lee, 2014). AD can give rise to partner-, self-, and relationship-focused sources of ambiguity. Each source is described in detail in the following paragraphs.

Care recipient changes and partner uncertainty. AD alters the spouse with the condition. For example, as cognitive function declines, there may be changes in the care recipient's personality, communication skills, role function, and ability to maintain the marital relationship (National Institute on Aging, 2012). AD may negatively impact everyday conversations between spouses, interests that they share, and mutual support (Evans & Lee, 2014). Care recipients may not remember their life with caregivers and may even fall in love with someone else (Alzheimer's Association, 2014). As a result of these numerous changes, spousal caregivers may question care recipients' participation in the marriage.

Caregiver changes and self uncertainty. Caregivers may be troubled by the changes in their spouse caused by AD. For example, caregivers may view the situation as their spouse becoming a stranger to them or as the loss of the person whom they had married (Evans & Lee, 2014). Wuest, Ericson, and Stern (1994) documented the experience of caregivers and their deteriorating relationships with care recipients; they found that the original emotional commitment to the person with AD increasingly became detached as the relative continued to change and digress into a seemingly different person. These findings suggest caregivers interact with care recipients on a continuum that ranges from high intimacy, positive evaluation of the relationship, and low levels of uncertainty in the early stages of disease, to low intimacy, negative evaluation of the relationship, and high levels of uncertainty as alienation increases over the course of the disease.

Marital relationship changes and relationship uncertainty. Caregivers may experience growing doubts about the status of their marriage that accompany their concerns about losing their spouse. For example, caregivers have to deal with the contradiction between a spouse's physical presence and cognitive absence. Kaplan (2001) labelled the different degrees of separation caused by AD as "unmarried-marrieds" and "husbandless-wives"/"wifeless-husbands." Baxter, Braithwaite, Golish, and Olsen (2002) examined interviews with spousal caregivers of persons with late-stage AD. Caregivers expressed how they loved their spouse and were married to them, but felt as if the person they married was gone or slowly passing away. Caregivers were classified as "married widows" (Rollins, Waterman, & Esmay, 1985) who felt obligated to perform marital duties, such as providing care while simultaneously pre-grieving the loss of their spouse. Based on the research described in the foregoing text, the following research question is proposed:

RQ1: How does relational uncertainty manifest among spousal caregivers coping with AD?

Alzheimer's Disease and Interference from a Partner

As AD progresses, care recipients' behaviors change, as does the role of caregiver. Caring for a person with AD can be physically, emotionally, and financially challenging. The demands of day-to-day care, changing family roles, and difficult decisions about placement in a care facility can be challenging to handle (Alzheimer's Association, 2014). Each challenge is described in detail in the following paragraphs.

Providing day-to-day care. On analyzing nationwide data of 1,247 care-givers, the Alzheimer's Association and the National Alliance for Caregiving (2004) concluded, "Caregivers of persons with AD shoulder a particularly heavy burden of care. Compared with other caregivers, the type of care they provide is more physically and emotionally demanding and more time con-suming, and it takes a heavier toll on work and family life" (p. i). Caregivers of persons with AD are more likely than caregivers of other older adults to assist with activities of daily living (Alzheimer's Association, 2013). Increased phy-sical strain becomes more pronounced as the care recipient's disease gradually progresses and memory and motor functions continue to diminish (Austrom & Lu, 2009). Georges et al. (2008) surveyed more than 1,000 AD caregivers and found that as the disease progresses and symptoms become more severe, 50% of informal caregivers of persons with AD spend more than 10 hours per day providing care.

Caregivers may take on new roles and responsibilities as the care recipi-ent's memory declines, including balancing the checkbook, doing the taxes, shopping, cooking, and managing legal and financial affairs (Alzheimer's Association, 2013). Caring for persons with AD also means managing symp-toms that caregivers of persons with other diseases may not face, such as neuropsychiatric symptoms and severe behavior problems (Alzheimer's Association, 2013).

Making difficult decisions. When persons with AD move to a residential care facility, the role of caregiver usually changes from hands-on activities of daily living types of care, to visiting, providing emotional support to the relative in residential care, interacting with facility staff, and advocating for appropriate care for their relative (Garity, 2006). AD caregivers may experi-ence psychological burden and emotional distress associated with taking on the responsibility of speaking for care recipients when they can no longer speak for themselves. In late-stage AD, caregivers often assume responsibility for advocating for care recipients first by identifying their physical and emotional concerns and then by informing health care providers (Caron, Griffith, & Arcand, 2005). In addition to becoming a voice for persons with AD regarding pain and emotional concerns, caregivers must also make decisions regarding end-of-life care preferences (Caron et al., 2005). Difficult decisions such as these often contribute to a great deal of psycholo-gical burden as emotions surface when caregivers are unclear about specifics of their loved one's preferences.

Experiencing social isolation. Providing care for a person with AD has been linked to various forms of social isolation, including, but not limited to, relational strain with the care recipient, lack of time for social engagement, and seclusion due to geographical distance from family and friends (Alzheimer's Association, 2014). AD caregivers often worry about their own limitations and about being embarrassed by the behavior of care recipients. These insecurities and fears may lead to a self-imposed exile in which caregivers limit social outings and forgo pleasurable activities (Austrom & Lu, 2009). Even caregivers who wish to escape and socialize often cannot because of the round-the-clock supervision required to care for a person with AD, which makes it difficult to leave the house (Czaja & Rubert, 2002).

Beyond AD caregiver behaviors, family and friends may withdraw from the relationship (Alzheimer's Association, 2014; Czaja & Rubert, 2002). Caregivers' family and friends may hesitate to spend time with them and the person with AD because they worry about not knowing what to do or say. Family and friends also may not understand the behavior changes caused by the disease or might not be able to accept that the person has AD.

Experiencing decline in physical and mental health. Persons with AD may require greater levels of supervision and personal care as the disease progresses, which can be associated with various physical and mental health consequences for care providers. Informal caregivers of persons with AD are at greater risk of chronic disease, physiological impairments, increased health care utilization, and mortality (Vitaliano, Zhang, & Scanlan, 2003). In addition, AD caregivers have increased levels of anxiety, depression, and grief (Alzheimer's Association, 2013). Spousal caregivers, in particular, are at high risk for depression due to a loss of relational intimacy, loss of communication, the end of future planning, and a loss of both social and recreational interactions (Austrom & Lu, 2009). Prioritizing care recipient needs over individual needs may impede caregivers from maintaining their personal health. Moreover, compromised personal health may make it more difficult for caregivers to participate in leisure activities.

Changes in employment. Providing care for persons with AD is also associated with lost wages due to disruptions in employment, and depleted income and finances (Liu & Gallagher-Thompson, 2009). Surveys of employed AD caregivers revealed their having to make major changes to their work schedules such as going in late, leaving early, or taking time off (65%) and taking a leave of absence (20%) because of caregiving responsibilities. Moreover, spousal caregivers were at the highest risk of quitting work because of caregiving responsibilities. In fact, more than 10% reported leaving their job to provide care, compared to 4% of the other caregiving spouses (Metlife Mature Market Institute, 2006). Based on the research described in the foregoing text, the following research question is proposed:

RQ2: How does partner interference manifest among spousal caregivers coping with AD?

METHOD

Sample

Spousal caregiver blogs were identified by exploring an online search engine, Google, using the search terms "Alzheimer's disease and blogs," "Alzheimer's disease caregivers and blogs," and "Alzheimer's disease spousal caregivers and blogs." Blogs are online journals that individuals maintain (Thurlow, Lengel, & Tomic, 2004). In the present study, each blog entry was treated as one unit. Criteria for inclusion of a blog entry in the study were: (a) they were written by a spousal caregiver and (b) they referenced either relationship or partner issues. This process yielded a total sample of 400 units (20 female bloggers and 20 entries each).

Data Analysis

Data were analyzed by three undergraduate coders blind to the study's purpose, in order to avoid a priori expectations for themes. The coders immersed themselves in a line-by-line reading and rereading of blog entries; then, they conducted open and axial coding (Strauss & Corbin, 1998). Open coding is an interpretive process designed to identify, name, and categorize emergent themes. Axial coding involves searching for similar data and relating categories to each other. During several meetings with the author, coders discussed emergent patterns in the data, and worked to refine and collapse patterns. Disagreements about the findings were resolved through discussion. Finally, the author conducted selective coding in which she interpreted and compared emergent themes to the RTT (Solomon et al., 2016). This process revealed five relational uncertainty themes (RQ1) and four partner interference themes (RQ2).

RESULTS

Data are organized by research question. Emergent themes within spousal caregiver blog entries are described, with illustrative quotes.

Relational Uncertainty

RQ1 sought to identify sources of relational uncertainty within spousal caregivers' experiences coping with AD. Five categories are particularly relevant for relational uncertainty in these data: (a) revisiting memories, (b) resentment instead of commitment, (c) moments of partner clarity, (d) mourning loss of the relationship, and (e) relationship redefinition.

Revisiting memories. Caregivers expressed revisiting the past in order to preserve personal commitment in the present. One caregiver described the benefits of watching old home movies, "It was very cool to be reminded of the man he was when we met and who so quickly faded away to the person he is now. Most days now it's very hard to remember that fellow. Today, for just a bit, I was reminded. Nice." In addition, caregivers evaluated relationship worth by focusing on the "good times together," before AD. One caregiver shared, "We have lived all of these years with a bond that has allowed us to know what is in each other's hearts and minds. AD is slowly taking that ability from you, but it has not taken it from me. It is because I understand you so well that my tears are as much for you as for me." In summary, caregivers attempted to manage uncertainty about their changing partner and marriage by remembering the spouse they once knew and the relationship they once had.

Resentment instead of commitment. For other caregivers, personal commitment to their marriage was replaced with feelings of obligation. One caregiver described her frustration in failing to uphold her marriage vows, "How can you resent your spouse? How can you resent caring for the love of your life? The marriage vows say – 'for better or worse'. Yes, they do. But they don't tell you how to handle 'the worse'. And no vow can tell you how to 'feel.'" Another caregiver expressed emotional distress associated with disliking the current version of her husband, "What could I do with the guilt and shame I felt about not liking this stranger, who bore no resemblance to my precious husband?" Thus, AD-related changes prompted caregivers to question the reasons they remained in their marriage. Caregivers expressed guilt about their changing feelings and increasing resentment toward their partner.

Moments of partner clarity. Caregivers described frequency of partner awareness and responsiveness that influenced expressions of intimacy. One early-stage caregiver reported her husband's daily displays of affection, "What AD has not changed is his love and concern for me. Not a day goes by that he does not take me in his arms and tell me how much he loves and appreciates me – how he hurts to see me have to bear the burden of so much." One mid-stage caregiver described clinging to the fleeting moments of partner lucidity, "My husband sort of woke up enough that in his semi-sleeping state, he knew who I was and said, 'Oh there you are.' Since he knew me, I crawled up on the bed with him and snuggled up and he snuggled back so that was cool that he was sort of his usual old self." One late-stage caregiver discussed the lack of partner recognition based on disease progression exacerbated by distance due to nursing home placement, "He has lost touch with who I am to an extent which will become more and more obvious, I'm sure. That's one of the things that made it so hard to make the decision to have him so far away. He still knows I'm important to him but just how is not clear." As AD progressed, moments of partner clarity decreased, which, in turn, shaped caregivers' assessment of partners' participation in the relationship and expression of affection. Early-stage AD was characterized by low levels of partner uncertainty, whereas late-stage AD was characterized by high levels of partner uncertainty.

Mourning loss of the relationship. Caregivers expressed how they loved their spouses and were married to them, but felt as if the person they married was gone or slowly passing away. One caregiver described relationship loss as, "When that realization hits you, the mourning period begins. You mourn the loss of the person you knew, surely as if that person had physically died. You mourn the loss of the relationship you treasured." Another caregiver shared the grieving process as, "When the realization hit – that the husband I adored, although still living, was gone; that the marital relationship I cherished was gone; and neither was coming back, my heart shattered." In addition to death, caregivers described AD-related changes in spouses as slipping away, "Marv, the man I met and fell in love with, slipped away a long time ago," and being kidnapped, "Where is my husband? AD crept into his head when my back was turned, and kidnapped him. I miss him so desperately." Despite the emotional toll associated with mourning the loss of the relationship, caregivers described this as a necessary step in creating a new, meaningful relationship. One caregiver summarized the process as, "We must go through this mourning period in order to come out on the other side and make a new and different life for ourselves and our 'different' spouses." In summary, AD-related changes resulted in caregivers questioning what happened to the spouse they used to know. Caregivers searched for signs that their "old" spouse was still present. Once the spouse had entered into late-stage AD and was no longer recognizable, caregivers expressed concern about how to relate to their "new" spouse.

Relationship redefinition. Caregivers discussed how AD-related changes in their spouse required them to reestablish or revisit the foundations of their intimacy in ways that either increased or decreased uncertainty about the future of their marriage. One caregiver described how she formed a new relationship with her husband, "No, he is not the person he was; we do not have the same relationship we had; but through AD education and our support system, we have worked to forge a new relationship." Another caregiver reported lowering relational expectations and settling for even a few moments of intimacy, "How sweet to have him or her hold you and tell you how much you are loved, how sorry they are that this disease shreds the relationship. How sweet to hold hands, lay your head on their shoulder, engage in a meaningful conversation, maybe even make love again. Treasure every single second of it. The reality of AD is that it may never come again." In addition, caregivers promoted relational well-being by focusing on and being grateful for the life they once had. One caregiver summarized this coping mechanism as:

But let's not forget the person inside that stranger's body. No matter the stage of the disease, that exceptional, distinctive individual you fell in love with is hidden deep inside the brain of the person you are looking at. Be forever thankful that you were given however many number of years with him/her – years to laugh together, make passionate love, travel, hold hands in the moonlight, share pillow talk, raise children, share joys and tragedies. If you were lucky enough to have shared those moments with someone, then you are truly blessed. Not everyone is afforded such opportunities in life.

Caregivers described strategies for managing uncertainty and moving forward in their marriage such as creating a new relationship that acknowledges AD, lowering expectations about what late-life marriage is when one spouse has AD, and focusing on the spouse they once knew despite AD-related changes.

Interference from a Partner

Beyond relational uncertainty, RQ2 identified sources of interference from a partner within spousal caregivers' experiences coping with AD. Spousal caregivers reported four categories of partner interference: (a) assuming additional roles, (b) overwhelming responsibility, (c) social isolation, and (d) ruined plans. Each type of partner interference is described next.

Assuming additional roles. Caregivers reported assisting with activities of daily living and taking on new roles and responsibilities as the care recipient advanced from early- to mid- and, finally, to late-stage AD. One caregiver highlighted the main tasks performed, "As caregivers to our spouses, we worry about their mental and physical health; we drive them to all of their doctor and testing appointments; we talk to all the doctors about the progression of their disease; we monitor their medications. We worry; we watch; we give care." Another caregiver echoed the responsibilities associated with caregiving, "We have to tell them what to do; how to do it; when to do it. We have to explain directions one at a time; organize their day; give them lists – on top of all the other things we have to do, including go to work, for us younger caregivers." Caregivers complained about the number and variety of roles and responsibilities they were forced to perform as a result of the gradual deterioration of their spouse.

In addition, caregivers expressed feeling more like they were in a parent–child relationship rather than a marriage. One caregiver described preparing a diaper bag prior to leaving the house, "So the new plan is to have always a change of clothes, Depends*, wipes, a washcloth in a baggy, a couple of bags to put the mess in and a fresh resolve to always make him go to the toilet before we leave the house. Who knew it would be like having a giant toddler?" Another caregiver summarized this relationship transition as, "Being married to someone with AD is like being married to a child, instead of a partner." Caregivers were dissatisfied with the types of tasks they had to perform as well as the nature of the relationship shifting to one partner being dependent on the other.

Overwhelming responsibility. AD caregivers manage a particularly heavy burden of care by providing more physically and emotionally demanding, as well as time-consuming tasks. One caregiver described full-time caregiving as, "Life as a full-time caregiver sucks the juice out of you. It's not so much that the work is hard but that it is relentlessly ongoing. You can't turn your back for a moment and even in sleep I find myself alert to anything unusual." The unrelenting nature of caregiving led to needing rest and relaxation. One caregiver shared, "I know that he is in a childlike stage in which he is afraid of losing me; I am his lifeline; his protector; his memory; his support system. I just need some breathing room."

The increasing caregiving demands as AD progresses from the mid to late stage prompts caregivers to consider residential care placement. One late-stage caregiver discussed her decision to admit her husband, "I am not superhuman. I have done all I could possibly do, and the time just came when I could not be awake 24 hours a day to give my loved one the care he needs. It was time to turn him over to the professionals." Another caregiver humorously described this transition as, "The train is heading out of Dementiaville into Poopytown, next stop Nursinghomeland."

When care recipients move to a residential care facility, the role of caregiver usually changes from hands-on involvement in enacting the mundane tasks of daily life to visiting and providing emotional support to the relative in residential care. Despite decreasing the number and physically demanding nature of caregiving tasks, caregivers experience guilt regarding relinquishing their caregiving duties. One caregiver shared, "I started crying at the Care Center and I haven't been able to stop since. I just want someone to go, 'It's okay, you can do it and it will be okay.'"

In summary, the number and types of tasks differed based on AD stage, with greatest amount of interference reported by caregivers of spouses transitioning from mid- to late-stage AD. As AD progressed, the amount of work became unmanageable and caregivers were forced to move spouses to a residential care facility. Caregivers experienced a decrease in the number of physical tasks to be performed and an increase in providing emotional support and managing guilt about no longer being able to care for their spouse.

Social isolation. Caregivers reported being abandoned by friends when they needed them the most. Caregivers' friends hesitated to spend time with them and the person with AD because they worried about not knowing what to do or say. One caregiver described the situation as, "My friends have started to exclude me and my husband from their group because he is no longer able to participate in the activities we once enjoyed together and they 'can't bear to see him like that.' All while I lose the companionship of my lifelong lover, and buckle under the crushing responsibilities of caregiving and financial stress." Another caregiver shared a similar experience, "My friends have stopped calling, stopped coming over to visit, stopped socializing with me and my husband. These are the people I never expected to let me down and abandon me when AD strikes." Caregivers sacrificed personal needs and opportunities to interact with others in order to care for their spouse.

Ruined plans. Caregivers expressed disappointment and frustration regarding changes in retirement plans and growing old together because of the progressive nature of AD. One caregiver reported not being able to rekindle their marriage and participate in joint activities like others in their age group, "For those of us in the retirement years, I watch in envy and sadness as my friends retain their marital closeness, travel together, enjoy activities with other friends." Another caregiver summarized dissatisfaction with their current life situation and inability to achieve pre-AD personal and relational goals, "You look around, anger and resentment festering, and you say, 'Wait a minute. What is going on here? This isn't the life we are supposed to be leading. We have been robbed of the life we planned.'" Caregivers lamented not being able to fulfill long-term marital goals because of their partners' AD. Ultimately, AD shattered caregivers' dreams about their future with their partner including travel, leisure activities, and spending quality time together.

DISCUSSION

This study examined changes to late-life marital relationships during the transition from care partner to caregiver, and partner interdependence to dependence. Blog entries were examined to identify examples of relational uncertainty (RQ1) and partner interference (RQ2). Spousal caregiver postings point to both coping with and being frustrated by relational changes during this transition. Study findings suggest important implications for extending the RTT and enhancing caregiver–care recipient relationships.

Theoretical Implications for the Relational Turbulence Theory

On a theoretical level, this study extends the RTT to a previously unexamined relationship context. The theory has been applied to relationship transitions that occur within dating (Solomon & Knobloch, 2001, 2004) and marital relationships, such as adding (Theiss et al., 2013) and launching children (Nagy & Theiss, 2013). The present study applies the RTT to examine the implications of a partner's deteriorating cognitive health for late-life marriages. Most people report being happier with their marriages in later life than in midlife (Goodman, 1999). Carstensen, Gottman, and Levenson (1995) found that compared to middle-aged couples, older couples displayed less negative affect and more affection. Dickson and Walker (2001) concur that many spouses become more emotionally expressive over time. AD caregiving disrupts the relational gains associated with late-life marriages. Caregivers may pull away from the care recipient in both an emotional and physical sense. They may be upset by the demands of caregiving while simultaneously mourning the loss of the spouse they once knew and loved. Caregivers may develop coping mechanisms such as revisiting past memories and clinging to moments of partner clarity in order preserve relational meaning. Study findings suggest that the RTT may be a useful tool for understanding the relationship challenges faced by couples during late-life transitions such as AD caregiving.

Besides a new relational context, this study extends the RTT to a previously unexamined health context. The RTT has previously been used to identify the issues couples face when managing infertility (Steuber & Solomon, 2008), breast cancer (Weber & Solomon, 2008), weight management (Theiss, Carpenter, & Leustek, 2016), and type 2 diabetes (Leustek & Theiss, 2018). The present study applies the RTT to a stage-based, progressive disease. Persons with early-stage AD may experience mild changes in the ability to think and learn, but continue to participate in daily activities and give-and-take dialogue. Spouses function as care partners who provide mutual support and help plan for the future. Since levels of companionship and reciprocity are high, early-stage AD is characterized by low levels of relational uncertainty and interference.

The transition from early- to mid-stage AD is marked by persons with AD experiencing increased difficulty communicating and comprehending new information, as well as becoming more reliant on others to perform the tasks of daily living. Spouses' roles transform from care partner to caregiver. Mid-stage AD is described as a period of increasing relational uncertainty and interference. Spousal caregivers in the present study expressed resentment and feelings of obligation during this stage because of having to assume new roles and responsibilities. Bloggers recommended focusing on the past and reducing expectations about the relationship to cope with this transition.

Persons with late-stage AD lose the ability to recognize loved ones, places, and objects, can no longer communicate, and become bed-ridden and reliant on 24/7 care until death. This is the most physically and emotionally demanding phase of caregiving that often results in moving the person with AD into a residential care facility. Spousal caregivers in the present study identified changing responsibilities once care recipients were institutionalized. Performing physical tasks was replaced with providing emotional support to care recipients. Caregivers described feelings of guilt about having to move their spouse into a residential care facility. Changes in the person with AD resulted in caregivers mourning the loss of their spouse and their marriage.

Practical Implications for Spousal Caregivers

This study demonstrates that blogs are a promising resource for spouses coping with the challenges of AD caregiving. Blogging provides an outlet for caregivers to share their inner thoughts and feelings with others through writing, as well as providing opportunities for the blogger to receive social support from others (site visitors who leave comments and/or message each other) (Ko & Kuo, 2009). Self-disclosure is often, but not always, related to positive outcomes such as health and social support. For example, researchers have found that verbally discussing or writing about traumatic or upsetting life experiences is associated with lower illness rates (Pennebaker & O'Heeron, 1984), fewer physician visits (Pennebaker, Colder, & Sharp, 1990; Pennebaker, Kiecolt-Glaser, & Glaser, 1988), and less immune dysfunction (Pennebaker et al., 1988). Self-disclosure of distressing information is often linked to catharsis (Kelly, Klusas, von Weiss, & Kenny, 2001). Therefore, self-disclosure through blogging may serve as the basis of building supportive relationships to counter the social isolation experienced as a result of caregiving, as well as buffering physical and emotional health consequences associated with caregiving.

Besides blogs, aging organizations have the ability to provide assistance to couples coping with AD by educating them about the condition and preparing them for increased uncertainty and interference during this transition. The Alzheimer's Association and National Institute on Aging identify likely communication and intimacy challenges and provide general advice about spending time together in ways that bring the caregiver and care recipient closer and help them relate to each other. More attention needs to be paid to helping couples reduce doubts about relationship status and negotiate shifting roles and responsibilities.

Strengths and Limitations

Utilizing blogs as the study data source served as both a strength and a weakness. As a benefit, blogs provided access to the inner thoughts of spousal caregivers' moods and feelings about coping with AD. At the same time, the focus on blogs limits generalizability to those individuals with consistent access to the internet and, most likely, excludes the most elderly caregivers and those of lower socioeconomic status (Smith, 2014). These groups may experience unique issues such as age-related health issues or lack of finances to assist with provision of care, making them the more vulnerable and in need of catharsis. Relying solely on blogs also may limit the availability of participant demographic information and representation of diverse perspectives. The 20 blogs analyzed were written by wives in heterosexual marriages, which may have underrepresented the perspectives of husbands and individuals in homosexual relationships coping with AD caregiving demands. Because prevalence rates of AD are higher among women, future research needs to examine husbands' experiences (Alzheimer's Association, 2013). Lastly, future studies would benefit from analyzing accounts of both spouses in the caregiver–care recipient relationship and the larger family system (adult children–parent relationships, sibling relationships, and grandchildren relationships).

Directions for Future Research

The RTT proposes relational uncertainty and interference from a partner as the two mechanisms that promote heightened reactivity to events that occur in romantic relationships (Solomon et al., 2016). Because relational uncertainty arises from three sources (self, partner, and relationship), one would expect interference from a partner to arise from the same three sources. Future studies of AD caregiving should examine self interference (how AD interferes with the things the caregiver likes to do each day), partner interference (how AD interferes with the things the care recipient likes to do each day), and relationship interference (how the health condition interferes with their relationship). In particular, a dyadic study should be conducted to examine differences in how caregivers and care recipients experience interference from a partner and how appraisals of interference influence communication outcomes and AD management.

The RTT tends to focus on turbulence in romantic partnerships, but many AD caregivers are nonromantic partners and are equally likely to experience relational uncertainty and interference (Alzheimer's Association and National Alliance for Caregiving, 2004). Future studies should examine relational turbulence among adult child, sibling, and grandchild caregivers.

The RTT was developed to explain emotional, cognitive, and behavioral turmoil during times of transition in close relationships. For example, studies have examined relational outcomes such as conflict (Solomon & Knobloch, 2004; Theiss & Solomon, 2006b), negative emotion (Knobloch & Theiss, 2010), and hurt (Theiss et al., 2009). Future studies should consider the potential for more positive outcomes during the transition from care partner to caregiver. Caregivers may experience emotional distress and psychological satisfaction simultaneously (Beach et al., 2000; Harmell et al., 2011). Spousal caregivers in the present study reported positive aspects of their experience, including being present for moments of care and recipient clarity, and identifying new opportunities for spousal connection.

Care recipients' thoughts and feelings about the AD illness experience are absent in the existing literature, including the present study. Besides the linguistic analysis of persons with AD speech patterns, scholars know very little about how persons with AD renegotiate their relational lives when faced with the impending eventuality they will transition from partner interdependence to dependence owing to the progressive nature of the disease. Future studies would benefit from analyzing accounts of persons with early- and mid-stage AD when communication faculties remain mostly intact (Alzheimer's Association, 2013). Sources of relational uncertainty and interference from a partner may be different for care recipients than for caregivers coping with AD.

CONCLUSION

The present study identified how relational uncertainty and interference from a partner manifest among spousal caregivers coping with AD. Blog entries provided insight into the impact that AD has on each spouse and the marital relationship. Over time, the spouses with AD had to relinquish their roles and responsibilities, and the other spouse had to assume these roles and responsibilities. The decrease in reciprocity signified the shift in relationship type from marital partners to caregiver–care recipient. Changes in companionship, intimacy, and the spouse with AD led to increased doubts about the future of the marriage. During late-stage AD, spousal caregivers mourned the loss of their partner and their marriage.

REFERENCES

Alzheimer's Association. (2013). Alzheimer's association report: 2013 Alzheimer's disease facts and figures. *Alzheimer's & Dementia, 9,* 5–61. doi: 10.1016/j.jalz.2013.02.003

Alzheimer's Association. (2014). Alzheimer's and dementia caregiver center: Stages/behaviors. Retrieved from: www.alz.org/care/alzheimers dementia-stages-behaviors.asp

Alzheimer's Association and National Alliance for Caregiving. (2004). *Families care: Alzheimer's caregiving in the United States.* Chicago, IL: Author.

Austrom, M. G., & Lu, Y. (2009). Long term caregiving: Helping families of persons with mild cognitive impairment cope. *Current Alzheimer Research*, 6, 392–398. doi: 10.2174/156720509788929291

Baxter, L. A., Braithwaite, D. O., Golish, T. D., & Olsen, L. N. (2002). Contradictions of interaction for wives of elderly husbands with adult dementia. *Journal of Applied Communication Research*, 30, 1–26. doi: 10.1080/00909880216576

Beach, S. R., Schulz, R., Yee, J. L., & Jackson, S. (2000). Negative and positive health effects of caring for a disabled spouse: Longitudinal findings from the Caregiver Health Effects Study. *Psychology and Aging*, 15, 259–271. doi: 10.1037//0882-7974.15.2.259

Caron, C. D., Griffith, J., & Arcand, M. (2005). End-of-life decision making in dementia: The perspective of family caregivers. *Dementia*, 4, 113–136. doi: 10.1177/1471301205049193

Carstensen, L. L., Gottman, J. M., & Levenson, R. W. (1995). Emotional behavior in long-term marriage. *Psychology and Aging*, 10, 140–149. doi: 10.1037/0882-7974.10.1.140

Czaja, S. J., & Rubert, M. P. (2002). Telecommunications as an aid to family caregivers of persons with dementia. *Psychosomatic Medicine*, 64, 469–476. doi: 10.1097/00006842-200205000-00011

Derksen, E., Vernooij-Dassen, M., Gillissen. F., Olde Rikkert, M., & Scheltens, P. (2006). Impact of diagnostic disclosure in dementia on patients and carers: Qualitative case series analysis. *Aging and Mental Health*, 10, 525–531. doi: 10.1080/13607860600638024

Dickson, F. C., & Walker, K. L. (2001). The expression of emotion in later-life married men. *Qualitative Research Reports in Communication*, 2, 66–71.

Evans, D., & Lee, E. (2014). Impact of dementia on marriage: A qualitative systematic review. *Dementia*, 13, 330–349. doi: 10.1177/1471301212473882

Federal Interagency Forum on Aging-Related Statistics. (2008). *Older Americans 2008: Key indicators of well-being*. Washington, DC: Author.

Garity, J. (2006). Caring for a family member with Alzheimer's disease: Coping with caregiver burden post-nursing home placement. *Journal of Gerontological Nursing*, 32, 39–48. PMID:16773862

Gaugler, J. E., Kane, R. L., & Kane, R. A. (2002). Family care for older adults with disabilities: Toward more targeted and interpretable research. *International Journal of Aging and Human Development*, 54, 205–231. doi: 10.2190/FACK-QE61-Y2J8-5L68

Georges, J., Jansen, S., Jackson, J., Meyrieux, A., Sadowska, A., & Selmes, M. (2008). Alzheimer's disease in real life—the dementia carer's story. *International Journal of Geriatric Psychiatry*, 23, 546–551. doi: 10.1002/gps.1984

Goodman, C. C. (1999). Intimacy and autonomy in long term marriage. *Journal of Gerontological Social Work*, 32, 83–97. doi: 10.1300/J083v32n01_06

Harmell, A. L., Chattillion, E. A., Roepke, S. K., & Mausbach, B. T. (2011). A review of the psychobiology of dementia caregiving: A focus on resilience factors. *Current Psychiatry Reports*, 13, 219–224. doi: 10.1007/s11920-011-0187-1

Harwood, J. (2007). *Understanding communication and aging: Developing knowledge and awareness*. Los Angeles, CA: SAGE.

Hebert, L. E., Weuve, J., Scherr, P. A., & Evans, D. A. (2013). Alzheimer's disease in the United States (2010–2050) estimated using the 2010 Census. *Neurology*, 80, 1778–1783. doi: 10.1212/WNL.0b013e31828726f5

Hellstrom, I., Nolan, M., & Lundh, U. (2005). "We do things together": A case study of couplehood in dementia. *Dementia*, 4, 7–22. doi: 10.1177/1471301205049188

Hellstrom, I., Nolan, M., & Lundh, U. (2007). Sustaining "couplehood": Spouses' strategies for living with dementia. *Dementia, 6,* 383–409. doi: 10.1177/1471301207081571

Kaplan, L. (2001). A couplehood typology for spouses of institutionalized persons with Alzheimer's disease: Perceptions of "We"-"I". *Family Relations, 50,* 87–98. doi: 10.1111/j.1741–3729.2001.00087.x

Kelly, A. E., Klusas, J. A., von Weiss, R. T., & Kenny, C. (2001). What is it about revealing secrets that is beneficial? *Personality and Social Psychology Bulletin, 27,* 651–665. doi: 10.1177/0146167201276002

Knobloch, L. K., & Carpenter-Theune, K. E. (2004). Topic avoidance in developing romantic relationships: Associations with intimacy and relational uncertainty. *Communication Research, 31,* 173–205. doi: 10.1177/0093650203261516

Knobloch, L. K., & Solomon, D. H. (2002). Intimacy and the magnitude and experience of episodic relational uncertainty within romantic relationships. *Personal Relationships, 9,* 457–478. doi: 10.1111/1475–6811.09406

Knobloch, L. K., & Solomon, D. H. (2005). Relational uncertainty and relational information processing: Questions without answers? *Communication Research, 32,* 349–388. doi: 10.1177/0093650205275384

Knobloch, L. K., & Theiss, J. A. (2010). An actor-partner interdependence model of relational turbulence: Cognitions and emotions. *Journal of Social and Personal Relationships, 27,* 595–619. doi: 10.1177/0265407510368967

Knobloch, L. K., & Theiss, J. A. (2011). Depressive symptoms and mechanisms of relational turbulence as predictors of relationship satisfaction among returning service members. *Journal of Family Psychology, 25,* 470–478. doi: 10.1037/a0024063

Ko, H., & Kuo, F. Y. (2009). Can blogging enhance subjective well-being through self-disclosure? *CyberPsychology & Behavior, 12,* 75–79. doi: 10.1089/cpb.2008.016

Leustek, J., & Theiss, J. A. (2018). Factors that shape cognitive and behavioral coping among individuals with type 2 diabetes: Features of illness versus features of romantic relationships. *Health Communication, 33,* 1549–1559. doi: 10.1080/10410236.2017.1384346

Liu, W., & Gallagher-Thompson, D. (2009). *Impact of dementia caregiving: Risks, strains, and growth.* In S. H. Qualls & S. H. Zarit (Eds.), *Aging families and caregiving* (pp. 85–112). Hoboken, NJ: John Wiley & Sons.

Metlife Mature Marketing Institute. (2006). *The MetLife study of Alzheimer's disease: The caregiving experience.* Westport, CT: Author.

Nagy, M. E., & Theiss, J. A. (2013). Applying the relational turbulence model to the empty-nest transition: Sources of relationship change, relational uncertainty, and interference from partners. *Journal of Family Communication, 13,* 280–300. doi: 10.1080/15267431.2013.823430

National Institute on Aging. (2012). Changes in intimacy and sexuality. Retrieved from: www.nia.nih.gov/alzheimers/intimacy-sexuality-and-alzheimers-disease-resourcelist

Pennebaker, J. W., Colder, M., & Sharp, L. K. (1990). Accelerating the coping process. *Journal of Personality and Social Psychology, 58,* 528–537. doi: 10.1037/0022–3514.58.3.528

Pennebaker, J. W., Kiecolt-Glaser, J. K., & Glaser, R. (1988). Disclosure of traumas and immune function: Health implications for psychotherapy. *Journal of Consulting and Clinical Psychology, 56,* 239–245. doi: 10.1037/0022-006X.56.2.239

Pennebaker, J. W., & O'Heeron, R. C. (1984). Confiding in others and illness rate among spouses of suicide and accidental death victims. *Journal of Abnormal Psychology, 93,* 473–476. doi: 10.1037/0021-843X.93.4.473

Rollins, D., Waterman, D., & Esmay, D. (1985). Married widowhood. *Activities, Adaptation, and Aging, 7,* 67–71. doi: 10.1300/J016v07n02_08

Sanders, S., & Power, J. (2009). Roles, responsibilities and relationships among older husbands caring for wives with progressive dementia and other chronic conditions. *Health and Social Work, 34,* 41–51. doi: 10.1093/hsw/34.1.41

Schulz, R., & Martire, L. M. (2004). Family caregiving of persons with dementia: Prevalence health effects, and support strategies. *American Journal of Geriatric Psychiatry, 12,* 240–249. doi: 10.1176/appi.ajgp.12.3.240

Smith, A. (2014). Older adults and technology use. Retrieved from: www.pewinternet .org/2014/04/03/older-adults-and-technology-use/

Solomon, D. H., & Knobloch, L. K. (2001). Relationship uncertainty, partner interference, and intimacy in dating relationships. *Journal of Social and Personal Relationships, 18,* 804–820. doi: 10.1177/0265407501186004

Solomon, D. H., & Knobloch, L. K. (2004). A model of relational turbulence: The role of intimacy, relational uncertainty, and interference from partners in appraisals of irritations. *Journal of Social and Personal Relationships, 21,* 795–816. doi: 10.1177/0265407504047838

Solomon, D. H., Knobloch, L. K., Theiss, J. A., & McLaren, R. M. (2016). Relational turbulence theory: Explaining variation in subjective experiences and communication within romantic relationships. *Human Communication Research, 42,* 507–532. doi: 10.1111/hcre.12091

Steuber, K. R., & Solomon, D. H. (2008). Relational uncertainty, partner interference, and infertility: A qualitative study of discourse in online forums. *Journal of Social and Personal Relationships, 25,* 831–855. doi: 10.1177/0265407508096698

Strauss, A., & Corbin, J. (1998). *Basics of qualitative research: Techniques and procedures for developing grounded theory* (2nd ed.). Thousand Oaks, CA: SAGE.

Theiss, J. A., Carpenter, A. M., & Leustek, J. (2016). Partner facilitation and partner interference in individuals' weight loss goals. *Qualitative Health Research, 26,* 1318–1330. doi: 10.1177/1049732315583980

Theiss, J. A., Estlein, R., & Weber, K. M. (2013). A longitudinal assessment of relationship characteristics that predict new parents' relationship satisfaction. *Personal Relationships, 20,* 216–235. doi: 10.1111/j.1475-6811.2012.01406.x

Theiss, J. A., Knobloch, L. K., Magsamen-Conrad, K., & Checton, M. (2009). Relationship characteristics associated with the experience of hurt in romantic relationships: A test of the relational turbulence model. *Human Communication Research, 35,* 588–615. doi: 10.1111/j.1468-2958.2009.01364.x

Theiss, J. A., & Solomon, D. H. (2006a). Coupling longitudinal data and hierarchical linear modeling to examine the antecedents and consequences of jealousy experiences in romantic relationships: A test of the relational turbulence model. *Human Communication Research, 32,* 469–503. doi: 10.1111/j.1468-2958.2006.00284.x

Theiss, J. A., & Solomon, D. H. (2006b). A relational turbulence model of communication about irritations in romantic relationships. *Communication Research, 33,* 391–418. doi: 10.1177/0093650206291482

Thurlow, C., Lengel, L., & Tomic, A. (2004). *Computer mediated communication: Social interaction and the Internet.* London: SAGE.

Vitaliano, P. P., Zhang, J., & Scanlan, J. M. (2003). Is caregiving hazardous to one's physical health? A meta-analysis. *Psychological Bulletin, 129,* 946–972. doi: 10.1037/0033-2909.129.6.946

Weber, K. M., & Solomon, D. H. (2008). Locating relationship and communication issues among stressors associated with breast cancer. *Health Communication, 23,* 548–559. doi: 10.1080/10410230802465233

Wuest, J., Ericson, P. K., & Stern, P. N. (1994). Becoming strangers: The changing family caregiving relationship in Alzheimer's disease. *Journal of Advanced Nursing, 20,* 437–443. doi: 10.1111/j.1365-2648.1994.tb02378.x

8

Communication as a Source of Misunderstanding and a Resource for Responding to the Stress of Parental Caregiving

TERESA KEELER

Studying communication exchanges between siblings in the context of elder care is necessary in today's aging society. In the United States, the number of adults aged 65 and older is expected to more than double over the next three decades (U.S. Census Bureau, 2010). The "oldest old," those 85 years old and older, are projected to be the fastest growing part of the senior population into the next century (U.S. Census Bureau, 2010). As the population ages, so does the need for personal assistance with everyday activities. The first line of assistance for aging individuals is often their immediate family, particularly their adult children. As such, the interactions of adult children are critical to preserving the health and well-being of the family (Kramer, Kavanaugh, Trentham-Dietz, Walsh, & Yonker, 2009; Lee, Netzer, & Coward, 1995; Lieberman & Fisher, 1999). Communication becomes both a resource for responding to a stressful event, as well as a source of misunderstanding and conflict around the event (Babrow, 1992).

All families experience conflict, the occurrence of which is neither good nor bad; rather, the response to conflict is what determines the long-term vitality and resilience of relationships (Sillars, Canary, & Tafoya, 2004). However, life events may occur that overwhelm family members. Caring for an aging parent may be a life transition that is seen as a normal event that occurs with the passage of time, or as a traumatic event that is unexpected or unwelcome and sends the family into crisis. Why some families manage this transition effectively and others do not has often been attributed to the characteristics, relationships, perceptions, and communication behaviors of its members (Boss, 2001; Hill, 1958; McCubbin & Patterson, 1985; Patterson, 1988).

This study set out to explore the communication behaviors of siblings to determine whether sibling communication is a help or a hindrance during elder care. Additionally, this study considered the type of communication enacted by the siblings and the level of care needed by the parents. To accomplish the goals of this research, interviews were conducted to explore the illness and relational uncertainties present during elder care. In addition, participants were asked to describe the information management behaviors that they exhibited with their siblings. The information management techniques of information sharing, topic avoidance, and secret keeping were used as proxies for communication responses to the stress of caregiving.

STRESSORS ASSOCIATED WITH ELDER CARE

The present research extended Gill and Morgan's (2011) work that illuminated the ways older adults make sense of the challenges of aging within the context of moving to a care-related facility, to how siblings confront uncertainty within the context of becoming a caregiver for an aging parent. As such, participants described their perceptions of uncertainties and communication behaviors related to their sibling relationship during elder care.

Communication about Caregiving

The roles and parts of the caregiving process are typically coordinated by a main care provider who directs the efforts of all subordinate caregivers. When one adult child has primary responsibility for caregiving, other siblings take secondary roles or completely remove themselves from caregiving (Merrill, 1996). Primary caregivers must then devise a number of strategies for involving siblings in care (Merrill, 1996). These include asking for respite care and occasional help, hinting that they could use help, demanding that their siblings help, attempting care for a period of time, or forgoing any further involvement. Caregivers stated that their challenge to involve others was greatest when the parent lived with the caregiver or when the caregiver volunteered for the role (Merrill, 1996).

When siblings attempt to negotiate among themselves about who will provide care for an aging parent and in what manner, conflict often arises (Connidis & Kemp, 2008). If the primary caregiver feels that there are inequalities in the division of labor among adult siblings, the caregiver may confront other siblings and ask them to contribute more (Ingersoll-Dayton, Neal, Ha, & Hammer, 2003) or avoid their siblings and change their perceptions of the situation. Children asked by their parents to be caregivers will have very different perceptions than those who volunteered or just "fell into" the position because no one else would provide care. Even if siblings find a way to equitably deal with their caregiving responsibilities, advance directives for health care that appoint one child as power of attorney, for example, may undermine sibling relationships (Khodyakov & Carr, 2009). For example, early patterns of cooperation may account for sharing responsibilities for parent care (Tonti, 1988), while the reactivation of early conflicts may account for conflicts that arise over parent care (Bedford, 1996). How siblings communicate with one another during adolescence is associated with the development and perception of relationships later in life (Rocca & Martin, 1998).

Families rarely have explicit discussions about end-of-life decisions, and little congruence exists between the caregiver's, the care recipient's, and other family members' perceptions of these issues (Pecchioni, 2001). Explicit discussions involve active problem solving through direct, conscious, and verbal agreements that require expressivity, self-disclosure, and proactive planning from participants. However, families tend to avoid open conflict and rely on silent arrangements in which decisions evolve without conscious, verbal discussions about the topic (Pecchioni, 2001). Problems arise when family members make caregiving decisions based on false assumptions that are not consistent with the care recipient's desires. With siblings, the matter is complicated because one sibling may have strong opinions about what should be done and others may have very different ideas, leading to difficulty as they attempt to integrate their ideas and make decisions.

Stress and Caregiving

An aging parent's need for assistance with daily activities raises many uncertainties and challenges in family relationships. For some siblings, this type of change is expected with the passage of time (Cowan, 1991) and may not prompt the same level of stress as an unexpected event, such as a fall requiring surgery and intense medical care. This type of event is more difficult to foresee because it seems to be somewhat random and does not occur in all families. Without any preparation, some siblings may be shocked by the sudden changes and experience heightened uncertainty about the event. Family stressors can also be classified along the dimensions of temporary versus permanent, or voluntary versus involuntary (Adams, 1975). The care needed after a fall may be only for a short period of time; however, the care needed for a parent developing Alzheimer's disease is for a much longer duration. The resulting uncertainty can produce varied individual reactions and alter the communication behaviors of family members (Segrin & Flora, 2005), especially between siblings.

In addition, family members sometimes willingly enter into situations that can be stressful. A son or daughter may feel an obligation to care for an aging parent and volunteer for the task. Segrin and Flora (2005) note that many individuals conclude that voluntary stressors are easier to cope with than those that are involuntary. However, voluntary stressors carry with them more personal responsibility as well as more uncertainty about the role of others. This can create considerable emotional distress within the family (Segrin & Flora, 2005). For example, one adult child might volunteer to care for a parent, expecting that siblings will help. If those expectations are not met, the caregiver is likely to be left with more uncertainty about the caregiving situation and his or her sibling relationships than might otherwise have occurred (e.g., why are my siblings not helping?; how will our relationship adapt to this situation?).

Defining the stressor. Older parents' need for assistance often results in complex role transitions that are challenging for family members to navigate (Gill & Morgan, 2011). These transitions may be further complicated if the assistance required is highly personal or time intensive. In this study, participants were asked to describe their parent's current health status and the caregiving tasks they and their sibling(s) enacted. The purpose of these questions was to gauge the participant's perceptions (including whether the caregiving situation was possible to manage successfully or overwhelming to the individual or family unit). Individuals exhibit different communication behaviors depending on whether caring for an aging parent is seen as a challenge or a threat (Babrow, Kasch, & Ford, 1998). Therefore, the definition of the stressor as manageable or burdensome may influence sibling interactions and perceptions of problematic integration.

RQ1: Does the type or level of care needed by a parent influence the perceived level of stress during caregiving?

PERCEPTIONS OF UNCERTAINTY

A seeming contradiction exists between notions that communication between people is (a) virtually automatic and effortless and carried out with only minimal forethought and planning, and (b) the product of considerable conscious deliberation and effort (see Berger, 1997; Kellerman, 1992; Langer, 1992; Reddy, 1979). This contradiction exists because even routine social encounters involving individuals who are well acquainted with each other can have the shared knowledge underlying their relationship disrupted (Berger, 1997). Individuals, their relationships, and the contexts in which they are interacting can all change. Dramatic events may be associated with even more striking changes, creating conditions of considerable uncertainty.

Uncertainty exists when "details of situations are ambiguous, complex, unpredictable, or probabilistic; when information is unavailable or inconsistent; and when people feel insecure in their own state of knowledge or the state of knowledge in general" (Brashers, 2001, p. 478). Uncertainty is primarily a perception about one's own knowledge and ability to derive meaning from that knowledge (Brashers, 2001). Therefore, lacking knowledge is different from one's perception about knowledge, and one individual's perception may be very different from another person's perception. Perceptions about uncertainty can be so different because there are numerous sources of uncertainty (Babrow, 1998, 2001; Berger, 1997), such as questions about the abilities, goals, and emotions of the parties involved. The communication exchanges between siblings associated with an aging parent's injury or illness are filled with emotion and turmoil, and the complexities of caregiving and its numerous possibilities and outcomes create highly uncertain scenarios. A lens for examining the various facets of uncertainty is the problematic integration theory (Babrow, 1992, 1998).

Problematic Integration Theory

Whereas uncertainty reduction theory (Berger & Calabrese, 1975) proposes that humans strive to reduce uncertainty, problematic integration theory (Babrow, 1992, 2001) proposes that alternative responses to uncertainty include avoiding information or altering probabilistic or evaluative assessments (Dennis, Kunkel, & Keyton, 2008). These alternative responses may be considered because reducing uncertainty is not always possible (Brashers, 2001) or desirable and, even if it is, reducing uncertainty on one issue may give rise to a cascading sequence of other uncertainties about other issues (Babrow & Kline, 2000). Alternatively, some individuals may even seek to sustain or create additional uncertainty (Babrow, 1995; Lazarus, 1983).

Problematic integration theory (Babrow, 1992) considers the relationship between expectations and desires (Dennis et al., 2008) and presumes that humans need both probabilistic (will it happen?) and evaluative (will it be good?) understandings of their world. Babrow (1992) notes how humans must ultimately integrate these two orientations, a process involving the shared effects and the linking of each "to broader complexes of knowledge, feelings, and behavioral intentions" (p. 96). As a result, this integration often becomes problematic as behavioral intentions may muddy an individual's understanding of a given event or situation. Siblings' orientations and intentions may become more difficult to understand and communicate within the complex context of caregiving. This difficulty may leave siblings to employ counterproductive communication behaviors.

Identifying the problem. According to Babrow et al. (1998), variations in the meanings of uncertainty mandate different courses of action by an individual and different responses from those around him or her. For example, uncertainty due to personal ignorance or lack of knowledge may require an individual to search for additional information. Uncertainty due to protective avoidance may need a greater understanding of one's motivations (Babrow et al., 1998). Even if a sibling understands another's uncertainties, that person may fail to understand the form or the source of the uncertainty and compromise well-intentioned efforts (Babrow et al., 1998). Or, put another way, even if one sibling finds a meaning behind another sibling's uncertainty, that may not match the sibling's understanding and may mean that the siblings cannot agree on a mutual course of action. Communication about serious illness or approaching death may necessitate the need to talk with others who may misjudge the uncertainties that another finds of most concern (Babrow et al., 1998). Therefore, caregivers must consider the possible meaning behind the challenges with their siblings.

RQ2: How do participants perceive the challenges and uncertainties associated with a sibling relationship during elder care?

INFORMATION MANAGEMENT STRATEGIES

While caring for aging parents, some of the common communication behaviors that may be employed are the information management strategies of topic avoidance, secret keeping, or information sharing. An additional aspect to be investigated in this study is how siblings manage the information associated with caregiving decisions relative to perceptions of ambiguity, ambivalence, and divergence. When discussing an issue openly, such as the need for additional help with caregiving, siblings take the risk of displaying some weakness, revealing hidden information, or challenging their relationship. During the discussion, siblings may recognize that they are at risk of personal or financial loss (Roloff, 1976) or that their relationship is at risk (Greene, 2009). Siblings may decide to use the potentially antisocial communication strategy of keeping information about themselves or their position hidden in order to manage the situation. Information sharing, topic avoidance, and secret keeping provide ways by which individuals can manage privacy in relationships (Guerrero & Afifi, 1995a) and the stress of caregiving.

INFORMATION SHARING

Information sharing may involve self-disclosure, relational disclosure, or informational disclosure. Greene, Derlega, and Mathews (2006) define self-disclosure as "an interaction between at least two individuals where one intends to deliberately divulge something personal to another" (p. 411). Even though self-disclosure is usually studied in terms of verbal messages, nonverbal messages may also be examples of self-disclosure if the goal is to reveal something personal (Greene et al., 2006). An abundance of communication research has focused on high-stress, potentially stigmatizing disclosures, most notably HIV infection (e.g., Derlega, Metts, Petronio, & Margulis, 1993; Greene, Carpenter, Catona, & Magsamen-Conrad, 2013), but also heart conditions (e.g., Checton & Greene, 2012), cancer (e.g., Venetis et al., 2012), and infertility (Steuber & Solomon, 2011). This research has concentrated on how significant life events, such as medical diagnoses or family-planning information, affected patients' revealing or concealing private information about such events (Durham, 2008).

Greene et al. (2006) distinguish between personal self-disclosure (disclosure about oneself) and relational self-disclosure (disclosure about a relationship with another person). Both personal and relational disclosures may simultaneously be occurring in sibling relationships. During caregiving, one sibling may disclose to another sibling, "I am worried about Mom being home alone," or may share, "I am behind at work from taking Dad to so many doctor appointments." These are examples of personal disclosures. At the same time, one sibling may reveal to another during caregiving, "You never help me. You only think of yourself," or "We have to find a way to pay for more care for dad." These relational disclosures are a negative relational statement and filled with considerable risk to their future affiliation. Both forms of disclosure have consequences for the development and maintenance of personal relationships (Derlega, Winstead, Wong, & Greenspan, 1987; Greene et al., 2006; Petronio, 2002). However, owing to the high level of risk to the relationship, a relational disclosure may require considerably more deliberation than one about a parent's health.

TOPIC AVOIDANCE

One means of limiting damage to relationships is to restrict the expression of dissimilarity or, rather, avoid communicating about issues of disagreement. Roloff and Ifert (1998) argue that romantic partners should not be assumed to have identical interests, and siblings also do not necessarily share identical interests. Adult siblings may have different interests, priorities, and viewpoints as a result of different life experiences, and so develop ways of interaction that avoid conflict and overt rivalry (Cicirelli, 1991). Individuals may choose to avoid conflict by withholding their complaints about another, by suppressing arguments or preventing elaborate discussions, and/or by negotiating an agreement to stop talking about the source of conflict (Roloff & Ifert, 2000). However, a family crisis may require communication about these once avoided topics, such as a sibling's lack of responsibility or a spouse's interference in family affairs. Early rivalries and aggression between siblings may be reactivated in later adulthood at times of crisis or stress, leading to conflicts and aggressive actions with siblings (Cicirelli, 1991).

Avoiding topics with family members is different from knowingly keeping information from family members. During caregiving, certain adult children may develop alliances with their parents to withhold information from their siblings, or siblings may form coalitions with one another to keep information from their parents or other siblings. Family secrets require greater levels of negotiation than "taboo topics" over who owns the information, who gets to share that information, and what level of information they get to share.

SECRET KEEPING

Secrets are distinct from more general private or nondisclosed information. Secrets are composed of information that is purposefully hidden, typically viewed as negative (Vangelisti, 1994), and usually involve the secret keeper (Kelly & McKillop, 1996). In addition, secrets are held within a social context, and secret keepers may believe that other people may have some claim to the hidden information (Kelly, 2002). For example, people's daily bathing rituals are considered to be private but not secret because people agree that these practices are not for public display. However, hiding a dangerous contagious disease from a sexual partner is considered a "secret" because the partner may perceive a right to know this information in such a case (Derlega & Chaikin, 1977; Kelly, 2002). The difficulty in a family setting may lie in knowing how different family members categorize information, for example, as private, secret, or "open."

Keeping information secret can serve beneficial and even necessary functions for interpersonal relationships (e.g., Petronio, 1991). For example, keeping a secret can protect the other person emotionally, maintain the other person's respect, and preserve a level of relational satisfaction that may not exist once the information is revealed (Derlega et al., 1987; Derlega, Winstead, Mathews, & Braitman, 2008). Family secrets can maintain illusions about family relationships by managing from whom a secret is withheld (e.g., some family members, all family members), which secret is withheld (e.g., relationship status, health diagnosis), or why a secret is withheld (Vangelisti, 1994).

Choosing the strategy. The integration of uncertainty becomes more difficult when there is decreasing clarity about the probability of an event occurring or increasing conflict regarding expectations (Bradac, 2001). These difficulties may manifest in the information management behaviors of information sharing, topic avoidance, and secret keeping. When discussing an issue openly, siblings take the risk of displaying some weakness, revealing a secret, or challenging their relationship. Avoiding topics and keeping information secret provide ways by which individuals can maintain privacy in relationships (Guerrero & Afifi, 1995a) and protect against personal risk. Therefore, this study investigates whether an individual will avoid or keep secret information when that individual does not know how a sibling will respond to information or feels that the sibling will respond negatively.

RQ3: To what extent do siblings enact the information management behaviors of topic avoidance or secret keeping when interacting with their siblings during the caregiving process?

METHOD

A purposive sample of adults who had recently negotiated care for an aging parent with their sibling(s) was solicited from the national and local chapters of various professional and networking organizations, such as the National Communication Association, the National Council on Family Relations, and the National Association of Women Business Owners, with whom the researcher was affiliated. Additional participants were recruited via the researcher's personal and professional contacts (including senior housing executives, social work professionals, and home health care organizations in New Jersey), as well as through social media accounts and email listservs. There were multiple criteria for inclusion in the study. Consistent with Merrill (1996) and Checkovich and Stern (2001), participants included adults older than the age of 35, with up to three living siblings, and at least one unmarried parent (i.e., divorced, widowed, or never married) to whom the participant or a sibling had provided direct assistance (versus advice or information). The number of siblings a participant may have was limited to three in this study in order to limit variation in family size for this initial exploration. Provision of direct assistance was identified as activities of daily living (Fillenbaum, 1987), health care decisions, financial matters, or living arrangements within the past 12 months. For this study, the aging parent needed to be receiving assistance solely from his or her adult children (and not a spouse, niece, nephew, sibling, or other extended family member). At least one sibling had to provide assistance (virtually or face-to-face) to the aging parent no less than once per month during the previous year.

Sample

Participants included 22 adults (21 females and one male) from across the United States, but primarily in the Northeast region. Ages ranged from 38 to 72 years, with a mean of 56.7 years ($SD = 9.19$). Nearly all participants were caring for one unmarried parent; however, one participant was involved in the care of two aging parents, another participant was caring for an unmarried parent living with a partner, and a third was caring for a parent but not involved in the care of the parent's spouse. The ages of the parents receiving care ranged from 77 to 97 ($M = 88.5$, $SD = 5.92$). Five participants lived with the parent (either in their or their parent's home), eight participants were within an hour drive of the parent, and nine participants were at a farther distance from the parent. Those participants living with or geographically close to the parent tended to be the primary caregiver.

One participant reported a race of African American; all other participants reported Caucasian (n = 21). More than half of the participants identified as Christian (n = 12), while the others identified as Jewish (n = 5), Unitarian (n = 2), or no specific religious affiliation (n = 3). More than half of the participants reported being married (n = 13); others were single (n = 5), divorced (n = 3), or widowed (n = 1). Participants reported between zero and three children (M = 1.41, SD = 1.05). The mean age of those children was 27.70, with a range from 5 to 41 years old (SD = 14.20). All participants reported being college educated, and 15 reported earning graduate degrees. The mean participant annual income was more than \$75,000, with a range from \$20,000 to \$150,000 (three participants declined to report income).

Procedure

Data collection occurred either face-to-face (n = 3) or via phone (n = 19). The face-to-face meetings took place at a public location convenient for the participant (e.g., his or her office or a restaurant). At the outset of the meeting, participants were given a consent form with an audiotape addendum to review and sign. If a potential participant lived at a distance, interviews took place via phone and the consent forms were emailed in advance of the call. All interviews were conducted by the same interviewer (a Caucasian woman age 40–45) and were audio-recorded. No patterns of difference were noted between the face-to-face and the phone interviews, and thus they were combined for analysis.

Individuals were first asked to provide answers to general demographic questions. Following completion of the demographic section, each participant was then asked about caring for the aging parent. Following Matthews and Rosner's (1988) loosely structured format, participants were asked to respond to a series of questions describing the current health or living situation of their parent, caregiving roles and tasks being completed by them and their sibling(s), and the resources available to cope with this transition. In addition, participants were asked to describe any uncertainties they had about the parent's illness or injury, possible care alternatives for the parent, or their expectations for relating with their sibling(s). Finally, participants were asked to describe the information management tactics displayed by them or their sibling(s); for example, did they share information, avoid certain topics, or keep pieces of information secret?

Analyses

The interview data were initially transcribed by an undergraduate research assistant who was blind to study hypotheses and research questions. A second undergraduate research assistant read the interview transcript to verify that all aspects of the interview had been captured completely and accurately. A total of four trained and Institutional Review Board-certified undergraduate research assistants were randomly assigned the initial transcriptions and the second reads of the interviews. The researcher conducted final reads of the transcripts, formatted the transcripts, and removed references to any names or places in order to de-identify the transcripts. A total of 847 minutes of audio-recordings were transcribed (M = 40.34 minutes, SD = 13.85 per interview, ranging from 14.34 to 63.03 minutes), resulting in 256 pages of interview text (M = 12 pages, SD = 2.77 per interview, ranging from 7 to 19 pages).

Each transcript was coded using an abductive technique (Miles & Huberman, 1994). This approach calls for starting with concepts from the existing literature and then adding any ideas that emerge from the data in an effort to extend a conceptual framework. Abductive coding was used because problematic integration theory has been previously explored in other health contexts (i.e., Babrow & Kline, 2000; Hines, 2001; Matthias, 2009), but not within the framework of elder care. Similarly, the information management behaviors of topic avoidance, secret keeping, and information sharing have been well documented in social relationships (i.e., Afifi & Guerrero, 1998; Caughlin & Vangelisti, 2009; Greene et al., 2013; Petronio, 2002) and family relationships (i.e., Checton & Greene, 2012; Guerrero & Afifi, 1995a, 1995b; Vangelisti, 1994); however, researchers have yet to explore the narrower context of adult sibling communication behaviors.

RESULTS

Stressors Experienced by Adult Children

RQ1 asked whether the type or level of care needed by a parent influences the perceived level of stress during caregiving. The responses from participants suggested that the type of illness does influence the perceived level of stress. This is because different illnesses require different types of care. Chronic illnesses more often require assistance with instrumental activities of daily living (IADLs) such as transportation, shopping, medication management, or maintaining a home. Cognitive illness, however, more often require assistance with activities of daily living (ADLs), such as feeding, bathing, dressing, and toileting. When these more personal, physically intensive tasks are combined with the behavior changes associated with advanced stages of dementia, stress levels often rise for the caregiver.

For some adult children, the stress associated with caregiving came from the responsibility they placed on themselves for ensuring their parent's well-being. As one female participant stated, "I was calling her every day and I was, you know, I was starting to get a little over the edge, stressed out and I needed to have this check in with her." This participant was stressed from the amount of time she spent monitoring her mother's daily activities and fulfilling her mother's personal and medical needs. Other caregivers were stressed about the amount of money needed to ensure quality care living arrangements for their parents. "There's always stress about whether or not I'll [work] enough ... for the month to be able to um cover her expenses in uh this type of independent living situation because it's quite pricey." For this participant, financial stresses were affecting her own health and well-being. She complained of being tired all the time, because she was constantly working in an effort to pay for her mother's housing.

Many caregivers found the changes in behavior caused by Alzheimer's disease to be the most challenging and distressing effect of the illness, consistent with findings from the Alzheimer's Association (ALZ, 2014). A 65-year-old female summed up the challenge of caring for someone with a cognitive illness: "My father's dementia has been difficult for all of us." Part of this difficulty is the intense hands-on, physical activities required of caregivers: "My mother deteriorated enough that her personal hygiene could not be taken care of by herself." The caregiving situation becomes even more stressful when siblings do not comprehend the behaviors associated with the disease. For example, a 43-year-old female lamented her brother's lack of understanding and what it meant for her: "My mother's personality and the dementia have just compounded [everything]; so that's a lot of stress here for me. My brother just has no idea, because he doesn't live with it on a day to day basis, he deals with it for an hour and then leaves." This participant's mother lived with her and she worried that her brother did not know "the stress of living with this and that it's only going to get worse."

Although caring for someone with dementia requires considerable assistance with physical activities, it also necessitates a considerable emotional shift to "meet the parent where he or she is." Those adult children who could adjust their thinking about how to interact with their parent felt less frustrated with the caregiving process. A 45-year-old female and her sister decided to do creative activities with their ailing mother: "We like doing some collaging ... and just sitting sometimes with my mom and saying let's make some backgrounds ... just kind of painting loosely with watercolors ... she can actually manage to focus on it for sometimes as long as an hour which is a really long time for her."

However, another participant and her brother were having difficulties because her brother wanted to communicate with his mother as he had in the past: "He has a very hard time talking to her, cause every time he calls, he cannot understand what she's saying ... she jumps from one thing to another." The stressor was greater in this situation because one sibling could accept the cognitive change in the parent, but the other sibling could not. Stress and perceptions of uncertainty were often closely aligned.

Perceptions of Uncertainty

RQ2 asked how siblings perceive the challenges and uncertainties associated with their parent's needs during elder care. Participant uncertainty centered on two key areas: uncertainty about the parent and uncertainty about the self. Each of these areas included specific concerns related to mental and physical health, housing, and finances. Uncertainty about self included an additional concern about levels of personal knowledge and information, the one result reflecting the traditional literature on uncertainty reduction (Berger & Calabrese, 1975). Consistent with other health communication studies, uncertainty played a prominent role during the caregiving situation (e.g., Babrow, 2007; Checton & Greene, 2012; Dennis et al., 2008; Matthias, 2009).

Uncertainty about the parent. The uncertainties highlighted by participants generally surrounded questions about the parent's mental or physical health (e.g., will the symptoms worsen?; how will we continue to provide care?). As one participant noted, "What I was mostly concerned about was the early stages of dementia and my mom not remembering, just not remembering certain things or how to do simple things like how to work the CD player, just turning the heat up and down, or . . . how to work the toaster oven." Another participant commented, "I am worried about my mom's physical health. We worry that she's gonna trip and fall, break her hip, the classic thing that would happen to an older person."

Uncertainty also surrounded the parent's housing and finances (e.g., where will our parent have to move?; when will he or she have to move?; will she or he have enough money for the care he or she needs?). One participant was really at a loss for what was coming next. "What are we going to do? Where is she going to live? She won't be able to stay here forever. [We] will have to get her into some kind of assisted living. I don't really know what that entails." Others knew what was coming, but did not know how to tell their parents. A female caregiver commented, "At some point there could be a conflict between our desire to get [our mother] into a place we feel might be more helpful and [the] desire to keep her in the home for a longer period of time." However, regardless of the changes coming as a result of the age or health of the parent, money was always a concern. A female caregiver summed up the feelings of many participants when she said, "The only concern I had was whether mom's money would last to the end of her life."

Uncertainty about self. Participants also experienced uncertainty about their own mental and physical health, their own housing and financial matters, and their own knowledge. "I'm always afraid I won't be able to handle whatever comes next. I mean physically I just won't be able to handle it." Other participants felt uncertain about their plans for the future because of the responsibilities of caregiving: "At some point, I would like to be able to move. I would only live here if there's gonna be [further] decline." Another female participant also noted how she and her family put their house search on hold: "When we were looking at houses, I just kind of stopped and said I don't see the point. If we sell [my mother's] house, it makes sense for her to move in with us. But nobody wants to have that discussion." Finally, caregivers commented on uncertainty they experienced about their parent's medical issues: "I've tried to understand what's going on medically and just sort of know a lot of Google sites. But there's really no way to know." These results highlight what a difficult time individuals have defining the problematic areas of caregiving. For some, the problems center on their parents, for others the problems concern themselves, and for still others the problems involve their siblings' actions or their siblings' response to the parent's problems. Having a situation filled with such a multitude of problems leaves little room to clearly discuss a parent's care.

Communicative Behaviors between Siblings

RQ3 explored the information management behaviors that siblings enact in the course of providing elder care for a parent. The results of the study described how siblings employed various communication strategies to manage the flow of information about the caregiving situation and about their relationship with sibling(s) and others in the family. Most participants chose to avoid conflict with the sibling in an attempt not to "make things worse" for themselves or their parent. This avoidance occurred either directly, by limiting contact and/or communication with a sibling, or indirectly, by avoiding conversation about particular issues or by holding back personal feelings. A smaller number of participants chose to keep secrets from their sibling(s) or others within the family.

Avoidance. Seventeen participants reported using primarily one of three strategies to avoid conflict with their sibling(s): curtailing interaction, restricting topics, and suppressing thoughts. The results of this study revealed a tendency by participants to avoid what one participant labeled "poking the bear": "there are things I just avoid with him, like politics; we have different views on that." Years of previous interactions with their siblings provided participants a sense of certainty about how their siblings would react to particular topics or behave in specific situations.

Curtailing interaction. *Curtailing interaction* was choosing to limit face-to-face contact and other means of communication (including phone calls, emails, or text messages) with their siblings. As one participant stated, "I don't really interact with him a lot to be honest with you, because he's very combative. I just don't need to deal with it, so honestly I try to interact with him as little as possible." This participant felt that she needed to limit interaction to save her energy for caregiving. Other participants chose to curtail interaction in an effort to more broadly define personal relationships: "I just look at [brother] as someone I don't get along with, who I don't agree with most of the time and that's someone I don't wanna [associate] with."

Restricting topics. Another way that participants set out to control conversations with a sibling and to focus on the parent was by restricting topics open for discussion. This strategy was employed when participants had a strong sense of how their siblings would react to certain issues such as property, "[The cottage] is an elephant in the room for sure and a lot of it also has to do with my mother creating a lot of emotional upset around it"; sibling addiction, "[My sister] went to [Alcoholics Anonymous] and has stopped drinking. I don't think she has had a drink in 20 years. We sure couldn't talk about that for a long time"; or personal successes, "I never discuss anything that's happening to our house in terms of how [son] is excelling. I know that will not be received well."

Even more interesting were the participants who restricted talking about the gender issues often associated with caregiving. One female, who was the youngest of the siblings, talked about how expectations around family roles were creating conflict: "Maybe the whole tension that we had was that I saw them as being male and older and that they should step in. And maybe they saw it as me being the female of the family and that I should be stepping into a certain role."

Another female participant wanted her brother to understand that "just because I'm a single woman does not mean I'm gonna go down [and] take care of my mother," but knew that discussing the topic would strain their relationship even further.

Suppressing thoughts. The third type of avoidance strategy enacted was to suppress thoughts. Participants most often concealed thoughts and feelings about siblings' caregiving efforts following a process of calculating the risks in a situation. "I might feel a little disappointed in my brother or my sister in terms of what they're doing. I'll say some things, but I won't say that much and I won't say it that clearly." Although one participant was frustrated with her brother's caregiving efforts, she knew she could not raise the topic, "Every time we go down that road, it takes a bad turn."

A number of participants told of situations in which they held back personal feelings about others in family because they knew voicing such opinions would cause conflict. One participant suppressed thoughts about her sibling: "Oh, I keep my mouth shut when my mother starts talking how wonderful her other daughter is, how perfect and how hardworking. I just sit there and you know don't say a word." Other participants suppressed thoughts about their siblings' spouses. One commented, "I would never say to [brother], 'Gee your first wife was actually one of the nastiest people I've ever met and don't you see that your second wife is doing something similar.'"

Another participant evoked a strategy of never talking about her sister's spouse: "We don't talk about him, we only talk about her." Another participant still talked to her brother-in-law, even though she was angry with him: "I do feel some strain with my brother in law, I'm still a little angry maybe at the way he treated [mother]. But I've never said that to him." Other participants took suppressing thoughts a step further into secret keeping.

Secret keeping. Secret keeping involves actively hiding private information from others (Kelly, 1999, 2002). Secrecy has also been related to self-concealment (a personality trait) and active inhibition of disclosure (Kelly, 1999, 2002). In this study, some family members chose to hide particular pieces of information from one another. Results showed that some participants kept secrets from their parent(s): "My mother is really nervous about money, I mean really nervous about money. I decided that I'm hiring someone to come in that my mother knows already and telling her that the county is paying for it." Other participants kept secrets from their sibling(s), "I don't tell him she has these episodes that all of a sudden people are saying they are mild seizures," and their extended family, "We're probably gonna move in about a year and a half, two years ... I don't wanna worry anybody." But parents and siblings often jointly kept secrets from the larger family as well. In one instance, parents began contemplating a move without telling the larger family: "[My mother] got frightened thinking that my father had died when he'd gone to sleep one afternoon ... they started planning [a move] without even including us." In some instances, these secrets were kept to protect oneself, but in other instances information was kept secret to protect others in the family. Regardless of the reason, the outcome was usually the same: family members expressed hurt or anger once the information was discovered.

DISCUSSION

The results of this study support Babrow's (1992) contention that uncertainty is a broad construct comprising multiple, overlapping concepts. Each concept poses different levels of information needs and different responses from individuals (Babrow, 1992; Babrow et al., 1998; Mishel, 1988). Even as participants were uncertain about their parents' changing caregiving needs, they were also uncertain as to what the future would hold for themselves and the relationship with their sibling(s). This study extends the claim that there are "many meanings of uncertainty" (Babrow et al., 1998). An event or situation may be interpreted in many different ways. Although individuals may be able to "put words" to their perceptions of their parent's health condition, the results of this study revealed that they might not want to put words to their expectations or opinions of their siblings.

A great difficulty for many participants was how their opinions of the responsibilities associated with caregiving and their expectations of family involvement were so different from those of their siblings. "This isn't what families are supposed to be like," was a frequent sentiment expressed by participants. The participants wanted their siblings to take a direct role caring for the parent, or the participants wanted the siblings to offer verbal support or gratitude for the care the participants were providing. For unknown reasons, however, participants did not know or did not agree with the reasons siblings gave for not doing what was expected. As a result, participants and siblings struggled to share information and communicate effectively while co-managing their parent's care.

Participants reported using a number of communication behaviors and information management strategies to manage the interpersonal exchanges with their siblings during caregiving. The avoidance strategies of curtailing interaction, restricting topics, and suppressing thoughts were most often used, but the strategy of secret keeping was also utilized. Although avoidance strategies were used to prevent conflict-inducing topics from being reintro-duced within the family, the secret keeping strategy was more often used to protect the participant from disapproval about his or her caregiving methods. These results aligned with those of prior research on topic avoidance (e.g., Guerrero & Afifi, 1995a, 1995b) and secret keeping (Kelly, 1999), which suggest that individuals manage information to protect themselves from criticism. Reducing personal attacks was one way of reducing the stress associated with caregiving.

Implications for Practice

The results of this study have numerous implications for those serving the aging population, including health and communication educators, health care and aging professionals, and family and family service providers. Understanding components of the underlying tensions and how those ten-sions translate into specific communication behaviors is difficult. Even more challenging is how to design interventions that neutralize years of family dynamics. During elder care, differences in perception may depend on the ways that family members construct uncertainty and "problems" around caregiving and family relationships.

Health and aging professionals. One important result from this research is the confirmation that different players in the caregiving process bring different perspectives to the situation. These different perspectives come from various frames of reference and result in various opinions about caregiving. For example, one sibling may be focused on the logistics of caring for the parent (i.e., getting the parent to appointments); another may be focused on the financial cost of fulfilling the care needs of the parent, all while the health care provider is focused on the medical diagnosis of the parent. These multiple points of focus result in many areas in which the family members and the professional staff may experience problematic integration. Those in the caregiving process may be unable or unwilling to acknowledge that others have alternative viewpoints, thereby heightening interpersonal tensions.

Reminding caregivers and service providers of potential differences is a step forward in reducing tensions and caregiving burden and enhancing positive communication behaviors. An ultimate goal of this line of research is to preserve the family as a critical "unit of care" for the aging adult. This research provides support for developing dyadic interventions that help siblings manage relational issues, caregiving burdens, and problematic integrations. These interventions could be between the provider and the cooperative sibling, or the provider and the uncooperative sibling.

Limitations

A number of limitations are present in this study. These include the sample (demographics and the sample size), the structure (the single versus dyadic perceptions and the cross-sectional nature of the studies), and the operationalization of a complex process. By recruiting participants from the national and local chapters of various professional organizations, the respondents were primarily Caucasian women with college and professional degrees. This group of respondents may not experience the same challenges with their siblings during the caregiving process as do other groups. In addition, the sample was biased toward those siblings with more productive relationships (i.e., those more willing to discuss the state of their family relationships.) This study included 22 participants, which is consistent with the sample size of many qualitative studies. Although qualitative analysis did reach saturation in this study, a more diverse group of participants may yield additional insights into the caregiving topics explored. Finally, a dyadic study would have allowed the opportunity to examine if sibling perceptions regarding the problematic aspects of caregiving aligned or diverged, and whether communication behaviors were consistent across sibling groups.

Future Directions

The results of this study suggested that participants whose parents were suffering a chronic illness were at different places in terms of perceptions of caregiving burden and problematic integration than participants whose parents were suffering a cognitive illness such as Alzheimer's disease. Future research should further test the differences in caregiving burden and problematic integration among family caregivers whose loved one is suffering a chronic versus cognitive illness. With the rapid increase in diagnoses of Alzheimer's disease and other forms of dementia, health professionals need additional information to support families in this caregiving situation. To date, education and support are focused on the individual caregiver, such as Understanding Dementia, Legal and Financial Planning for Persons with Dementia (ALZ.org/NYC). Research should further investigate the relational dimensions of dementia caregiving as a means for supporting the primary caregiver, as well as the family unit as a whole. In general, the severity and types of illness and disease progression would be important to further understand in relation to caregiving burden, information management, and problematic integration.

Regardless of the parent's health, a sibling's decision to assist with caregiving tasks may be viewed as a provision of social support, an interaction that provides assistance (Hobfoll, 1988). An avenue for future research is exploring the association between social support (Burleson, Albrecht, Goldsmith, & Sarason, 1994; Campbell, Marsden, & Hurlbert, 1986; Haines, Hurlbert, & Beggs, 1996; House, 1981; Walker, Wasserman, & Wellman, 1993; Wellman, 1992), caregiving burden, and problematic integration. Another aspect of caregiving burden to explore in the future is feelings of caregiving burden and ambiguity of the primary family caregiver versus the ancillary family caregiver(s). There were frequent comments from primary caregivers in Study 1 alluding to the thought that "my sibling does not understand." However, the study did not explore whether this misunderstanding was related to differences in communication behaviors or differences in caregiving perceptions. A dyadic study of caregiving burden could address this question.

Additional revelations in family research could come from following adult sibling caregivers over time. A longitudinal study would align with Babrow's arguments that perceptions of problems (i.e., problematic integration) change continuously. A cross-sectional study only captures one point in time and misses the chaining (how one event influences perceptions of the next, and the next, etc.) that occurs. Feelings of caregiving burden, perceptions of sibling relational quality, perceptions of problematic integration, and information management behaviors could be very different at the start of caregiving versus the height of caregiving versus soon after caregiving has ended or even later.

SUMMARY

Family and psychology scholars describe the sibling relationship as one of the most important interpersonal relationships, for it is a lifelong affiliation that spans other well-documented relationships such as those of parents, friends, and married couples (Cicirelli, 1995). Most research on siblings, however, has focused on their interactions during childhood or adolescence. Less is known about the communication exchanges of siblings in middle to late adulthood. This research increases understanding of the communication strategies utilized by adult siblings as they manage the complexities of caring for an aging parent while negotiating their adult sibling relationships. Communication acted as a resource to the caregiver, as it allowed the caregiver to manage information exchange and interaction levels with siblings in order to manage the caregiver's overall stress levels.

REFERENCES

Adams, B. N. (1975). *The family: A sociological interpretation* (2nd ed.). Chicago, IL: Rand McNally.

Afifi, W. A., & Guerrero, L. K. (1998). Some things are better left unsaid II: Topic avoidance in friendships. *Communication Quarterly, 46,* 231–249. doi: 10.1080/01463379809370099

Alzheimer's Association. (2014). Alzheimer's disease facts and figures. *Alzheimer's & Dementia, 10,* 1–80. Retrieved from: www.alz.org/downloads/Facts_Figures_2014.pdf

Babrow, A. S. (1992). Communication and problematic integration: Understanding diverging probability and value, ambiguity, ambivalence, and impossibility. *Communication Theory, 2,* 95–130. doi: 10.1111/j.1468-2885.1992.tb00031.x

Babrow, A. S. (1995). Communication and problematic integration: Milan Kundera's "lost letters" in *The book of laughter and forgetting. Communication Monographs, 62,* 283–300. doi: 10.1080/03637759509376364.

Babrow, A. S. (1998). Colloquy: Developing multiple process theories of communication. *Human Communication Research, 25,* 152–155. doi: 10.1111/j.1468-2958.1998.tb00440.x

Babrow, A. S. (2001). Uncertainty, value, communication, and problematic integration. *Journal of Communication, 51,* 553–573. doi: 10.1111/j.1460-2466.2001.tb02896.x

Babrow, A. S. (2007). Problematic integration theory. In B. B. Whaley & W. Samter (Eds.), *Explaining communication: Contemporary theories and exemplars* (pp. 181–200). Mahwah, NJ: Lawrence Erlbaum Associates.

Babrow, A. S., Kasch, C. R., & Ford, L. A. (1998). The many meanings of "uncertainty" in illness: Toward a systematic accounting. *Health Communication, 10,* 1–24. doi: 10.1207/s15327027hc1001_1

Babrow, A. S., & Kline, K. N. (2000). From "reducing" to "coping with" uncertainty: Reconceptualizing the central challenge in breast self-exams. *Social Science & Medicine, 51,* 1805–1816. doi: 10.1016/S0277-9536(00)00112-X

Bedford, V. H. (1996). Sibling relationships in middle and old age. In V. H. Bedford & R. Blieszner (Eds.), *Aging and the family: Theory and research* (pp. 201–222). Westport, CT: Praeger Publishers.

Berger, C. R. (1997). Producing messages under uncertainty. In J. Greene (Ed.), *Message production: Advances in communication theory* (pp. 221–244). Mahwah, NJ: Lawrence Erlbaum Associates.

Berger, C. R., & Calabrese, R. (1975). Some explorations in initial interaction and beyond: Toward a developmental theory of interpersonal communication. *Human Communication Research, 1*, 99–112. doi: 10.1111/j.1468-2958.1975.tb00258.x

Boss, P. (2001). *Family stress management: A contextual approach* (2nd ed.). Thousand Oaks, CA: SAGE.

Bradac, J. J. (2001). Theory comparison: Uncertainty reduction, problematic integration, uncertainty management, and other curious constructs. *Journal of Communication, 51*, 456–476. doi: 10.1111/j.1460-2466.2001.tb02891.x

Brashers, D. (2001). Communication and uncertainty management. *Journal of Communication, 51*, 477–497. doi: 10.1111/j.1460-2466.2001.tb02892.x

Burleson, B. R., Albrecht, T. L., Goldsmith, D. J., & Sarason, I. G. (1994). The communication of social support. In B. R. Burleson, T. L. Albrecht, & I. G. Sarason (Eds.), *Communication of social support: Messages, interactions, relationships, and community* (pp. xi–xxx). Thousand Oaks, CA: SAGE.

Campbell, K. E., Marsden, P. V., & Hurlbert, J. S. (1986). Social resources and socio-economic status. *Social Networks, 8*, 97–117. doi: 10.1016/S0378-8733(86)80017-X

Caughlin, J. P., & Vangelist, A. L. (2009). Why people conceal or reveal secrets: A multiple goals theory perspective. In T. D. Afifi & W. A. Afifi (Eds.), *Uncertainty and information regulation in interpersonal contexts: Theories and applications* (pp. 279–299). New York, NY: Routledge.

Checkovich, T. J., & Stern, S. (2001). Shared caregiving responsibilities of adult siblings with elderly parents. *The Journal of Human Resources, 37*, 441–478. doi: 10.2307/3069678

Checton, M. G., & Greene, K. (2012). Beyond initial disclosure: The role of prognosis and symptom uncertainty in patterns of disclosure in relationships. *Health Communication, 27*, 145–157. doi: 10.1080/10410236.2011.571755

Cicirelli, V. G. (1991). Sibling relationships in adulthood. In S. K. Pfeifer & M. B. Sussman (Eds.), *Families: Intergenerational and generational connections* (pp. 291–310). Binghamton, NY: Haworth Press.

Cicirelli, V. G. (1995). *Sibling relationships across the lifespan*. New York, NY: Plenum Press. doi: 10.1007/978-1-4757-6509-0

Connidis, I. A., & Kemp, C. L. (2008). Negotiating actual and anticipated parental support: Multiple sibling voices in three-generation families. *Journal of Aging Studies, 22*, 229–238. doi: 10.1016/j.jaging.2007.06.002

Cowan, P. A. (1991). Individual and family life transitions: A proposal for a new definition. In P. A. Cowan & M. Herrington (Eds.), *Family transitions* (pp. 3–30). Hillsdale, NJ: Lawrence Erlbaum Associates.

Dennis, M. R., Kunkel, A., & Keyton, J. (2008). Problematic integration theory, appraisal theory, and the bosom buddies breast cancer support group. *Journal of Applied Communication Research, 36*, 415–436. doi: 10.1080/00909880802094315

Derlega, V. J., & Chaiken, A. L. (1977). Privacy and self-disclosure in social relationships. *Journal of Social Issues, 33*, 102–115. doi: 10.1111/j.1540.4560.1977.tb01885.x

Derlega, V. J., Metts, S., Petronio, S., & Margulis, S. (1993). *Self-disclosure*. Newbury Park, CA: SAGE.

Derlega, V. J., Winstead, B. A., Mathews, A., & Braitman, A. (2008). Why does someone reveal highly personal information? Attributions for and against self-disclosure in close relationships. *Communication Research Reports, 25*, 115–130. doi: 10.1080/08824090802021756

Derlega, V. J., Winstead, B. A., Wong, P. T. P., & Greenspan, M. (1987). Self-disclosure and relational development: An attributional analysis. In M. E. Roloff & G. R. Miller (Eds.), *Interpersonal processes: New directions in communication research* (pp. 172–187). Newbury Park, CA: SAGE.

Durham, W. T. (2008). The rules-based process of revealing/concealing the family planning decisions of voluntarily child-free couples: A communication privacy management perspective. *Communication Studies, 59*, 132–147. doi: 10.1080/10510970802062451

Fillenbaum, G. G. (1987). Multidimensional functional assessment. In G. L. Maddox (Ed.), *The encyclopedia of aging* (pp. 460–464). New York, NY: Springer Publishing.

Gill, E., & Morgan, M. (2011). Home sweet home: Conceptualizing and coping with the challenges of aging and the move to a care facility. *Health Communication, 26*, 332–342. doi: 10.1080/10410236.2010.551579

Greene, K. (2009). An integrated model of health disclosure decision-making. In T. D. Afifi & W. A. Afifi (Eds.), *Uncertainty and information regulation in interpersonal contexts: Theories and applications* (pp. 226–253). New York, NY: Routledge.

Greene, K., Carpenter, A., Catona, D., & Magsamen-Conrad, K. (2013). The Brief Disclosure Intervention (BDI): Facilitating African Americans' disclosure of HIV. *Journal of Communication, 63*, 138–158. doi: 10.1111/jcom.12010

Greene, K., Derlega, V. J., & Mathews, A. (2006). Self-disclosure in personal relationships. In A. Vangelisti & D. Perlman (Eds.), *Cambridge handbook of personal relationships* (pp. 409–427). New York, NY: Cambridge University Press. doi: 10.1017/CBO9780511606632.023

Guerrero, L. K., & Afifi, W. A. (1995a). Some things are better left unsaid: Topic avoidance in family relationships. *Communication Quarterly, 43*, 276–296. doi: 10.1080/01463379509369977

Guerrero, L. K., & Afifi, W. A. (1995b). What parents don't know: Topic avoidance in parent-child relationships. In T. J. Socha & G. H. Stamp (Eds.), *Parents, children, and communication: Frontiers of theory and research* (pp. 219–245). Mahwah, NJ: Lawrence Erlbaum Associates.

Haines, V. A., Hurlbert, J. S., & Beggs, J. J. (1996). Exploring the determinants of support provision: Provider characteristics, personal networks, community contexts, and support following life events. *Journal of Health and Social Behavior, 37*, 252–264. doi: 10.2307/2137295

Hill, R. (1958). Generic features of families under stress. *Social Case Work, 49*, 139–150.

Hines, S. C., Babrow, A. S., Badzek, L., & Moss, A. (2001). From coping with life to coping with death: Problematic integration for the seriously ill elderly. *Health Communication, 13*, 327–342. doi: 10.1207/S15327027HC1303_6.

Hobfoll, S. E. (1988). *The ecology of stress.* Washington, DC: Hemisphere.

House, J. S. (1981). *Work stress and social support.* Reading, MA: Addison-Wesley.

Ingersoll-Dayton, B., Neal, M. B., Ha, J. H., & Hammer, L. B. (2003). Redressing inequity in parent care among siblings. *Journal of Marriage and the Family, 65*, 201–212. doi: 10.1111/j.1741-3737.2003.00201.x

Kellerman, K. (1992). Communication: Inherently strategic and primarily automatic. *Communication Monographs, 59*, 288–300. doi: 10.1080/03637759209376270

Kelly, A. E. (1999). Revealing personal secrets. *Current Directions in Psychological Science, 8*, 105–109. doi: 10.1111/1467-8721.00025

Kelly, A. E. (2002). *The psychology of secrets.* New York, NY: Kluwer Academic/Plenum Publishers. doi: 10.1007/978-1-4615-0683-6

Kelly, A. E., & McKillop, K. J. (1996). Consequences of revealing personal secrets. *Psychological Bulletin, 120*, 450–465. doi: 10.1037/0033-2909.120.3.450

Khodyakov, D., & Carr, D. (2009). The effect of late life parental death on adult sibling relationships: Do parents' advance directives help or hurt? *Research on Aging, 31*, 1–25. doi: 10.1177/0164027509337193

Kramer, B. J., Kavanaugh, M., Trentham-Dietz, A., Walsh, M., & Yonker, J. A. (2009). Predictors of family conflict at the end of life: The experience of spouses and adult children of persons with lung cancer. *The Gerontologist, 50*, 215–225. doi: 10.1093/geront/gnp121

Langer, E. J. (1992). Interpersonal mindlessness and language. *Communication Monographs, 59*, 324–327. doi: 10.1080/03637759209376274

Lazarus, R. S. (1983). The costs and benefits of denial. In S. Breznitz (Ed.), *The denial of stress* (pp. 1–30). New York, NY: International Universities Press.

Lee, G. R., Netzer, J. K., & Coward, R. T. (1995). Depression among older parents: The role of intergenerational exchange. *Journal of Marriage and the Family, 57*, 823–833. doi: 10.2307/353935

Lieberman, M. A., & Fisher, L. (1999). The effects of family conflict resolution and decision making on the provision of help for an elder with Alzheimer's disease. *The Gerontologist, 39*, 159–166. doi: 10.1093/geront/39.2.159

Matthews, S. H., & Rosner, T. T. (1988). Share filial responsibility: The family as the primary caregiver. *Journal of Marriage and the Family, 50*, 185–195. doi: 10.2307/352438

Matthias, M. S. (2009). Problematic integration in pregnancy and childbirth: Contrasting approaches to uncertainty and desire in obstetric and midwifery care. *Health Communication, 24*, 60–70. doi: 10.1080/10410230802607008

McCubbin, H. I., & Patterson, J. M. (1985). Adolescent stress, coping, and adaptation: A normative family perspective. In G. K. Leigh & G. W. Patterson (Eds.), *Adolescents in families* (pp. 256–276). Cincinnati, OH: Southwestern.

Merrill, D. M. (1996). Conflict and cooperation among adult siblings during the transition to the role of filial caregiver. *Journal of Social and Personal Relationships, 13*, 399–413. doi: 10.1177/0265407596133006

Miles, M. B., & Huberman, A. M. (1994). *Qualitative data analysis*. Thousand Oaks, CA, SAGE.

Mishel, M. H. (1988). The measurement of uncertainty in illness. *Nursing Research, 30*, 258–263. doi: 10.1097/00006199-198109000-00002

Patterson, J. (1988). Families experiencing stress: The family adjustment and adaptation response model. *Family Systems Medicine, 5*, 202–237. doi: 10.1037/h0089739

Pecchioni, L. L. (2001). Implicit decision making in family caregiving. *Journal of Social and Personal Relationships, 18*, 219–237. doi: 10.1177/0265407501182004

Petronio, S. (1991). Communication boundary management: A theoretical model of managing disclosure of private information between married couples. *Communication Theory, 1*, 311–335. doi: 10.1111/j.1468-2885.1991.tb00023.x

Petronio, S. (2002). *Boundaries of privacy: Dialectics of disclosure*. Albany, NY: SUNY Press.

Reddy, M. J. (1979). The conduit metaphor: A case of frame conflict in our language about language. In A. Ortony (Ed.), *Metaphor and thought* (pp. 284–324). Cambridge: Cambridge University Press.

Rocca, K. A., & Martin, M. M. (1998). The relationship between willingness to communicate and solidarity with frequency, breadth, and depth of communication in the sibling relationship. *Communication Research Reports, 15*, 82–90. doi: 10.1080/ 08824099809362100

Roloff, M. E. (1976). Communication strategies, relationships and relational change. In G. R. Miller (Ed.), *Explorations in interpersonal communication* (pp. 173–195). Thousand Oaks, CA: SAGE.

Roloff, M. E., & Ifert, D. E. (1998). Antecedents and consequences of explicit agreements to declare a topic taboo in dating relationships. *Personal Relationships, 5*, 191–205. doi: 10.1111/j.1475–6811.1998.tb00167.x

Roloff, M. E., & Ifert, D. E. (2000). Conflict management through avoidance: Withholding complaints, suppressing arguments, and declaring topics taboo. In S. Petronio (Ed.), *Balancing the secrets of private disclosures* (pp. 151–163). Mahwah, NJ: Lawrence Erlbaum Associates.

Segrin, C., & Flora, J. (2005). *Family communication*. Mahwah, NJ: Lawrence Erlbaum Associates.

Sillars, A., Canary, D. J., & Tafoya, M. (2004). Communication, conflict, and the quality of family relationships. In A. Vangelisti (Ed.), *Handbook of family communication* (pp. 413–446). Mahwah, NJ: Lawrence Erlbaum Associates.

Steuber, K. R., & Solomon, D. H. (2011). Factors that predict married partners' disclosures about infertility to social network members. *Journal of Applied Communication Research, 39*, 250–270. doi: 10.1080/00909882.2011.585401

Tonti, M. (1988). Relationships among adult siblings who care for their aged parents. In M. D. Kahn & K. G. Lewis (Eds.), *Siblings in therapy: Life span and clinical issues* (pp. 417–434). New York, NY: W. W. Norton.

Vangelisti, A. L. (1994). Family secrets: Forms, functions and correlates. *Journal of Social and Personal Relationships, 11*, 113–135. doi: 10.1177/0265407594111007

Venetis, M. K., Greene, K., Magsamen-Conrad, K., Banerjee, S. C., Checton, M. G., & Bagdasarov, Z. (2012). "You can't tell anyone but . . .": Exploring the use of privacy rules and revealing behaviors. *Communication Monographs, 79*, 344–365. doi: 10.1080/03637751.2012.697628

U.S. Census Bureau (2010). Summary of population and housing. Retrieved from: www.census.gov/prod/www/decennial.html

Walker, M. E., Wasserman, S., & Wellman, B. (1993). Statistical models for social support networks. *Sociological Methods and Research, 22*, 71–98. doi: 10.1177/ 0049124193022001004

Wellman, B. (1992). Which types of ties and networks provide what kinds of social support? *Advances in Group Processes, 9*, 207–235. Retrieved from: https://pdfs .semanticscholar.org/1cd0/ab172b7afbfabb5dfef52df480c984c17fb9.pdf

9

Examining Uncertainty and Interference with Cardiology Patients: Applying a Relational Turbulence Perspective in Health Contexts

AMANDA CARPENTER, KATHRYN GREENE, MARIA
G. CHECTON, AND DANIELLE CATONA

Heart disease is the leading cause of death in the United States (Centers for Disease Control and Prevention [CDC], 2015). It is the leading cause of death for both men and women of most races and ethnicities, and approximately 600,000 people die of heart disease every year (CDC, 2015). Managing a heart condition can be difficult because of the significant lifestyle changes required to cope effectively with such a diagnosis. Owing to the severity of heart disease, understanding the psychosocial factors that contribute to successfully managing heart disease can lead to significant benefits.

Specific factors in social and romantic relationships have been documented as a risk factor to health (Burman & Margolin, 1992; House, Landis, & Umberson, 1988), especially in relation to chronic health conditions. There is evidence that marital stress worsens the prognosis for women diagnosed with coronary heart disease (Orth-Gomer et al., 2000). In fact, marital stress was associated with an almost three times increased risk for recurrent coronary heart disease events after controlling for other factors, including age, estrogen levels, education, smoking, diagnosis, diabetes, blood pressure, and triglyceride level (Orth-Gomer et al., 2000). In this study, work stress did not predict any recurrent events related to coronary heart disease (Orth-Gomer et al., 2000), highlighting the key role of marital stress rather than stress generally. In related research, cardiac patients who experienced high levels of stress from either family or work had further disease progression than did patients who experienced low stress generally (Wang et al., 2007), suggesting that added stress from relationships, combined with or aside from work, influenced patients managing a cardiac diagnosis. Further, loneliness and marital quality were both found to influence recovery and health outcomes of patients undergoing cardiac rehabilitation (Dafoe & Colella, 2016). The literature also suggests the psychological traits of the patient and spouse affect the patient's psychological well-being after undergoing coronary artery bypass surgery (Ruiz, Matthews, Scheier, & Schulz, 2006). For example, higher presurgical neuroticism from the spouse predicted higher levels of patient depression, which has been identified as a risk factor for cardiac patients (Rozanski, Blumenthal, Davidson, Saab, & Kubzansky, 2005).

The findings from this review suggest that romantic partners, specifically spouses, can make it difficult for patients diagnosed with a cardiac condition to manage their disease effectively. This study draws upon the logic of relational turbulence theory (RTT; Solomon et al., 2016) to identify features of the illness experience that influence outcomes related to health management. Specifically, this study examines illness uncertainty and partner interference in health behavior as predictors of health-related topic avoidance and perceptions that one's health condition is a burden. Theoretically, the current study advances the literature on the RTT by examining health as a context in which a romantic partner's influence may be relevant to managing a chronic health condition. Pragmatically, this study identifies features of illnesses and romantic relationships that may serve as barriers to successfully managing a cardiac condition so that they can be targeted to improve treatment and adherence. In the sections that follow, we outline the RTT and explain how managing a heart condition is subject to a partner's influence. Finally, we report the results of a study designed to assess the ways in which romantic partners might influence cardiac patients' disease management.

RELATIONAL TURBULENCE THEORY AND HEALTH MANAGEMENT

RTT (Solomon et al., 2016) focuses on the challenges that arise when established relationships experience transitions. The theory highlights two features of close relationships, relational uncertainty and partner interference, that are heightened during transitions and predict heightened emotional, cognitive, and behavioral reactivity in relationships (e.g., Solomon & Knobloch, 2004; Solomon & Theiss, 2008). The RTT has been applied to health-related transitions in established relationships including depression (Knobloch & Knobloch-Fedders, 2010; Knobloch, Knobloch-Fedders, & Durbin, 2011), infertility (Steuber & Solomon, 2008, 2011), breast cancer (Weber & Solomon, 2008), type 2 diabetes (Leustek & Theiss, 2018), and weight loss (Theiss, Carpenter, & Leustek, 2016). Although previous applications of RTT in health contexts have examined how ambiguity about the relationship and disruptions to interdependence are implicated in health transitions, they have not considered how uncertainty and interference related to the illness itself may exacerbate experiences of relational turbulence. This study invokes the logic of RTT, but shifts the focus of uncertainty and interference to consider sources of ambiguity and goal disruptions stemming from the health condition. Accordingly, the sections that follow define illness uncertainty and health interference and describe their anticipated associations with health outcomes of topic avoidance and perceived burden.

UNCERTAINTY AND INTERFERENCE AS MECHANISMS OF TURBULENCE

The first mechanism in RTT that is responsible for heightened reactivity in close relationships is *relational uncertainty*, which reflects a lack of confidence in people's perceptions of their relationship (Solomon et al., 2016). Relational uncertainty encompasses doubts about one's own involvement in the relationship (*self uncertainty*), the partner's involvement in the relationship (*partner uncertainty*), and the nature of the relationship as a whole (*relationship uncertainty*). Whereas relational uncertainty indexes ambiguity about relationship involvement, it does not capture ambiguity, confusion, or doubt about the broader context or external factors that might be influencing the relationship. In the context of acute or chronic illness, uncertainties about the diagnosis and prognosis of one's illness are likely to permeate the relational climate. This study extends the sources of uncertainty that may invoke relational turbulence to include *illness uncertainty*, which reflects people's inability to determine the meaning of illness-related events (Mishel, 1988).

The second mechanism in RTT that predicts reactivity during relationship transitions is the degree of influence between partners (Solomon et al., 2016). As part of establishing interdependence, relationship partners have an increasing amount of influence over one another's goals and routines. In some cases, a partner's influence can help to facilitate individuals' personal goals and routines, which is referred to as *facilitation from partners*. More often, creating interdependence leads to missteps, barriers, and disruptions to personal goals and routines, which is referred to as *interference from partners*. Most empirical tests of RTT have considered how mundane disruptions to personal routines in the execution of daily life contribute to frustration, irritation, and turbulence for romantic partners (e.g., Knobloch & Theiss, 2010; Solomon & Knobloch, 2001; Theiss & Knobloch, 2009). Coping with a health condition creates unique opportunities for a romantic partner to interfere with the treatment and management of one's illness. Thus, this study adds *health interference* as a unique source of partner interference that reflects a perceived disruption in health management caused by a relational partner (Greene et al., 2012).

Although the RTT has been applied to consider the potential for relational turbulence in a number of different health contexts (e.g., Leustek & Theiss, 2018; Knobloch, Knobloch-Fedders, & Durbin, 2011; Steuber & Solomon, 2008; Theiss et al., 2016; Weber & Solomon, 2008), these investigations have primarily considered how people's appraisals of the relationship both shape and reflect their experiences with a health condition. Given that relationship mechanisms have been the main focus of this research, these studies overlook specific features of the health context that may be driving reactivity to interpersonal events. Focusing on illness uncertainty and health interference brings elements of the illness experience into the forefront as possible predictors of relational turbulence. Based on the logic of the RTT, we expect illness uncertainty and health interference to predict indicators of turbulence. We also expect illness uncertainty and health interference to covary, such that increased illness uncertainty is positively associated with higher health interference. The management of a chronic health condition provides increased opportunities for partner involvement in care and treatment, which can give rise to interference and raise questions about the impact of one's health condition on relationship quality. Therefore, our first hypothesis follows the logic of the RTT to suggest that illness uncertainty and health interference covary.

H1: Perceptions of illness uncertainty and health interference are positively associated.

MARKERS OF TURBULENCE IN THE CONTEXT OF CHRONIC ILLNESS

The RTT argues that relational uncertainty and interference from partners heighten people's emotional, cognitive, and communicative reactivity to relationship events (Solomon et al., 2016). Prior tests of the theory have linked these mechanisms to a variety of outcomes, including irritations (e.g., Solomon & Knobloch, 2004; Theiss & Knobloch, 2009), negative emotion (e.g., Knobloch & Theiss, 2010), jealousy (e.g., Theiss & Solomon, 2006), hurt (e.g., Theiss, Knobloch, Checton, & Magsamen-Conrad, 2009), perceived turmoil (e.g., Knobloch, 2007), indirect communication (e.g., Theiss & Knobloch, 2009), and topic avoidance (e.g., Knobloch & Carpenter-Theune, 2004). Notably, most of the outcomes that have been considered in previous tests of RTT examine variables that are important features of close relationships. In this study, we consider two markers of turbulence that are especially relevant to the management of chronic illness: topic avoidance and perceived partner burden.

Topic Avoidance as a Marker of Turbulence in Chronic Illness

Topic avoidance is an intentional decision to evade certain topics in relationships, either by an individual or both parties (Afifi & Guerrero, 1998). Several studies have documented a positive association between relational uncertainty and avoidance of communication about taboo topics or the relationship in general (e.g., Knobloch & Carpenter-Theune, 2004; Knobloch & Theiss,

2011; Theiss & Estlein, 2014; Theiss & Nagy, 2012). Several studies have also documented associations between relational uncertainty and topic avoidance in various health contexts. For example, Knobloch, Sharabi, Delaney, and Suranne (2016) found that relational uncertainty mediated the relationship between depressive symptoms and topic avoidance in couples in which one or both partners was experiencing depression. In addition, Donovan-Kicken and Caughlin (2010) identified sources of and reasons for topic avoidance in a sample of women diagnosed with breast cancer, and the association between topic avoidance and relationship quality was moderated by several factors stemming from uncertainty about avoidance, such as self-protection and social constraints. A dyadic study about cancer communication indicated that increased open communication between partners predicted less topic avoidance about the illness (Venetis, Magsamen-Conrad, Checton, & Greene, 2014). Interestingly, a study specific to cardiology patients found that patients perceived that they shared more information with their partner than they actually did share (Checton & Greene, 2014). Taken together, this evidence suggests that, like relational uncertainty, illness uncertainty should render people more reluctant to talk to their partner about their cardiac health because they may lack sufficient information about their condition to be able to discuss it with a partner, or they may worry about how their health condition affects the partner or the relationship. Therefore, we propose the following hypothesis:

H2: Perceptions of illness uncertainty are positively associated with topic avoidance about a cardiac condition.

Health interference should also increase people's topic avoidance when it comes to discussing their cardiac health with a partner. Some tests of RTT have indicated that interference from partners is associated with less open and direct communication about a variety of topics (e.g., Theiss & Knobloch, 2013; Theiss & Solomon, 2006), as well as being indirectly associated with increased topic avoidance about taboo topics such as sexual intimacy (e.g., Theiss & Estlein, 2014). Although tests of the RTT have tended to focus on the influence of partner interference in everyday goals and activities, some research has considered the impact of interference related to health goals. For example, in couples in which one partner was trying to lose weight, interference in weight loss behavior from a partner resulted in topic avoidance about weight loss (Theiss, Carpenter, & Cox, 2015). The health interference scale (Greene et al., 2012) has received limited empirical attention, but the logic of RTT provides guidance for hypothesizing about the association between health interference and topic avoidance. Individuals are unlikely to want to discuss their health condition with a partner who is frequently making it more difficult to manage their illness or accomplish health-related goals. Thus, we propose the following hypothesis:

H3: Perceptions of health interference are positively associated with topic avoidance about a cardiac condition.

Perceived Burden as a Marker of Turbulence in Cardiac Health

The second marker of turbulence that we consider as a downstream outcome of illness uncertainty and health interference is the perceived burden of managing the illness on one's partner. *Perceived partner burden* is defined as the degree to which chronically ill individuals feel that they are a hindrance to their romantic partner (Cousineau, McDowell, Hotz, & Hebert, 2003). We anticipate that illness uncertainty and health interference both influence perceived partner burden through their effect on health-related topic avoidance. Prior research demonstrates that topic avoidance can have negative consequences for individuals and their relationships, such as increased levels of depression and anxiety (Donovan-Kicken & Caughlin, 2011), as well as decreased relationship satisfaction and intimacy (e.g., Theiss & Estlein, 2014; Theiss & Nagy, 2012). In health contexts, topic avoidance can have additional consequences. For example, in a study of cancer patients, Venetis et al. (2014) examined cancer-related communication, partner burden, and topic avoidance. Results indicated that topic avoidance from both patients and partners predicted an increase in the patient's perceived level of partner burden, as well as reports of the partner's experienced burden. Therefore, our final hypothesis considers the association between topic avoidance and perceived partner burden as a marker of turbulence.

H4: Topic avoidance is positively associated with perceived partner burden.

METHOD

To examine these hypotheses, we conducted a cross-sectional study in which patients completed surveys while waiting for their appointment in a cardiology office. Participants were approached by members of the research team to participate in the study. Individuals were eligible to participate if they were (a) 18 years of age or older, (b) diagnosed with a heart condition, and (c) received assistance in managing their heart condition from another individual. Eligible cardiac diagnoses included coronary artery disease, arrhythmias, hypercholesteremia, hypertension, heart failure, congenital heart failure, and cerebrovascular disease.

Procedure

After patients signed in for their appointments and were in the waiting room, they were approached to participate. We excluded patients at the office for an initial consultation or for cardiac preoperative clearance for an unrelated condition. After consenting to and before beginning the survey, participants were asked to complete the survey while thinking about a specific person who helped manage their cardiac condition. Based on this response, they received either a survey worded for a spouse or romantic partner, or a survey worded for another person (e.g., friend, child, parent, sibling, etc.)

Participants

We asked participants to think of a specific person who helped manage their care when completing the survey. Most participants completed the survey about their spouse (n = 161, 72.2%), while others completed the survey about their daughter (n = 33, 14.8%), friend (n = 11, 4.9%), son (n = 10, 4.5%), or sister (n = 5, 2.2%). For the purposes of this study, we utilized only spousal data for analyses, and these spouse-specific data (N = 161) are presented in this section and the results. Our sample included 112 males (69.6%) and 46 females (28.6%). Average age was 67.3 years (SD = 10.9, range = 47–93 years). Length of diagnosis ranged from 1 to 44 years (M = 11.3 years). Participants reported visiting the cardiologist between one and eight times annually. The average length of the relationship reported by participants was 36.4 years (SD = 13.6, range = 6 – 65 years). The majority of participants self-identified as Caucasian/white (n = 138, 85.7%), followed by African American/black (n = 3, 1.9%), Hispanic/Latino(a) (n = 2, 1.2%), multiracial (n = 2, 1.2%), and Middle Eastern (n = 2, 1.2%). Five participants did not report race or ethnicity. Reported education level ranged from college (n = 62, 38.5%), high school (n = 40, 24.8%), master's degree (n = 27, 16.8%), some college (n = 18, 11.2%), professional school [including law, medical, or PhD] (n = 6, 3.7%), to associate degree (n = 3, 1.9%).

Measures

Study variables used 5-point Likert-type scales. All scales underwent exploratory factor analysis (EFA). The scales used in the study have previously received validation in other health contexts, but never in a sample of cardiology patients. Therefore, the EFA (Varimax rotation) was employed for all model variables. Items loaded above .50, and all loaded onto a primary factor. Variables were computed by averaging responses. Information for each of the variables included in the model is presented in the following section.

Illness uncertainty. To measure illness uncertainty, we used a shortened version of Mishel's (1997) illness uncertainty scale. Instructions asked participants to indicate their agreement, on a 5-point scale (1 = *strongly disagree* to 5 = *strongly agree,* with an additional option, 0 = *not applicable*), with statements about uncertainty regarding their heart condition. Higher scores indicated increased concerns about the illness and effective illness management. Sample items included "Because of the unpredictability of my heart condition, I cannot plan for the future" and "My symptoms continue to change unpredictably." Results suggested a one-factor scale (eigenvalue = 5.50, 34.40% variance explained, 10 items loading above 0.60 onto this factor, $\alpha = 0.90$, $M = 1.86$, $SD = 0.79$).

Health interference. To tap into the health interference construct, we used a modified version of Knobloch and Solomon's (2004) partner interference scale. Checton, Greene, Magsamen-Conrad, and Venetis (2012) and Greene et al. (2012) tailored the original Knobloch and Solomon (2004) scale to measure patient perceptions of health interference. Instructions asked participants how they viewed their heart condition, how the other person viewed the heart condition, and how participants viewed their relationship and heart condition. Items were measured on a 5-point scale (1 = *strongly disagree* to 5 = *strongly agree*), with higher scores indicating increased interference from partners. Sample items include "My heart condition negatively affects my life" and "My heart condition interferes with the things my spouse likes to do each day." Results indicated a one-factor solution (eigenvalue = 5.01, 55.64% variance explained, nine items loading above 0.60, $\alpha = 0.89$, $M = 2.02$, $SD = 0.83$).

Topic avoidance. Measurement of topic avoidance was adapted from Donovan-Kicken and Caughlin's (2010) scale that was developed for health-specific perceptions of avoidance. Instructions asked participants what they avoided discussing with their spouse. Items were measured on a 5-point scale (1 = *strongly disagree* to 5 = *strongly agree*, with an additional option, 0 = *not applicable*). Higher scores indicated greater avoidance about a particular issue. Sample items included those pertaining to "sexual issues," "health issues," and "fear of dying." Results pointed to a one-factor solution (eigenvalue = 7.08, 41.67% variance explained, 16 items loading above 0.50, $\alpha = 0.91$, $M = 2.17$, $SD = 0.64$).

Perceived partner burden. Perceived partner burden was measured using items from the Cousineau et al. (2003) scale for medical patients. Instructions asked participants to think about their heart condition and how it affected their spouse. Items were measured on a 5-point scale (1 = *none of the time* to 5 = *all of the time*), with higher scores indicating greater perceptions of burden. Sample items included "I worry that [my spouse] is overextending him/herself in helping me" and "I feel guilty about the demands that I make on [my spouse]." Results indicated a single factor (eigenvalue = 4.65, 46.47% variance explained, eight items loading above 0.60, $\alpha = 0.89$, $M = 1.55$, $SD = 0.66$).

RESULTS

This section outlines analyses and results from the hypotheses and research question we presented. The section begins with a review of the preliminary analyses, followed by a description of the use of structural equation modeling to examine the research question.

Preliminary Analyses

To begin our analyses, we examined bivariate correlations between the variables in the model (see Table 9.1). Our first hypothesis asked about the relationship between illness uncertainty and health interference. Results indicated that uncertainty and interference were positively correlated, such that increased uncertainty was related to increased interference, $r = 0.64$, $p < 0.01$. Neither illness uncertainty nor health interference was associated with topic avoidance as predicted. Finally, topic avoidance and perceptions of burden were positively associated, such that increased topic avoidance was associated with increased perceptions of burden ($r = 0.16$, $p < 0.05$).

Substantive Analyses

To examine our remaining research question, we used structural equation modeling (SEM). Factor variances and covariances were freely estimated, and we used indirect latent factor scaling (i.e., fixing the factor loading of items within each latent factor). Results of the SEM revealed good model fit, χ^2 (56) = 109.30, $p < 0.05$, CFI = 0.94, RMSEA = 0.08 (see Figure 9.1 for final model with path coefficients). Consistent with H1, illness uncertainty and illness interference were positively associated. As predictors of topic avoidance, however, neither illness uncertainty (H2) nor illness interference (H3) was significantly associated with the avoidance of communication about one's health condition.

TABLE.9.1 *Zero-order correlations between model variables*

Measure	Uncertainty	Interference	Topic Avoidance	Perceptions of Burden
Uncertainty	—			
Interference	0.64**	—		
Topic Avoidance	0.12	−0.03	—	
Perceptions of Burden	0.59**	0.48**	0.16*	—

*$p < 0.05$. **$p < 0.01$.

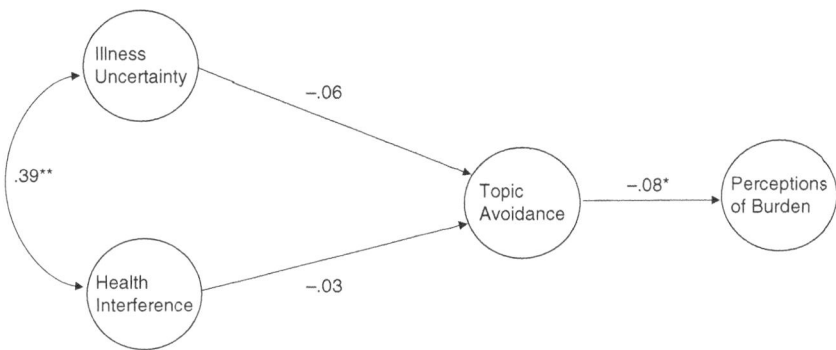

FIGURE 9.1   Final model with path coefficients.
*p < 0.05. **p < 0.01.

Finally, although H4 predicted a positive association between topic avoidance and partner burden, results indicated that avoiding communication about one's health condition decreased, rather than increased, perceptions of partner burden.

DISCUSSION

This study explored health-specific variables and their relationship to an indicator of relational turbulence, topic avoidance. Our results extend the assumptions of the RTT as it relates to health management and point to aspects of chronic illness that may serve as a barrier to managing a chronic health condition effectively. Our first hypothesis was supported, as illness uncertainty and health interference were positively associated. Neither our second nor third hypothesis was supported, because neither illness uncertainty nor health interference was associated with topic avoidance. Our fourth hypothesis found a negative association between topic avoidance and perceptions of partner burden, contrary to what we hypothesized. Results suggest that the modified mechanisms stemming from the logic of RTT may not be suitable for predicting markers of turbulence in an ongoing health management context. Although the model yielded a good fit overall, the main pathways linking illness uncertainty and health interference were not significant. With regard to application, these results point to topic avoidance as a significant factor that can hinder effective health management. The rest of this section discusses the implications of the results of this study, as well as its strengths, its limitations, and suggestions for future research.

Theoretical Implications

As a starting point, this research considered sources of illness uncertainty and types of health interference that impede conversations about health management with a relational partner. With regard to H1, illness uncertainty and health interference were positively correlated, indicating that within a framework of chronic health management, higher levels of uncertainty are related to higher levels of interference from a spouse. H2 and H3 predicted that illness uncertainty and health interference would be positively associated with topic avoidance. Although the model fit our data, neither illness uncertainty nor health interference significantly predicted topic avoidance, and the effects were in the opposite direction of what was predicted. We identify two possible explanations for the lack of association. First, the average relationship length for the couples in this study was 36.4 years; thus, given that these were established relationships, there might be few topics that patients are unwilling to discuss with their spouse. Second, perhaps patients are more motivated to communicate about their illness when they are trying to reduce uncertainty about their illness or more effectively coordinate their actions with a spouse. Theoretical perspectives on uncertainty management and uncertainty reduction point to information seeking as the primary means through which individuals reduce their uncertainty (Berger & Calabrese, 1975; Brashers, 2001); thus, it is possible that people are less likely to avoid conversations about this topic to the extent that they desire uncertainty reduction. Similarly, when a partner is regularly interfering in efforts to manage a health condition, more direct communication might be necessary to avoid misunderstandings and forestall disruptions. Additional research is needed to examine the potential for illness uncertainty and health interference to predict health outcomes in the context of chronic illness.

Our results also highlight a significant association between topic avoidance and perceptions of partner burden, although the effect was not in the predicted direction. We found that topic avoidance was negatively associated with perceived partner burden for cardiology patients, suggesting that less communication about managing their illness was related to decreased burden on the spouse. Although this finding is not what we expected, in hindsight it seems logical that individuals will feel less burdened by their partner's illness to the extent that the partner withholds information about their health. When individuals avoid discussing their health condition, partners are unlikely to feel burdened because they lack awareness of what the patient is going through. In fact, one explanation for this finding is that preventing partner burden might actually serve as a motivation for individuals to avoid communicating about topics related to their illness. In this way, topic avoidance may be a protective action designed to buffer a romantic partner from the stress and burden of co-managing the illness. This result also points to the potential for bidirectional effects between these variables. Although we positioned topic avoidance as a mediator in our model based on evidence that the mechanisms of relational turbulence predict more avoidant communication behaviors (e.g., Knobloch & Carpenter-Theune, 2004; Theiss & Nagy, 2012), an alternative possibility is that partner burden is a more proximal outcome of uncertainty and interference that predicts topic avoidance. When relationship partners share the burden of managing illness, they are likely unable to avoid conversations about a partner's health condition. Thus, individuals may be less likely to avoid talking about a cardiac condition if they are willingly trying to help their partner manage the illness. Additional research is needed utilizing different types of designs to further explore the potential for bidirectional effects.

Practical Implications

The findings from this study also offer several practical implications for couples co-managing a chronic health condition. First, illness uncertainty and health interference were positively related, suggesting that romantic partners may struggle to collectively manage a chronic condition long term. One interpretation of this finding is that when people have ambiguity about a health condition, it can make it difficult for partners to identify the best ways to provide assistance or support. Consequently, partners might struggle to effectively coordinate their actions if they are unsure about what actions would be most appropriate or effective for managing the illness. An alternate interpretation is that when a partner is perceived as interfering in efforts to manage a chronic health condition, individuals may experience more questions about their ability to cope with their illness. Thus, illness uncertainty and health interference likely exert mutual influence on one another in the process of coping with a health diagnosis.

Our findings also point to interesting implications regarding the role of interpersonal communication in managing a chronic health condition. There tends to be a positive bias in people's assumptions about the role and impact of communication in relational and health contexts, with individuals endorsing the belief that open communication will result in closer relationships and more effective health management. Our results challenge this notion that increased openness will produce more relational and health benefits by showing that avoiding communication about one's health condition can mitigate the burden on partners to help manage a health condition. Particularly in the context of a chronic health condition, constant openness about the condition over the long term may contribute to chronic fatigue. Our findings suggest that although there are certainly times to promote openness about one's health, there are also times when it may be beneficial for the patient to exercise some restraint for the benefit of the relationship and/or the partner. The challenge, of course, is navigating the fine line between appropriate levels of openness and privacy. Additional research is needed to determine the point at which topic avoidance becomes problematic rather than beneficial.

Limitations

This study has some limitations. First, we asked for the perspective of only one partner in the relationship, specifically the patient with a cardiac condition. Although understanding how cardiac patients perceive their health condition and the support they receive from a relationship partner in managing their condition is crucial, it is equally important to understand how the partner of individuals with a chronic health condition might cope with that partner's illness. Helping a romantic partner manage the health condition can contribute to uncertainty about one's feelings toward a partner or the future of the relationship, and it can interfere in one's ability to pursue and achieve personal goals and routines. Dyadic data would be beneficial for providing insight into the experiences of both the patient and the partner when managing a chronic health condition. Moreover, dyadic data would make it possible to examine how partners collectively manage and cope with the illness.

Attempting to extend the RTT beyond the scope of the original theory is another limitation of this study. The RTT is concerned with features of relationships that are heightened during relationship transitions, specifically relational uncertainty and general partner interference. We attempted to extend the theory by examining sources of uncertainty and partner interference that stem from illness. Although it is likely that relationship and health processes work in tandem by affecting partners' perceptions of uncertainty, interference, and other communicative behaviors, our results suggest that the mechanisms in RTT may not have been effectively translated into variables specific to this health context. Future RTT studies should compare models with solely relationship or health variables to explore which process might be more pertinent.

Finally, a more robust study would examine these processes over time to observe how relationships and health are interconnected and evolve over the course of a chronic illness. Longitudinal studies would measure changes in the relationship and health management behaviors. Additionally, studying a relationship from initial diagnosis through the course of disease progression would extend the RTT literature. Our study examined patients in couples who had been married long term and generally diagnosed with their heart condition for an extended period of time. Perhaps couples who were in developing relationships or managing an initial diagnosis would experience increased turbulence over time. These are areas ripe for future research.

REFERENCES

Afifi, W. A., & Guerrero, L. K. (1998). Some things are better left unsaid II: Topic avoidance in friendships. *Communication Quarterly, 46*, 231–249. doi: 10.1080/01463379809370099

Berger, C. R., & Calabrese, R. J. (1975). Some explorations in initial interactions and beyond: Toward a developmental theory of interpersonal communication. *Human Communication Research, 1*, 99–112. doi: 10.1111/j.1468–2958.1975.tb00258.x

Brashers, D. E. (2001). Communication and uncertainty management. *Journal of Communication, 51*, 477–497. doi: 10.1111/j.1460–2466.2001.tb02892.x

Burman, B., & Margolin, G. (1992). Analysis of the association between marital relationships and health problems: An interactional perspective. *Psychological Bulletin, 112*, 39–63. doi: 10.1037/0033–2909.112.1.39

Centers for Disease Control and Prevention (CDC). (2015). *Heart disease facts.* Retrieved from: www.cdc.gov/heartdisease/facts.htm

Checton, M. G., & Greene, K. (2014). "I tell my partner everything . . . (or not)": Patients' perceptions of sharing heart-related information with their partner." *Journal of Family Nursing, 20*, 164–184. doi: 10.1177/1074840714521320

Checton, M. G., Greene, K., Magsamen-Conrad, K., & Venetis, M. K. (2012). Patients' and partners' perspectives of chronic illness and its management. *Families, Systems, & Health, 30*, 114–129. doi: 10.1037/a0028598

Cousineau, N., McDowell, I., Hotz, S., & Hebert, P. (2003). Measuring chronic patients' feelings of being a burden to their caregivers. *Medical Care, 41*, 110–118. doi: 10.1097/01.MLR.0000039832.32412.7D

Dafoe, W. A., & Colella, T. J. F. (2016). Loneliness, marriage, and cardiovascular health. *European Journal of Preventive Cardiology, 23*, 1242–1244. doi: 10.1177/2047487316643441

Donovan-Kicken, E., & Caughlin, J. P. (2010). A multiple goals perspective on topic avoidance and relationship satisfaction in the context of breast cancer. *Communication Monographs, 77*, 231–256. doi: 10.1080/03637751003758219

Donovan-Kicken, E., & Caughlin, J. P. (2011). Breast cancer patients' topic avoidance and psychological distress: The mediating role of coping. *Journal of Health Psychology, 16*, 596–606. doi: 10.1177/1359105310383605

Greene, K., Magsamen-Conrad, K., Venetis, M. K., Checton, M. G., Bagdasarov, Z., & Banerjee, S. C. (2012). Assessing health diagnosis disclosure decisions in relationships: Testing the disclosure decision-making model. *Health Communication, 27*, 356–368. doi: 10.1080/10410236.2011.586988

House, J. S., Landis, K. R., & Umberson, D. (1988). Social relationships and health. *Science, 241*, 540–544. doi: 10.1126/science.3399889

Knobloch, L. K. (2007). Perceptions of turmoil within courtship: Associations with intimacy, relational uncertainty, and interference from partners. *Journal of Social and Personal Relationships, 24*, 363–384. doi: 10.1177/0265407507077227

Knobloch, L. K., & Carpenter-Theune, K. E. (2004). Topic avoidance in developing romantic relationships. *Communication Research, 21*, 173–205. doi: 10.1177/0093650203261516

Knobloch, L. K., & Knobloch-Fedders, L. M. (2010). The role of relational uncertainty in depressive symptoms and relationship quality: An actor-partner interdependence model. *Journal of Social and Personal Relationships, 27*, 137–159. doi: 10.1177/0265407509348809

Knobloch, L. K., Knobloch-Fedders, L. M., & Durbin, C. E. (2011). Depressive symptoms and relational uncertainty as predictors of reassurance-seeking and negative feedback-seeking in conversation. *Communication Monographs, 78,* 437–462. doi: 10.1080/03637751.2011.618137

Knobloch, L. K., Sharabi, L. L., Delaney, A. L., & Suranne, S. M. (2016). The role of relational uncertainty in topic avoidance among couples with depression. *Communication Monographs, 83,* 25–48. doi: 10.1080/03637751.2014.998691

Knobloch, L. K., & Solomon, D. H. (2004). Interference and facilitation from partners in the development of interdependence within romantic relationships. *Personal Relationships, 11,* 115–130. doi: 10.1111/j.1475-6811.2004.00074.x

Knobloch, L. K., & Theiss, J. A. (2010). An actor-partner interdependence model of relational turbulence: Cognitions and emotions. *Journal of Social and Personal Relationships, 27,* 595–619. doi: 10.1177/0265407510368967

Knobloch, L. K., & Theiss, J. A. (2011). Relational uncertainty and relationship talk within courtship: A longitudinal actor-partner interdependence model. *Communication Monographs, 78,* 3–26. doi: 10.1080/03637751.2010.542471

Leustek, J., & Theiss, J. A. (2018). Factors that shape cognitive and behavioral coping among individuals with type 2 diabetes: Features of illness versus features of romantic relationships. *Health Communication, 33,* 1549–1559. doi: 10.1080/10410236.2017.1384346

Mishel, M. H. (1988). Uncertainty in illness. *Journal of Nursing Scholarship, 20,* 225–232. doi: 10.1111/j.1547-5069.1988.tb00082.x

Mishel, M. H. (1997). Uncertainty in illness scales manual. Available from M. Mishel at the University of North Carolina-Chapel Hill, School of Nursing.

Orth-Gomer, K., Wamala, S. P., Horsten, M., Schenck-Gustafsson, K., Schneiderman, N., & Mittleman, M. A. (2000). Marital stress worsens prognosis in women with coronary heart disease. The Stockholm female coronary risk study. *Journal of the American Medical Association, 284,* 3008–3014. doi: 10.1001/jama.284.23.3008

Rozanski, A., Blumenthal, J. A., Davidson, K. W., Saab, P. G., & Kubzansky, L. (2005). The epidemiology, pathophysiology, and management of psychosocial risk factors in cardiac practice. *Journal of the American College of Cardiology, 45,* 637–651. doi: 10.1016/j.jacc.2004.12.005

Ruiz, J. M., Matthews, K. A., Scheier, M. F., & Schulz, R. (2006). Does who you marry matter for your health? Influence of patients' and spouses' personality on their partners' psychological well-being following coronary artery bypass surgery. *Journal of Personality and Social Psychology, 91,* 255–267. doi: 10.1037/0022-3514.2.255

Solomon, D. H., & Knobloch, L. K. (2001). Relationship uncertainty, partner interference, and intimacy within dating relationships. *Journal of Social and Personal Relationships, 18,* 804–820. doi: 10.1177/0265407501186004

Solomon, D. H., & Knobloch, L. K. (2004). A model of relational turbulence: The role of intimacy, relational uncertainty, and interference from partners in appraisals of irritations. *Journal of Social and Personal Relationships, 21,* 795–816. doi: 10.1177/0265407504047838

Solomon, D. H., Knobloch, L. K., Theiss, J. A., & McLaren, R. M. (2016). Relational turbulence theory: Explaining variation in subjective experiences and communication within romantic relationships. *Human Communication Research, 42,* 507–532. doi: 10.1111/hcre.12091

Solomon, D. H., & Theiss, J. A. (2008). A longitudinal test of the relational turbulence model of romantic relationship development. *Personal Relationships, 15,* 339–357. doi: 10.1111/j.1475–6811.2008.00202.x

Steuber, K. R., & Solomon, D. H. (2008). Relational uncertainty, partner interference, and infertility: A qualitative study of discourse within online forums. *Journal of Social and Personal Relationships, 25,* 831–855. doi: 10.1177/0265407508096698

Steuber, K. R., & Solomon, D. H. (2011). Factors that predicted married couples' disclosures about infertility to social network members. *Journal of Applied Communication Research, 39,* 250–270. doi: 10.1080/00909882.2011.585401

Theiss, J. A., Carpenter, A., & Cox, J. (2015, May). *Relationship characteristics that predict communication about weight loss and efficacy to achieve weight loss goals.* Paper presented at the annual meeting of the International Communication Association, San Juan, Puerto Rico.

Theiss, J. A., Carpenter, A. M., & Leustek, J. (2016). Partner facilitation and partner interference in individuals' weight loss goals. *Qualitative Health Research, 26,* 18–30. doi: 10.1177/1049732315583980

Theiss, J. A., & Estlein, R. (2014). Antecedents and consequences of the perceived threat of sexual communication: A test of the relational turbulence model. *Western Journal of Communication, 78,* 404–425. doi: 10.1080/10570314.2013.845794

Theiss, J. A., & Knobloch, L. K. (2009). An actor-partner interdependence model of irritations in romantic relationships. *Communication Research, 36,* 510–536. doi: 10.1177/0093650209333033

Theiss, J. A., & Knobloch, L. K. (2013). A relational turbulence model of military service members' relational communication during reintegration. *Journal of Communication, 63,* 1109–1129. doi: 10.1111/jcom.12059

Theiss, J. A., Knobloch, L. K., Checton, M. G., & Magsamen-Conrad, K. (2009). Relationship characteristics associated with the experience of hurt in romantic relationships: A test of the relational turbulence model. *Human Communication Research, 35,* 588–615. doi: 10.1111/j.1468–2958.2009.01364.x

Theiss, J. A., & Nagy, M. E. (2012). A cross-cultural test of the relational turbulence model: Relationship characteristics that predict turmoil and topic avoidance for Koreans and Americans. *Journal of Social and Personal Relationships, 29,* 545–565. doi: 10.1177/0265407512443450

Theiss, J. A., & Solomon, D. H. (2006). Coupling longitudinal data and multilevel modeling to examine the antecedents and consequences of jealousy experiences in romantic relationships: A test of the relational turbulence model. *Human Communication Research, 32,* 469–503. doi: 10.1111/j.1468–2958.2006.00284.x

Venetis, M. K., Magsamen-Conrad, K., Checton, M. G., & Greene, K. (2014). Cancer communication and partner burden: An exploratory study. *Journal of Communication, 64,* 82–102. doi: 10.1111/jcom.12069

Wang, H. X., Leineweber, C., Kirkeeide, R., Svane, B., Schenck-Gustafsson, K., Theorell, T., & Orth-Gomer, K. (2007). Psychosocial stress and atherosclerosis: Family and work stress accelerate progression of coronary disease in women. The Stockholm female coronary angiography study. *Journal of Internal Medicine, 261,* 245–254. doi: 10.1111/j.1365–2796.2006.01759.x

Weber, K. M., & Solomon, D. H. (2008). Locating relationship and communication issues among stressors associated with breast cancer. *Health Communication, 23,* 548–559. doi: 10.1080/10410230802465233

10

Uncertainty Management in Bereavement: Parent and Child Uncertainty Sources and Management Strategies

BRANDI N. FRISBY, JACOB M. MATIG, AND
CHRISTINA J. HARRIS

The turbulence that occurs following the loss of a loved one is "one of the most challenging and overwhelming circumstances an individual must face" (Bosticco & Thompson, 2005, p. 257). This loss is undeniably a source of stress, emitting an "aura of fear and uncertainty" (Reif, Patton, & Gold, 1995, p. 292). Indeed, some individuals who experience loss are more resilient than others in the face of the uncertainty and stress that accompany grief. However, understanding what makes some individuals more resilient than others is an understudied concept, as the "field of grief continues to remain in its infancy" (Kaplow, Layne, Saltzman, Cozza, & Pynoos, 2013, p. 324; Nader & Layne, 2009). This is especially true in the literature on children's grief, which has not advanced at the same rate as the literature on adult grievers (Kaplow et al., 2013) or in the communication literature (Hastings, 2000). Thus, this study examined the sources of uncertainty for both parents and children following the death of a family member and illuminated uncertainty management strategies.

UNCERTAINTY AND STRESS

Uncertainty is a source of stress (Greco & Roger, 2003; Monat, Averill, & Lazarus, 1972). Stress can manifest physically (e.g., headaches, weight loss, insomnia) and psychologically (e.g., rumination, mood swings, anxiety; Casarett, Kutner, & Abraham, 2001; Chiriboga, Brierton, Krystal, & Pierce, 1982; Mancini & Bonanno, 2009) and damage physical and psychological health (Reif et al., 1995). Prolonged uncertainty and stress have also been linked to parental posttraumatic stress disorder (PTSD; Santacroce, 2003). The link between uncertainty and these reactions can be explained by communibiology, which asserts that communication affects the stress hormone cortisol (Floyd, Mikkelson, & Hesse, 2008). The link between uncertainty and stress has been supported in other studies, ranging from those discussing hurtful messages (Priem & Solomon, 2011) to those discussing financial uncertainty (Afifi et al., 2015).

Uncertainty can be especially stressful for individuals who are intolerant of uncertainty and perceive "future negative events as stressful, believe that uncertainty is negative, reflects badly on a person, should be avoided, and have difficulties functioning well in uncertain situations" (Boelen, 2010, p. 471). While some individuals are intolerant of uncertainty, others may develop context-specific intolerance, including when the details of a situation are complex or ambiguous, when information is unavailable or conflicting, when individuals feel insecure about the knowledge they possess, and when the probability of an event directly affecting them is high (DeLorme & Huh, 2009). The death of a loved one represents one scenario under which uncertainty and, in turn, stress can thrive within parents and their children (Reif et al., 1995).

UNCERTAINTY AND STRESS IN BEREAVED PARENTS AND CHILDREN

For parents, uncertainty may progress along several trajectories. Although some individuals experience improved outcomes after the death of a loved one (Bonanno et al., 2002), most experience some decline in functioning, even if only temporary. Others experience prolonged or delayed grief. The grief process may be especially complicated for surviving caregivers (Shapiro, Howell, & Kaplow, 2014) who are struggling to manage the daily functioning of the family while simultaneously coping with their own grief or identity changes (Hastings, 2000; Toller, 2011; Wolchik, Ma, Tein, Sandler, & Ayers, 2008). For example, a parent may be thrust into a new familial role or filling the role of both parents in the event of a loss, and this role adjustment may distract the parent from attending to the child(ren)'s grief.

Outcomes for children are also differentiated by multiple trajectories. In the long term, children who experience death of a loved one may suffer from depression, anxiety, underdeveloped social skills, negative emotions, chronic stress, low self-esteem, uncertainty, academic issues, or substance abuse (Avelin, Gyllensward, Erlandsson, & Radestad, 2014). These negative outcomes are compounded when the surviving caregiver is also grieving (Avelin et al., 2014), or when the child and surviving caregiver have a poor relationship (Kaplow et al., 2013). In fact, Avelin et al. (2014) reported that children whose parent had died also experienced grief over the lost relationship and lack of emotional closeness with the surviving parent. Part of the challenge for children is that they are continuing to develop physically, emotionally, and cognitively. As children transition into each developmental phase, they are forced to reexperience, renegotiate, and reinterpret parental death (Biank & Werner-Lin, 2011). Some children return to relatively normal functioning within two months, while others begin to display the more serious symptoms of grief beginning as late as two years after the loss (Biank & Werner-Lin, 2011). Children also experience stress related to having their basic needs unmet (Wolchik et al., 2008). For example, children may recognize changes in resources, changes in housing and contact with friends and family, or new responsibilities and expectations (Wolchik et al., 2008).

It appears, then, that the stress experienced by each griever is attributable to the uncertainty experienced following the death of a loved one. However, further investigation of the causes of uncertainty following death of a loved one is needed. Thus:

RQ1: What are the sources of uncertainty for (a) parents and (b) children following the loss of an immediate family member?

The need for a communication-centric approach to how parents and children cope with uncertainty-induced stress is salient, as communication processes are central in buffering individuals against the negative effects of stress influenced by uncertainty (Mishel, 1988). We address this by focusing on the uncertainty management strategies (Brashers, 2001) of bereaved individuals.

UNCERTAINTY AND STRESS APPRAISAL AND MANAGEMENT

Although uncertainty reduction may remain a goal in many situations, Brashers (2001) conceptualized a more complex uncertainty management theory (UMT), arguing that individuals may find ways to manage, rather than reduce, uncertainty. Moreover, uncertainty management is dependent on individual preference, cultural norms for uncertainty avoidance, the context, and anticipated outcomes (Bradac, 2001; Brashers, 2001; Goldsmith, 2001). Reflective of this paradigmatic shift, Babrow and Kline (2000) argued that managing uncertainty is preferable to reducing uncertainty.

When an individual experiences uncertainty, he or she will appraise the uncertainty and select a response to fit the uncertainty level and source. The response is highly individualistic and will depend on the personal relevance, personal goals, coping abilities, and resources (Brashers, 2007; Delorme & Huh, 2009). If uncertainty becomes a cause of stress or distress, individuals will attempt to reduce it by using passive, active, or interactive strategies. Individuals who employ passive strategies make observations or notice information without actually seeking it. By gaining information, uncertainty can be managed. In the active strategy, people intentionally seek information about the source of uncertainty. Interactive strategies include communicating directly with another person or expert on the subject (Berger, 1979; Berger & Calabrese, 1975). Despite the choices available, communication through information seeking and information exchange is the central component to management (Brashers et al., 2000; Goldsmith, 2001).

UNCERTAINTY MANAGEMENT STRATEGIES IN BEREAVED PARENTS AND CHILDREN

Parents may passively manage uncertainty by using observations of others who have grieved or by using observations of their children's behavior to assess their grieving process. Some may seek to maintain a high level of uncertainty or even avoid uncertainty related to death. For example, Reif et al. (1995) argued that bereaved individuals may try to ignore intrusive thoughts, deny the event, or even avoid feelings or information related to the loss. This avoidant approach can be considered maladaptive and prevents the completion of the stress response. However, the individual may reappraise the situation on a different grief timeline (Reif et al., 1995).

Actively seeking grief support (Toller, 2011) could be categorized as an active strategy. It is only through the provision of support by others that the strategy would become interactive. Supportive communication involves behaviors that people use in an attempt to assist others who need help (Burleson & MacGeorge, 2002) and can have a buffering effect on the stress experienced by grieving parents and children (Cohen & Willis, 1985). Support intervenes to influence how the stress affects outcomes, often by reducing or eliminating stress outcomes (Cohen & Willis, 1985), reducing the stress hormones (Floyd et al., 2008), and allowing the uncertain individual to clarify and reappraise the situation (Mishel & Braden, 1987). Parents identify their family members, but especially their children, as sources of informal social support (Gear, 2014).

Although familial support is a critical coping strategy, this can prove difficult, as family members experience and respond to grief differently (Kaplow et al., 2013). Further, "these discordances in grief reactions can interfere with family members' capacity to communicate and empathize with one another's experiences and to support one another during stressful times" (p. 326).

Additionally, Wolchik et al. (2008) reported that parents dealing with stressors and task overload may spend less time with children or be less supportive. Even in cases of maternal support provision, Afifi, Afifi, Robbins, and Nimah (2013) found, in uncertainty related to being a refugee, uncertainty can "overwhelm the role of the mothers' supportive communication" (p. 495). In grief, disruption in social support between parent and child often leads to "reluctance to seek support for dealing with bereavement-related emotions and stressors" and "lead(s) to maintenance of high levels of grief" or even uncertainty maintenance (Wolchik et al., 2008, p. 599).

Support reduces "uncertainty about the situation, the self, the other, or the relationship," and can be expressed in many ways (Albrecht & Adelman, 1987, p. 19). Although emotional support is studied primarily in grief contexts (Toller, 2011), support can take many forms, including instrumental and informational support (Goldsmith, 2004). To illustrate the need to focus on a variety of forms of support, Gear's (2014) bereaved participants reported that feeling natural, showing a bond and commitment to the bereaved, offering practical help, being authentic, and distracting the bereaved was most helpful in supportive situations. Toller (2011) also found that tangible or practical aid (e.g., preparing meals) and informational support (e.g., advice on coping) were helpful for bereaved parents.

However, not all bereaved individuals receive support, as they may not have a strong support network or they may not receive what they consider to be helpful support (Goldsmith & Albrecht, 2011). Support providers may not provide support entirely and can come across to others as insensitive or threatening (Burleson, 2008; Burleson & MacGeorge, 2002; Coyne, Ellard, & Smith, 1990; Goldsmith, 2004; Holmstrom, Burleson, & Jones, 2005). Consequently, the role of support provider is important, but risky. It requires communication competence to recognize the other person's support needs and to match that type of support, which not all individuals possess (Goldsmith, 2004). For example, although children may prefer using informal social support (Szymanowska, 2014), incompetent support provision may drive bereaved individuals to formal social support groups to cope.

Given individual differences in experiences of uncertainty and stress, it is important to understand the ways parents and children communicatively manage grief-related uncertainty. Previous research suggested interventions should target stressors (Wolchik et al., 2008) and uncertainty (Boelen, 2010) in grief. As a result, we posit that individuals' ability to cope with grief and stress is likely informed by uncertainty management. Because there are commonalities and differences in resilience across the lifespan (Bonanno, 2004), it is necessary to understand how bereaved parents and children manage uncertainty. Thus:

RQ2: How do parents and children manage uncertainty associated with the death of an immediate family member?

METHOD

We conducted one-on-one interviews with key informants (Lindlof & Taylor, 2011) from Fernside, a nonprofit organization in Cincinnati, Ohio, that specializes in child grief support (Fernside, 2016). Fernside provides no-cost services, including grief support groups (for children and parents), community outreach, crisis response, in-school programs, camps, advocacy, and training and consultation (Fernside, 2016). The second author, who was previously affiliated with Fernside's parent organization, contacted the director of Fernside, who granted access. They asked to be named in all publications.

Participants

We used purposive and snowball sampling to recruit our participants. The sample is purposive in the sense that we entered into our research with a desire to speak to individuals who are well versed in the ways in which families cope with stress following death. Based on the initial contact, Fernside's director helped with snowball sampling, as she served "the dual role of interviewee and guide to potential new interviews" (Lindlof & Taylor, 2011, p. 115). This approach resulted in a sample of 19 participants, which included all of Fernside's staff members ($n = 5$) and volunteers ($n = 14$). These informants were uniquely positioned to talk about the stressors and communicative coping for both parents and children. As planners and facilitators of support groups for both parents and children, they receive disclosures regarding the uncertainty and stress surrounding the death that other family and friends may not be privy to knowing. As such, they are trained support providers who are knowledgeable about the ways in which various forms of support (e.g., emotional, tangible) can mitigate uncertainty and stress.

Participants' average age was 49.58 years ($SD = 14.20$ years, range = 23–69 years). They were predominantly white, non-Hispanic ($n = 17$, 89.5%), and predominantly female ($n = 17$, 89.5%). Participants had been involved with Fernside for an average of eight years ($SD = 6.72$ years, range = 0.5–22 years). Two participants (10.5%) were Fernside clients before they began working at or volunteering with the organization. In the Results section, participants are noted by their role (S = staff, V = volunteer) and by the order in which they were interviewed; thus, for example, participant S01 is the first staff member we interviewed.

Data Collection

Data collection took place from February to April 2015. On receiving Institutional Review Board approval, the first two authors collected data via one-on-one, semistructured interviews with staff and volunteers. Participants completed informed consent and a basic demographic questionnaire, and provided verbal consent to be audio recorded. Interviews lasted between 27 and 58 minutes ($M = 41.78$ minutes, $SD = 9.32$ minutes).

The interview protocol was semistructured and consisted of questions that we presented to all participants, including questions about their experience working at/volunteering with Fernside, the role of communication in their work, and the role of communication in the lives of Fernside's clients. It is important to note that we did not limit our questions to specific types or causes of death, but most of the participants discussed examples of parental loss and none of the participants discussed an expected death (i.e., terminal illness). Recognizing the fluid nature of semistructured interview protocols, the first two authors discussed findings following each day of interviews and augmented the protocol in order to probe into these findings in future interviews. We reached saturation in our findings by our eleventh interview. We continued collecting data until we interviewed everyone who had volunteered.

Data Analysis

In line with other qualitative inquiries of family communication processes (e. g., Baxter & Braithwaite, 2006; Baxter, Braithwaite, Bryant, & Wagner, 2004; Baxter et al., 2009), we made sense of our data via the process of analytic coding (Lindlof & Taylor, 2011). Analytic coding "is an inductive process in which a given datum is compared to prior data for its similarity or difference" (Baxter et al., 2004, p. 453). Moreover, analytic coding is iterative; through multiple rounds of analysis, categories are added, removed, and collapsed until they are mutually exclusive and capture all possible explanations.

First, we transcribed the interviews verbatim. The lead author then read through all the transcripts to become familiar with the data and to derive an initial codebook. This first stage of analysis entailed identifying instances of uncertainty and coping/support mentioned by the participants. At this stage, there were three primary themes identified, each with multiple subthemes, and were compiled into a codebook. The first and third authors independently analyzed five randomly selected transcripts to establish interrater reliability. The coders achieved high reliability (Cohen's $\kappa = 0.88$) across the five transcripts in the first round of coding.

Next, all three authors reread the transcripts in their entirety to determine whether there was any overlap between the primary themes or the subthemes. We recognized some overlap, which led us to "[cluster] together similar categories into a coherent analytic set ... [that produced] larger family networks of codes" (Baxter et al., 2009, pp. 471–472). Again, each researcher analyzed the randomly selected transcripts independently to confirm the presence of these refined themes. Following this second round of coding, differences in coding were minor.

We used triangulation to ensure the credibility of our findings (Lindlof & Taylor, 2011). First, we employed a multiple researcher approach in which all authors independently conducted analytic coding on the transcripts, triangulating our analysis through discussion at the conclusion of our coding and identifying representative exemplars for this manuscript (Braithwaite &

Baxter, 2006). Second, we employed member validation procedures by sharing an early version of our findings with Fernside's director and a former Fernside client and asking if the findings seemed accurate with their experiences (Lindlof & Taylor, 2011).

RESULTS

Our research questions inquired about the sources of stress/uncertainty for both parents (RQ1a) and children (RQ1b) following a death in the family, and the subsequent strategies that are implemented to cope with this uncertainty (RQ2).

RQ1a: Parental Uncertainty/Stress

Five themes emerged: parenting logistics, discussing death, behavior changes in the child, privacy/information management, and burdening others.

Parenting logistics. In addition to grieving the loss of a partner emotionally, parents also deal with burdens and responsibilities on a practical level. Factors such as guardianship/childcare, finances, and housing/school changes all represent uncertainties and stresses parents face. Participant V07 summarized this: "I think it totally disrupts their family's real life, whether it was a mother or a father. You know, roles change. Um, just keeping up with chores and, you know, running the household . . . [you are] missing a parent." In some cases, uncertainty about the parenting logistics appear to delay the grief process, as explained by V06:

> For adults who go through a loss, it's probably not until the following year that things really start to hit them. Because they're dealing so much with the day-to-day stuff just to keep things moving – legal issues, job issues, the kid now is down from two parents to one parent.

Discussing death. The next theme was the uncertainty/stress of discussing death with the child(ren). Participant V06 explained that with death often being considered a taboo topic in our society, parents struggle to discuss it: "They may have the capability, having great word capability to express themselves, but they still don't know how to do it." Participant S02 noted that Fernside can help with discussing death by "giv[ing] them the language to help their kids move forward too." Parents clearly are unsure of what and how to communicate about death with a child. The primary goal is to help the child understand the death in a way that allows them to move on, but finding the language to do so is full of uncertainty. This can also be particularly problematic if the child is dealing with behavioral issues, which is the third theme that emerged from the data.

Behavior changes in child. Following a death, parents face uncertainty when a child undergoes behavior changes as a result of his or her grief. Because children might not have the language or cognitive development to express their grief in a productive way, they sometimes respond in ways that are maladaptive. Participant S04 noted, "We get a lot of families who are bringing their kids here because teachers at school have said your child is struggling, quit doing their work, they just aren't themselves, they may be disrespectful and maybe getting in fights." Participant V04 noted that some behavioral issues can escalate: "A lot of the parents are definitely concerned about how their kids are dealing with it emotionally and behaviorally ... kids that have had issues further than just grief, like depression, cutting." These changes can manifest emotionally, such as a child developing depression, or in more overt ways, such as being expelled from school. Parents are thus faced with a child who may behave radically differently and must quickly overcome this uncertainty to figure out how best to help him or her.

Privacy/information management. The fourth theme of parental uncertainty/stress is the negotiation of private information. Participants frequently discussed this struggle, particularly in regard to concealing the cause of death or circumstances surrounding the death. For instance, some parents notified Fernside that they did not want their child to know how the other parent had died (often because it was due to stigmatizing suicide or drug-related circumstances), and were concerned that the child would find out from someone else. Participant V13 described this struggle:

And so not knowing how much the child can handle, so it's almost like it's very hard because you're hiding your feelings when you're hiding the truth, so it's very hard to handle those situations, I'm sure. Because especially little ones, you don't want to scare them and you don't know what they can cope with, so you try to be, you know, like cushion the story.

In addition to wanting to conceal the cause of death, parents may also feel unsure of what information the child can handle. Thus, managing this private information and/or concealing it from children is a source of stress for some parents.

Burdening others. The final theme dealt with parents' perceptions that they were burdening others with their struggles and/or feelings about the death of a loved one. A parent may feel that they are pushing the limit with others, even those who are close to them, by continuously discussing the deceased individual. Participant V04 expressed this sentiment by describing that "even though they still have a really great support system, after a while a lot of them feel like, 'is it appropriate to still bring this up after this much time, are people getting sick of hearing about my problems?'" It is evident that parents undergo uncertainty about whether or not they are burdening others by discussing their issues and also face uncertainty about how much time it should take for them to move on and no longer feel the need to discuss the loss.

RQ1b: Child Uncertainty/Stress

Five themes emerged: others' emotional reaction, mortality, new role in the family, being perceived as different, and privacy/information management.

Others' emotional reaction. The first theme that represented uncertainties/ stresses that children face following the death of a loved one is others' emotional reaction. This is often evidenced through interactions with a parent, in that the child is worried that discussing his or her grief will further complicate how the parent is feeling. For example, Participant V04 noted that "a lot of kids ... don't want to talk to their parents about how grief or how they're feeling in general because they don't want to upset their parent and they say they feel guilty bringing that stress on to the parent." Similarly, S02 said, "if the parent or guardian is grieving too, they don't want to upset them and they'll start to cry and the kids don't want to deal with that." Consequently, children feel uncertain as to how they should communicate with a parent.

Mortality. A second theme that emerged was child uncertainty/stress related to mortality. Following the death of a loved one, children are forced to confront the stark reality that all individuals eventually die, and subsequently question their own and others' mortality. S01 said,

A primary concern for every grieving child and probably even grieving adults, is who is going to die next. And when you are a child if your parent has died you have a lot of fears about what happens if my other parent dies and who is going to take care of me.

This can be a particularly traumatizing issue if the child had a sibling die. One participant said, "This one family, this preteen and his brother are afraid to sleep by themselves because the sister died in her sleep" (Participant V07). Thus, children are left feeling vulnerable and uncertain about their own and other family members' mortality.

New familial role. The third source of uncertainty for children is feeling as though they must adapt and take on a new role in the family. In the same way that parents must fulfill the role(s) previously taken on by the deceased, children are also faced with having to adapt to new roles in their family. This is especially true for older adolescents. Participant V03 expressed:I think the teens, the older kids, feel more like caretakers. They have people telling them, "You're the man of the family now" and crap like that, you know. And they feel more responsible for their little brothers and sisters, whereas the younger kids are kind of still kids. I mean, the older ones are still kids but they don't feel like they are.

Thus, children feel that they must shoulder the responsibility of the deceased parent and help the family by taking care of their sibling(s), or even the remaining parent. This source of stress/uncertainty can also be the result of well-intentioned, but ultimately unhelpful, individuals who tell the child they need to take on new roles.

Being perceived as different. Fourth, children dealt with worrying that others would view them as not "normal," especially by their peers at school. Some children experienced tension at Fernside because of this particular stress – they feel "normal" at Fernside because they are surrounded by those who have also experienced a loss, but their very presence at Fernside or school-based programs enhances awareness that they are there because of something that distinguishes them from their peers. Participant S02 noted:

It's a challenge to get some kids to want to be there because at school they just want to be normal. When you are pulled out of class you're not. People wonder where you are and why you weren't in gym. You are missing something that's going on.

Another participant noted that a benefit of Fernside was putting children with others in similar situations and eliminating the feeling of not "being normal," stating that it "gives the kids a place to feel comfortable and to be around other people, other kids, that have lost a parent and not feel weird or feel like they're getting pitied or anything all the time" (Participant V04). In the face of so much other uncertainty following a death, children crave a sense of normalcy.

Privacy/information management. Our final theme paralleled a theme identified for parents. Children struggled with managing private information regarding a family member's death and knowing what and how to explain what has happened. V02 described one child's need for privacy through deception: "The kid doesn't want to share what happened. I know a few cases where there's been a suicide but they don't share that it's a suicide – they make up something else that happened." Privacy management is particularly problematic because of the prevalence of social media and the tendency for individuals to engage in disclosures that may be viewed as hurtful or offensive, as noted by Participant V04:

Another big thing is now that social media is crazy everywhere, I think that some kids have had problems with people posting things about them or posting things about the death that they felt were inappropriate or made them uncomfortable.

Therefore, some children may feel uncertain about who or what to tell regarding the death because they are unsure of what will be shared with others, either online or offline. Related to the previous theme, children often maintained tight or nonpermeable information and privacy boundaries in an attempt to maintain feelings of normalcy.

RQ2: Coping Strategies

Four themes emerged: informational support, social support, expressive outlets, and negative coping tactics.

Informational support. One way in which individuals cope with death is by obtaining information. Informational support from Fernside was especially salient for parents as they were trying to navigate practical logistics or a child's behavioral issues. Participant S02 said:

I think it is our responsibility to provide information. We can't make them use it and we can't make them tell their kids but we can say this is what we've seen over the years and this is why we think it is important.

Participant S01 echoes this: "So we are really trying to impart knowledge and information, and specific help, to our parents and guardians." Fernside staff can offer recommendations to parents who are struggling based on past experience. This can range from giving advice to offering recommendations for other resources, such as child psychologists or doctors. However, advice and informational support can also be obtained from support group members, either other parents or other children. Participant V04 illustrated that often it is the other children in the group who can offer the best advice:

So a girl in the group is like "your loved one would really want you to be strong and we know it's really hard, but what if you tried to find a hobby you like, or what if you tried to do what you used to do with them with someone else, and tried to be brave for the rest of your family."

Participant V08 focused more on the children as information seekers, stating, "They're just, some of the questions they ask—we always give them the opportunity to ask questions. Some of them come out with some real good questions."

Social support. Social support also helped the bereaved to manage uncertainty and stress. Participant S02 even noted that at its core, Fernside is a "peer support agency," meaning that individuals often gain support from fellow group members, as seen in this observation from V05, "You can really visibly see a difference how the older members take on empathy and sympathy for the newer members." This type of support is further exemplified in Participant V04's excerpt about the children:

I love seeing the kids interact with each other. They're so supportive of each other, it's amazing. I work with the teenagers so they kind of open up more and have more in depth discussion I would think. So I think the best part is being able to guide the conversation, but they'll give each other advice on what to do in certain situations and reaffirm that "we're all here for you" and it's just a really neat thing to see.

It is clear from this excerpt that many times it is the other group members who will provide the best social and emotional support.

Expressive outlets. One way individuals, primarily the children, can cope with uncertainty/stress is through creative outlets. Fernside emphasizes activities that incorporate art as a form of therapy because it helps many of the children express their grief and feelings for the deceased. Participant V04 discussed one of the art-based activities and its benefits:

I know one time we made decorative vases where you could put a candle in and we just sat around and while they were doing it we had a discussion . . . I think sometimes it's easier too if you don't have to be sitting there actively making eye contact with everybody or feel pressure to talk.

Having the children actively engage in something can facilitate a more laid-back discussion to help them cope with the uncertainty or stressors they are experiencing. Expressive outlets can also be beneficial in getting children to open up and get in touch with their feelings if they are having trouble doing so with their parents.

Negative coping strategies. The final theme was the use of negative uncertainty management strategies. These strategies can range from avoiding topics and conversation, to more serious and destructive tactics, such as anger, blame, and self-harm. For instance, Participant V03 noted that her group members will discuss how their parent does not want to discuss the death and that they are busy with other things. "But, they'll say, 'My mom doesn't want to deal with it. She's busy at work,' or 'She has other things to do. I don't usually talk to her. She won't understand anyway.'" Thus, communication about the death is avoided and perceived negatively by the child striving to manage uncertainty and looking to the parent as a facilitator in that process. Another participant discussed a situation in which a child was cutting herself, likely because it was the only way she knew how to handle her grief. "Everybody knew this girl was cutting herself—and, I mean she told us that. That was a little deeper than what we're able to handle here" (Participant V07). Participant V08 felt that although anger was normal, it could be expressed negatively:

Anger, because anger is very much a part of grieving, very much. So, it isn't a mistake. It's a, it's an outlet, maybe, that possibly parents, in their anger, um, take it out on the kids, or transfer it to the kids. And that's not their fault. That's nobody's fault. It's just what anger does.

DISCUSSION

This study examined the sources of uncertainty experienced by both parents and children who experienced the death of a loved one and how they managed the stress that often accompanies this uncertainty. While previous research has examined sources of uncertainty and stress for parents, much less attention has been afforded to grieving children. Our research reveals that although parents and children do experience some of the same uncertainties (e.g., privacy management, changing roles), they also have different uncertainties and stressors to manage (e.g., parents are concerned about parenting logistics, whereas children are worried about their own or others' mortality). Each of the participants in our sample reported on families that had sought professional support to deal with these uncertainties, noting both adaptive uncertainty management strategies (e.g., informational support, emotional peer support) and maladaptive uncertainty management strategies (e.g., avoidance, self-harm). The findings have significant implications for communication theory and for the practical approaches to facilitating grief in bereaved parents and children.

THEORETICAL IMPLICATIONS

Uncertainty management theory. Our study was framed using uncertainty management theory (UMT). Indeed, the uncertainties experienced by parents were a source of stress for the parents. In some cases, it is impossible to reduce or eliminate uncertainty in a permanent situation such as death. Instead, adapting to the uncertainty that now existed seemed more prevalent and consistent with UMT. For example, adapting to a new role in the family does not reduce the uncertainty. Novelty in the situation, the new way of life, or in discussing a taboo topic such as death with children can be a source of uncertainty. However, how individuals choose to adapt to that uncertainty can go a long way toward how they cope with it (Mishel, 1988).

Our findings regarding strategies that are typically considered maladaptive (e.g., avoidance) is an important theoretical discussion. Wolchik et al. (2008) identified negative strategies for dealing with death including alcohol abuse, violence, and anger. These strategies may similarly be used to manage uncertainty, much like the experience of depression, and the cutting and avoidance strategies identified by our participants. Especially relevant to uncertainty management is avoidance. Bonnano (2004) calls this *repressive coping*, or an individual's attempt to avoid unpleasant thoughts, emotions, and memories. Howell et al. (2015) found that avoidant coping significantly predicted maladaptive functioning in children, and Santacroce (2003) argued that avoidance is a sign of PTSD in uncertain parents. However, although avoidance may appear to be a maladaptive uncertainty management strategy,

Bonnano (2004) found that it can also foster adaptation in extreme circumstances and lead to resilience and eventual recovery in the long term. This avoidance, and the theme regarding uncertainty about discussing death, is also consistent with DeLorme and Huh's (2009) finding that individuals experience uncertainty when they feel insecure about the knowledge they need, when details are complex, or when they are directly affected. In this case, parents are uncertain because they may feel insecure about discussing death with their child, especially in complex death situations (e.g., overdose) in which both parties are affected.

Communication privacy management. Although not included as an a priori framework, communication privacy management (CPM) emerged as a significant theme for both children and parents, and is consistent with findings by Toller and McBride's (2013) study. CPM focuses on "how people regulate the disclosure or concealment of private information" (Petronio, 2007, p. 219), which is particularly salient to parents. Parents struggled with what information to share with their children, often motivated by the need to protect children from harsh realities about causes of death, stigma, and unflattering views of the deceased. Parents avoided or intentionally deceived their children about the death. However, this decision to erect solid boundaries around the information may be detrimental to the relationship. For example, Thomas and Booth-Butterfield (1995) found in their study on divorce that when children felt deceived, they reported lower self-esteem and lower communication satisfaction. Maintaining privacy around the issue and potentially risking the information being leaked to the child from another source (i.e., boundary turbulence) creates a situation in which the uncertainty is pervasive and maintained, rather than reduced, for the parent.

Children struggled with both inner (i.e., parent) and outer (i.e., peers) privacy boundaries (Petronio, 2013). Even if the child chose to have permeable boundaries with the parents, the communication was not always reciprocated. Thus, boundary coordination within the parent–child relationship is critical. Interestingly, and only mentioned by our participants for the children, communication privacy management around a traumatic personal event has changed drastically with the introduction of social media, which in many cases threatens privacy control (Petronio, 2013). Although some research suggests that creating a memorial page on Facebook or posting positive memories of a deceased individual may foster positive coping (Carroll & Landry, 2010), this may be the case only when the information is intentionally co-owned with those who are directly affected (e.g., bereaved spouse or child). Otherwise, the sharing of information on social media may be a source of privacy turbulence that adds to the uncertainty and stress.

PRACTICAL IMPLICATIONS

Practically, understanding the sources of uncertainty that result in stress for parents provides a springboard for which support can be tailored. The support matching hypothesis suggests that support providers should provide the type of support the recipient wants to receive rather than the type of support they want to provide (Goldsmith, 2004). Therefore, when practical parenting logistics are the primary concern, parents need to receive practical support rather than emotional or informational support. The idea of tailored support will likely also shape where support is sought. A support group is meant to "enable persons to gain support from others having a similar loss, to reduce isolation, to challenge assumptions about grief and loss, and to provide an opportunity for grieving persona to give support to others" in a safe environment where the griever may engage in greater sensemaking (Supiano, 2012, p. 500). Thus, a support group, such as those facilitated at Fernside or other similar organizations, is an outlet where desired support can be received.

Similarly, parents and other adults should not assume that children want to receive the same types of support that they would like to receive when coping with a loss. To that end, understanding the sources of uncertainty for children may provide parents with specific talking points for discussing death and grief with their children. This information is also helpful for schools that may have children enrolled who have experienced familial loss. Although well intentioned in providing support to the grieving student, schools may be unaware of the harm they may cause by singling students out and threatening their need to feel "normal." By addressing their concerns in open and honest conversation, the children are more likely to receive the reassurance they are seeking (Bosticco & Thompson, 2005; Halne, Ayers, Sandler, & Wolchik, 2008; Rossetto, 2015; Toller & McBride, 2013) and potentially avoid additional uncertainties and stressors.

LIMITATIONS AND FUTURE DIRECTIONS

Although our data were collected from key informants with years of collective experience and observations, this limits the data to the perspective of an outsider. Future research should continue to explore the uncertainty and respective information management strategies associated with death and grief for all family members who are affected. Second, this sample was homogeneous and lacked cultural perspective; it was primarily composed of Caucasian/white females, although this was not the demographic of the clientele at Fernside. Cultural differences exist in grief, uncertainty tolerance, stigma, and supportive communication, and should be a focus of future research on this topic. Finally, information management and privacy, especially in a digital age, emerged as the primary theme of convergence for both parents and children. Understanding how social media may create uncertainty, but also create an outlet for managing uncertainty, is an important area of future research.

CONCLUSION

Taken together, the loss of an immediate family member is a traumatic event that can induce uncertainty and stress. This uncertainty and stress, along with the uncertainty management strategies used to cope, characterize the grieving process and outcomes of that process, whether maladaptive or adaptive. Importantly, although there are some common sources of uncertainty, these sources of uncertainty and stress vary widely across the lifespan, even within a single family unit grieving the loss of the same person. This context is a ripe arena for the application of communication theory (e.g., uncertainty management, communication privacy management) to better understand these phenomena and translate the research to help all individuals, whether parents or children, to be more resilient in this life-altering event.

REFERENCES

Afifi, W. A., Afifi, T. D., Robbins, S., & Nimah, N. (2013). The relative impacts of uncertainty and mothers' communication on hopelessness among Palestinian refugee youth. *American Journal of Orthopsychiatry, 83*, 495–504. doi: 10.1111/ajop.12051

Afifi, T. D., Davis, S., Merrill, A. F., Coveleski, S., Denes, A., & Afifi, W. A. (2015). In the wake of the great recession: Economic uncertainty, communication, and biological stress responses in families. *Human Communication Research, 41*, 268–302. doi: 10.1111/hcre.12048

Albrecht, T. L., & Adelman, M. B. (1987). *Communicating social support.* Newbury Park, CA: SAGE.

Avelin, P., Gyllenswärd, G., Erlandsson, K., & Rådestad, I. (2014). Adolescents' experiences of having a stillborn half-sibling. *Death Studies, 38*, 557–562. doi: 10.1080/07481187.2013.809034

Babrow, A. S., & Kline, K. N. (2000). From "reducing" to "coping with" uncertainty: Reconceptualizing the central challenge in breast self-exams. *Social Science & Medicine, 51*, 1805–1816. doi: 10.1016/S0277-9536(00)0012-X

Baxter, L. A., & Braithwaite, D. O. (2006). "You're my parent but you're not": Dialectical tensions in stepchildren's perceptions about communicating with the nonresidential parent. *Journal of Applied Communication Research, 34*, 30–48. doi: 10.1080/00909880500420200

Baxter, L. A., Braithwaite, D. O., Bryant, L., & Wagner, A. (2004). Stepchildren's perceptions of the contradictions in communication with stepparents. *Journal of Social and Personal Relationships, 21*, 447–467. doi: 10.1177/0265407504404481

Baxter, L. A., Braithwaite, D. O., Koenig Kellas, J., LeClair-Underberg, C., Normand, E. L., Routsong, T., & Thatcher, M. (2009). Empty ritual: Young-adult stepchildren's perceptions of the remarriage ceremony. *Journal of Social and Personal Relationships, 26*, 467–487. doi: 10.1177/02654070509350872

Berger, C. R. (Ed.). (1979). *Beyond initial interactions*: Oxford: Basil Blackwell.

Berger, C. R., & Calabrese, R. J. (1975). Some explorations in initial interaction and beyond: Toward a theory of interpersonal communication. *Human Communication Research, 1*, 99–112. doi: 10.1111/j.1468–2658.1975.tb00258.x

Biank, N. M., & Werner-Lin, A. (2011). Growing up with grief: Revisiting the death of parent over the life course. *Omega: Journal of Death and Dying, 63*, 271–290. doi: 10.2190/OM.63.3.e

Boelen, P. (2010). Intolerance of uncertainty and emotional distress following the death of a loved one. *Anxiety, Stress, & Coping, 23*, 471–478. doi: 10.1080/10615800903494135

Bonanno, G. A. (2004). Loss, trauma and human resilience: Have we underestimated the human capacity to thrive after extremely aversive events? *American Psychologist, 59*, 20–28. doi: 10.1037/0003-066X.59.1.20

Bonanno, G. A., Wortman, C. B., Lehman, D. R., Tweed, R. G., Haring, M., Sonnega, J., . . . Nesse, R. M. (2002). Resilience to loss and chronic grief: A prospective study from preloss to 18-months postloss. *Journal of Personality and Social Psychology, 83*, 1150–1164. doi: 10.1037/0022-3514.83.5.1150

Bosticco, C., & Thompson, T. (2005). The role of communication and story telling in the family grieving system. *Journal of Family Communication, 5*, 255–278. doi: 10.1207/s15327698jfc0504_2

Bradac, J. J. (2001). Theory comparison: Uncertainty reduction, problematic integration, uncertainty management, and other curious constructs. *Journal of Communication, 51*, 456–476. doi: 10.1111/j.1460-2466.2001.tb02891.x

Brashers, D. E. (2001). Communication and uncertainty management. *Journal of Communication, 51*, 477–497. doi: 10.1111/j.1460-2466.2001.tb02892.x

Brashers, D. E. (2007). Theory of communication and uncertainty management. In B. B. Whaley & W. Samter (Eds.), *Explaining communication: Contemporary theories and exemplars* (pp. 223–242). Mahwah, NJ: Lawrence Erlbaum Associates.

Brashers, D. E., Neidig, J. L., Haas, S. M., Dobbs, L. K., Cardillo, L. W., & Russell, J. A. (2000). Communication in the management of uncertainty: The case of persons living with HIV or AIDS. *Communication Monographs, 67*, 63–84. doi: 10.1080/03637750009376495

Burleson, B. R. (2008). What counts as effective emotional support? In M. T. Motley (Ed.), *Studies in applied interpersonal communication* (pp. 207–227). Thousand Oaks, CA: SAGE.

Burleson, B. R., & MacGeorge, E. L. (2002). Supportive communication. In M. L. Knapp & J. A. Daly (Eds.), *Handbook of interpersonal communication* (pp. 374–424). Thousand Oaks, CA: SAGE.

Carroll, B., & Landry, K. (2010). Logging on and letting out: Using social online networks to grieve and mourn. *Bulletin of Science, Technology, and Science, 30*, 341–349. doi: 10.1177/0270467610380006

Casarett, D., Kutner, J. S., & Abraham J. (2001). Life after death: A practical approach to grief and bereavement. *Annals of Internal Medicine, 134*, 208–215. doi: 10.7326/0003-4819-134-3-200102060-00012

Chiriboga, D. A., Brierton, P., Krystal, S., & Pierce, R. C. (1982). Antecedents of symptom expression during marital separation. *Journal of Clinical Psychology, 38*, 732–741. doi: 10.1002/1097–4679(198210)38:4<732::AID-JCLP2270380407>3.0.CO;2-3

Cohen, S., & Willis, T. A. (1985). Stress, social support, and the buffering hypothesis. *Psychological Bulletin, 98*, 310–357. doi: 10.1037/0003-066X.59.1.29

Coyne, J. C., Ellard, J. H., & Smith, D. A. (1990). Social support, interdependence, and the dilemmas of helping. In B. R. Sarason, I. G. Sarason, & G. R. Pierce (Eds.), *Social support: An interactional view* (pp. 129–149). New York, NY: John Wiley & Sons.

DeLorme, D. E., & Huh, J. (2009). Seniors' uncertainty management of direct-to-consumer prescription drug advertising usefulness. *Health Communication, 24*, 494–503. doi: 10.1080/10410230903104277

Fernside. (2016). Retrieved on June 9, 2016 from www.fernside.org/.

Floyd, K., Mikkelson, A. C., & Hesse, C. (2008). *The biology of human communication.* Mason, OH: Cengage Learning.

Gear, R. (2014). Bereaved parents' perspectives on informal social support: "What worked for you?" *Journal of Loss and Trauma, 19*, 173–188. doi: 10.1080/15325024.2013.763548

Goldsmith, D. J. (2001). A normative approach to the study of uncertainty and communication. *Journal of Communication, 51*, 514–533. doi: 10.1111/j.1460-2466.2001.tb02894.x

Goldsmith, D. J. (2004). *Communicating social support.* Cambridge: Cambridge University Press.

Goldsmith, D. J., & Albrecht, T. L. (2011). Social support, social networks, and health. In T. L. Thompson, R. L. Parrott, & J. F. Nussbaum (Eds.), *The Routledge handbook of health communication* (2nd ed., pp. 335–348). New York, NY: Routledge.

Greco, V., & Roger, D. (2003). Uncertainty, stress, and health. *Personality and Individual Differences, 34*, 1057–1068. doi: 10.1016/S0191-8869(02)00091-0

Halne, R. A., Ayers, T. S., Sandler, I. N., & Wolchik, S. A. (2008). Evidence-based practices for parentally bereaved children and their families. *Professional Psychology: Research and Practice, 39*, 113–121. doi: 10.1037/0735-7028.39.2.113

Hastings, S. O. (2000). Self-disclosure and identity management in bereaved parents. *Communication Studies, 51*, 352–371. doi: 10.1080/10510970009388531

Holmstrom, A. J., Burleson, B. R., & Jones, S. M. (2005). Some consequences for helpers who deliver "cold comfort": Why it's worse for women than men to be inept when providing emotional support. *Sex Roles, 53*, 153–172. doi: 10.1007/s11199-005-5676-4

Howell, K. H., Shapiro, D. N., Layne, C. M., & Kaplow, J. B. (2015). Individual and psychosocial mechanisms of adaptive functioning in parentally bereaved children. *Death Studies, 39*, 296–306. doi: 10.1080/07481187.2014.951497

Kaplow, J. B., Layne, C. M., Saltzman, W. R., Cozza, S. J., & Pynoos, R. S. (2013). Using multidimensional grief theory to explore the effects of deployment, reintegration, and death on military youth and families. *Clinical Child & Family Psychology Review, 16*, 322–340. doi: 10.1007/s10567-013-0143-1

Lindlof, T. R., & Taylor, B. C. (2011). *Qualitative communication research methods* (3rd ed.). Thousand Oaks, CA: SAGE.

Mancini, A., & Bonanno, G. (2009). Predictors and parameters of resilience to loss: Toward an individual differences model. *Journal of Personality, 77*, 1806–1831. doi: 10.1111/j.1467-6494.2009.00601.x

Mishel, M. H. (1988). Uncertainty in illness. *IMAGE: Journal of Nursing Scholarship, 20*, 225–231. doi: 10.1111/j.1547-5069.1988.tb00082.x

Mishel, M. H., & Braden, C. J. (1987). Uncertainty. *Western Journal of Nursing Research, 9*, 43–57. doi: 10.1177/019394598700900106

Monat, A., Averill, J. R., & Lazarus, R. S. (1972). Anticipatory stress and coping reactions under various conditions of uncertainty. *Journal of Personality and Social Psychology, 24,* 237–253. doi: 10.1037/h0033297

Nader, K. O., & Layne, C. M. (2009). Maladaptive grieving in children and adolescents: Discovering developmentally linked differences in the manifestation of grief. *Traumatic Stress Points, 23,* 12–15.

Petronio, S. (2007). Translational research endeavors and the practices of communication privacy management. *Journal of Applied Communication Research, 35,* 218–222. doi: 10.1080/00909880701422443

Petronio, S. (2013). Brief status report on communication privacy management theory. *Journal of Family Communication, 13,* 6–14. doi: 10.1080/15267431.2013.743426

Priem, J. S., & Solomon, D. H. (2011). Relational uncertainty and cortisol responses to hurtful and supportive messages from a dating partner. *Personal Relationships, 18,* 198–223. doi: 10.1111/j.1475–6811.2011.01353.x

Reif, L. V., Patton, M. J., & Gold, P. B. (1995). Bereavement, stress, and social support in members of a self-help group. *Journal of Community Psychology, 23,* 292–306. doi: 10.1002/1520–6629(199510)23:4<292::AID-JCOP2290230403>3.0.CO;2-Y

Rossetto, K. R. (2015). Developing conceptual definitions and theoretical models of coping in military families during deployment. *Journal of Family Communication, 15,* 249–268. doi: 10.1080/15267431.2015.1043737

Santacroce, S. J. (2003). Parental uncertainty and posttraumatic stress in serious childhood illness. *Journal of Nursing Scholarship, 35,* 45–51. doi: 10.1111/j.1547–5069.2003.00045.x

Shapiro, D. N., Howell, K. H., & Kaplow, J. B. (2014). Associations among mother–child communication quality, childhood maladaptive grief, and depressive symptoms. *Death Studies, 38,* 172–178. doi: 10.1080/07481187.2012.738771

Supiano, K. P. (2012). Sense-making in suicide survivorship: A qualitative study on the effect of grief support group participation. *Journal of Loss and Trauma, 17,* 489–507. doi: 10.1080/15325024.2012.665298

Szymanowska, J. (2014). A child in the face of a parent's death: Aspects of children's loneliness. *Progress in Health Sciences, 4,* 118–123.

Thomas, C. E., & Booth-Butterfield, M. (1995). Perceptions of deception, divorce disclosures, and communication satisfaction with parents. *Western Journal of Communication, 59,* 228–245. doi: 10.1080/10570319509374519

Toller, P. W. (2011). Bereaved parents' experiences of supportive and unsupportive communication. *Southern Communication Journal, 76,* 17–34. doi: 10.1080/10417940903159393

Toller, P. W., & McBride, M. C. (2013). Enacting privacy rules and protecting disclosure recipients: Parents' communication with children following the death of a family member. *Journal of Family Communication, 13,* 32–45. doi: 10.1080/15267431.2012.742091

Wolchik, S. A., Yue, M., Tein, J., Sandler, I. N., & Ayers, T. S. (2008). Parentally bereaved children's grief: Self-system beliefs as mediators of the relations between grief and stressors and caregiver-child relationship quality. *Death Studies, 32,* 597–620. doi: 10.1080/07481180802215551

PART IV

SUPPORT AND CAREGIVING IN HEALTH AND
RELATIONSHIPS

11

Family Reactions to Partner Stress and Depression in Same-Sex Couples: A Dyadic Examination of the Moderating Effects of Dyadic Coping

CHUN TAO, ASHLEY K. RANDALL, AND CASEY J. TOTENHAGEN

Sexual minority individuals – those who identify as gay, lesbian, and bisexual – are at a higher risk for mental health issues, including greater symptoms of mood disorders and substance use behaviors, compared to heterosexual individuals (for a review, see King et al., 2008). Minority stress theory (Meyer, 1995, 2003) posits that discrepancies in sexual minorities' well-being are associated with experiences of unique stress from their sexual orientation, such as discrimination from coworkers, friends, or family (Lewis, Derlega, Berndt, Morris, & Rose, 2001; Rostosky, Riggle, Gray, & Hatton, 2007). Stress due to individuals' family reactions to their disclosure of sexual orientation or introduction of a same-sex partner may be particularly challenging. For example, they may face conflicts with their parents or perceive lack of support from parents, which have been found to be directly related to greater psychological distress and lower levels of well-being across sexual minority individuals of different age groups (e.g., Freitas, D'Augelli, Coimbra, & Fontaine, 2016; Graham & Barnow, 2013). Moreover, as sexual minority individuals introduce and bring their same-sex partner around family, additive stress can originate from their families' reactions to their partner (hereafter referred to as "family reactions to partner stress"), such as complete rejection or internal denial (Béres-Deák, 2011), which is linked with greater symptoms of depression (Lewis et al., 2001).

Romantic partners are known to share their emotional experiences owing to their interdependence (Kelley, 1979; Schoebi & Randall, 2015; Thibaut & Kelley, 1959). Subsequently, when individuals experience stress as a result of family reactions to their partner, this stress may influence both their own symptoms (actor effect) as well as their partner's symptoms (partner effect) of depression (Papp, Kouros, & Cummings, 2010). Romantic partners can, however, cope together to help (or not) the partner experiencing stress (dyadic coping [DC]; Bodenmann, 1995, 2000, 2005). Specifically, partners can offer empathy and understanding (emotion-focused supportive DC) and provide new perspectives to help each other see the experience of stress from a new light (problem-focused supportive DC; Bodenmann, 2005). Conversely, they may also be reluctant to support or may invalidate each other's experiences (negative DC; Bodenmann, 2005).

Despite the abundance of research findings on actor and partner effects of stress (e.g., Neff & Karney, 2007; Totenhagen, Butler, & Ridley, 2012) as well as the moderating effects of partner DC behaviors in heterosexual couples (e.g., Falconier, Jackson, Hilpert, & Bodenmann, 2015; Falconier, Randall & Bodenmann, 2016), there remains a dearth of literature specifically examining how partners' use of DC strategies may mitigate (or exacerbate) stress associated with family reactions to one's partner (for exceptions see Randall, Tao, Totenhagen, Walsh, & Cooper, 2017; Randall, Totenhagen, Walsh, Adams, & Tao, 2017), and furthermore how this may be associated with reported symptoms of depression. To address this gap in the literature, we adopted a dyadic approach to examine both actor and partner effects of family reactions to partner stress and their association with depressive symptoms, as moderated by partner DC behaviors.

FAMILY REACTIONS TO A SAME-SEX PARTNER

The "coming out" process, or the act of disclosing one's sexual orientation to others, is important in the identity development of sexual minority individuals but can be stressful (Heatherington & Lavner, 2008). Although some members of sexual minorities may choose to "stay in the closet" or separate their social circles of those they have "come out" to from those to whom they have not, it becomes more difficult to conceal their sexual orientation from their family when they enter into a same-sex relationship (Béres-Deák, 2011). In fact, coming out to one's family may bring stress to both the individual and the family, as the family may not be aware of the individual's sexual orientation (Crosbie-Burnett, Foster, Murray, & Bowen, 1996). Individuals may feel pressure to facilitate harmonious interactions when their same-sex partner and family are in the same place, such as attending the same family event (Lewis et al., 2001). In a semistructured interview study of 21 same-sex couples in Hungary, Béres-Deák (2011) found families' reactions toward individuals' same-sex partners could range from direct rejection, creation of a "transparent closet" (e.g., ignoring the same-sex relationship, not talking to others about the relationship, being afraid of being blamed for the individual's sexual orientation), to "unconditional acceptance" (e.g., integrating the same-sex partner into the family as kin). Sexual minorities may feel discriminated against when their family does not acknowledge their partner, especially when their family acknowledges siblings' opposite-sex partners (Béres-Deák, 2011). Extant research has pointed to a positive association between family reactions to partner stress and symptoms of depression (Lewis et al., 2001).

Moreover, those in a same-sex relationship have also reported feeling unsupported when their partner concealed their relationship to their family or when their partner's family did not accept them (Béres-Deák, 2011). These findings suggest that experiences of family reactions to partner stress can influence not only sexual minority individuals' own but also their same-sex partners' well-being (stress crossover; Neff & Karney, 2007; Totenhagen, Randall, Cooper, Tao, & Walsh, 2017).

THE SYSTEMIC TRANSACTIONAL MODEL AND ROLE OF DYADIC COPING

The systemic transactional model (STM) of stress and coping (Bodenmann, 1995, 2005; Bodenmann, Randall, & Falconier, 2016) posits that partners' individual experiences of stress can be considered systemic insomuch as the feelings associated with stress can spill over into one's romantic relationship and cross over from one partner to the other (Buck & Neff, 2012; Totenhagen et al., 2017), which is based on interdependence theory (Kelley, 1979; Thibaut & Kelley, 1959). As an example, Pat's experience of stress stemming from her family's negative reactions to her partner becomes shared by her partner, Jamie. This is especially true when Pat communicates this stress to Jamie directly (i.e., verbally expressing the stress associated with this event) or nonverbally (i.e., disengaging from interaction with one's partner as a response to the stress). As Pat has expressed this stress, Jamie will then appraise the situation and respond accordingly (e.g., engage in DC). Partners' coping responses to stress can take the form of either positive or negative DC. Positive forms of DC include emotion-focused supportive DC (e.g., Jamie providing Pat empathy and understanding) and problem-focused supportive DC (e.g., Jamie helping Pat problem-solve about the current stressor). Negative forms of DC include displaying hostile or ambivalent behaviors, wherein the partner is reluctant to give support or does so unwillingly (e.g., Jamie invalidating the stress Pat communicates).

Robust empirical evidence has shown associations for both types of positive and negative DC with relational outcomes in the expected directions, across types of stress and cultures (for a review, see Falconier et al., 2015). Most research to date, however, has examined these associations among heterosexual couples, leaving unanswered questions regarding the use and beneficial (or detrimental) effects of same-sex partners' engagement in DC (for exceptions see Randall et al., 2017a, 2017b; Weaver, 2014). For example, Weaver (2014) examined the effects of gender and sexual orientation on individuals' perceived sexual minority stress, DC, and relationship satisfaction, yet did not further examine the association between sexual minority stress and relationship satisfaction, or the potential moderating effects of DC. Specific types of sexual minority stress (e.g., work discrimination, family reactions to partner) may exert differential effects on individual and relationship well-being (Lewis et al., 2001). Therefore, it is important to examine whether individuals' perceived family reactions to partner stress may be positively associated with their reported depressive symptoms, and moreover, their partner's reported depressive symptoms.

Similarly, more light can be shed on the specific types of DC that can moderate the association between family reactions to partner stress and depression. Notably, Bodenmann (2008) differentiated the types of DC not only by effectiveness (positive vs. negative) but also by agent of perceptions: perceived partner DC can be defined as an individual's perceptions of the DC behaviors of their partner (e.g., Pat perceived empathy from Jamie), whereas partner reported DC delineates a partner's perceptions of their DC behaviors toward the individual (e.g., Jamie reported that she showed empathy toward Pat). Although reports from the individual who demonstrates the DC behaviors (i.e., partner reported DC) and from the partner who perceives them (perceived partner DC) are often moderately correlated (Randall et al., 2015), comparable examinations of DC from both perspectives can offer insights into the type of DC that exerts a more salient moderating effect. In other words, it becomes possible to determine if the level of emotion-focused support (e.g., empathy and understanding) Pat perceives, as opposed to what Jamie thinks she offers, is more important in helping Pat cope with her stress. Although existing research on DC has focused predominantly on perceived partner DC (e.g., Landis, Peter-Wight, Martin, & Bodenmann, 2013; Randall et al., 2017a, 2017b; Regan et al., 2014), we aim to advance the literature by examining how partner reported DC moderates the (negative) association between stress and reported symptoms of depression, and whether moderating effects of partner reported DC are similar to that of perceived partner DC in this study.

GENDER DIERENCES IN FAMILY REACTIONS TO PARTNER STRESS, DEPRESSION, AND THE ROLE OF DYADIC COPING

Existing literature suggests potential gender differences in sexual minority individuals' experiences of stress, depression, and the effects of DC. Men and women from sexual minorities may experience stress differently (e.g., McCabe, Bostwick, Hughes, West, & Boyd, 2010) – for example, women perceive more general sexual minority stress than do men (Lewis et al., 2001; Weaver, 2014). As such, gender differences may exist regarding how men and women perceive and respond to stress associated with their family's reactions to their partner. In fact, women were found to report higher levels of family reactions to partner stress than men in a sample of 459 men and 333 women from sexual minorities (Lewis et al., 2001). Further, there have been mixed findings on gender differences in the prevalence of depression in men and women from sexual minorities. One study found no gender differences (King et al., 2008), while another national survey (Gilman et al., 2001) found that women, but not men, who had had a same-sex partner presented a higher 12-month prevalence of mood disorders (e.g., major depression) in comparison to women who had been only in heterosexual relationships. In another study on heterosexual couples' minority stress from immigration, the buffering effect of partner supportive DC was evidenced only for female but not male partners (Falconier, Nussbeck, & Bodenmann, 2013). These findings suggest that individuals from sexual minorities may respond to partner DC for one form of minority stressor differently across gender.

Although several of these studies (Falconier et al., 2013; Gilman et al., 2001; Lewis et al., 2001) found effects specific to, or stronger in, women as opposed to men, it is unclear whether family reactions to partner stress, and moderating effects of DC, operate differently for men and women in same-sex relationships. Thus, gender is examined as a moderator in this study.

PRESENT STUDY

Individuals' experiences of stress from their family's reaction to their same-sex partner can be negatively associated with their well-being (Béres-Deák, 2011; Lewis et al., 2001). This association may be moderated by their partner's engagement in DC, a well-documented buffering (or exacerbating) factor in relationship research among heterosexual couples (Falconier et al., 2015). The goal of the present study was to build upon existing literature and examine the association between family reactions to partner stress and reported symptoms of depression for individuals in a same-sex relationship. Both actor and partner family reactions to partner stress were expected to be positively associated with individuals' depressive symptoms (H1). Furthermore, we examined whether DC, assessed by partner reported DC (e.g., Jamie's report of her DC toward Pat) and perceived partner DC (e.g., Pat's perceptions of DC from Jamie), moderates this association. We hypothesized that both perceived partner and partner reported *positive* DC (emotion- and problem-focused supportive DC) would weaken the positive association between family reactions to partner stress and their own (i.e., actor effects) as well as their partner's (i.e., partner effects) depressive symptoms, whereas partner reported and perceived partner *negative* DC would strengthen these associations (for a proposed model, see Figure 11.1; H2). Lastly, we explored potential gender differences in the associations between family reactions to partner stress, DC, and depression (RQ1).

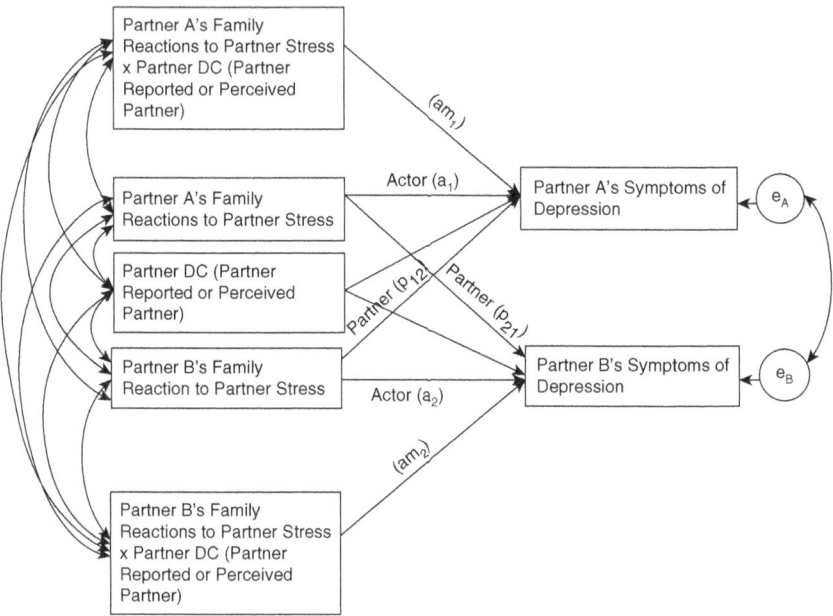

FIGURE 11.1   Hypothesized model.

METHOD

Procedure

These data were part of a larger project using the vulnerability–stress–adaptation model (Karney & Bradbury, 1995) and the STM (Bodenmann, 1995, 2005) to better understand the unique stressors, vulnerabilities, and resiliencies in same-sex couples. Same-sex couples were recruited from two states in the United States – one in the Southwest (Arizona) and one in the Southeast (Alabama). The research teams posted recruitment flyers in the respective communities, on social media, and disseminated recruitment to local LGBT organizations. Interested couples contacted the respective research team and were screened to ensure they met the eligibility criteria: whether they and their partner were adults, both willing to participate, and had been in a relationship together for at least two months. This choice of the minimum relationship length was based on prior research (e.g., Butler, Young, & Randall, 2010; Totenhagen, Curran, Serido, & Butler, 2013) that ensures partners had time to establish interdependence. Each partner was instructed to independently respond to an online survey that included a demographic questionnaire and measures related to the present study. Participants who completed all portions of the study were compensated up to $30 per person ($60 per couple) for their time. Duplicate entries were deleted and only couples in which both partners completed the measures of interest were retained for the present analyses.

Participants

Ninety-five same-sex couples participated (n = 21 male and 32 female dyads from Arizona; n = 10 male and 32 female dyads from Alabama). Participants ranged in age from 18 to 61 years old (M = 33.80, SD = 9.92). A majority of the sample self-identified as non-Hispanic white American (73.7%), followed by Hispanic or Latino(a) American (10.5%), Asian American (5.3%), African American (4.2%), Native American (3.2%), and other (3.2%). Most participants identified as lesbian (48.4%) or gay (33.7%), with 11.6% identifying as bisexual, 4.7% as queer, and 1.6% as pansexual. Participants were well educated, with 30.5% having completed a graduate degree, 27.9% an undergraduate degree, and 33.2% with some college education at the time of their participation.

Relationship length ranged from 2.5 months to 35 years (M = 5.33 years, SD = 5.82 years). Approximately half of the couples reported being in a committed relationship and living together with their partner (49.5%), followed by 19.7% engaged and living together, 18.1% married, and 11.7% in a committed relationship but not currently living together. Most couples reported not having children (79.4%), while 16.4% had children living with them full time and another 4.2% had children living with them part time.

Our sample is similar to the national population of married and unmarried same-sex couples regarding their racial makeup, educational background, and whether they had children in the household at the time of recruitment (U.S. Census Bureau, 2013).

MEASURES

Family reactions to partner stress. We used the 3-item *family reaction to my partner* subscale of the *Measures of Gay-Related Stress* (MOGS; Lewis et al., 2001) to evaluate individuals' perceptions of family reactions to partner stress. Types of situations captured in the items included introducing a new partner to family, having the lover and the family in the same place at the same time, and unwillingness of the family to accept the partner. Participants rated their experience of stress for each item using a 4-point Likert scale (0 = *no stress* to 3 = *severe stress*). Sum scores were computed, with higher scores indicating greater family reactions to partner stress. The *family reaction to my partner* subscale has shown good internal consistency, validity, and measurement invariance across gender and relationship status in prior studies among sexual minority individuals (e.g., Lewis et al, 2001). In the present study, which uses a similar sample, this subscale also showed good internal consistency (see Table 11.1).

TABLE 11.1 *Means, standard deviations, and t-tests of the main study variables by sex*

	Possible Range	M (SD)						t(df)	t
		Overall	α	Males	α	Females	α		
Depression	0–21	3.29 (3.57)	0.86	3.66 (3.95)	0.88	3.12 (3.38)	0.85	186	0.97
1. Depression (Transformed)	1–4.58	1.50 (1.02)	0.86	1.64 (1.00)	0.88	1.44 (1.02)	0.85	186	1.22
2. Family Stress	0–9	2.35 (2.50)	0.85	1.90 (1.92)	0.74	2.56 (2.71)	0.87	185	-1.71†
3. ESDC (PR)	1–5	4.17 (0.73)	0.66r	4.11 (0.71)	0.66r	4.20 (0.74)	0.64r	188	-0.80
4. ESDC (PP)	1–5	4.19 (0.78)	0.68r	4.08 (0.82)	0.77r	4.25 (0.75)	0.66r	188	-1.41
5. PSDC (PR)	1–5	3.69 (0.76)	0.30r	3.58 (0.80)	0.32r	3.75 (0.74)	0.29r	188	-1.44
6. PSDC (PP)	1–5	3.76 (0.92)	0.71r	3.58 (0.92)	0.70r	3.85 (0.91)	0.72r	188	-1.92†
7. NDC (PR)	1–5	1.78 (0.74)	0.78	1.96 (0.81)	0.76	1.70 (0.70)	0.78	188	2.89*
8. NDC (PR)	1–5	1.80 (0.78)	0.77	2.01 (0.87)	0.81	1.70 (0.71)	0.74	188	2.59*
9. Relationship Satisfaction	7–35	29.14 (2.58)	0.86	1.64 (1.00)	0.88	1.44 (1.02)	0.85	186	1.22

Note. A = actor; P = partner; Family Stress = family reactions to partner stress; PR = partner reported; PP = perceived partner; ESDC = emotion-focused supportive DC; PSDC = problem-focused supportive DC; NDC = negative DC. r Because there are only two items on these subscales, correlation coefficients are reported instead. † $p < 0.10$; * $p < 0.05$.

Symptoms of depression. Participants reported symptoms of depression using the 7-item *depression* subscale from the shortened version of the *Depression Anxiety Stress Scales* (DASS-21; Lovibond & Lovibond, 1995). Items assessed for depressive symptoms, including decreased interests and negative affect. Participants responded with their agreement to each item according to their experiences over the past week on a 4-point Likert scale (0 = *did not apply to me at all* to 3 = *applied to me very much, or most of the time*). Sum scores were computed, with higher scores indicating a greater amount of depressive symptoms. The depression subscale of DASS-21 has demonstrated good internal consistency from prior research with sexual minority samples (Cronbach's α = 0.86; Mereish & Poteat, 2015), which was comparable in this study for males and females in same-sex relationships specifically and overall (see Table 11.1).

Dyadic coping. We used the English-language version of the Dyadic Coping Inventory (DCI; Bodenmann, 2008; Randall, Hilpert, Jimenez-Arista, Walsh, & Bodenmann, 2015) to measure individuals' perceptions of DC from their partner as well as their own reports of DC toward their partner. Specifically, we used the 2-item *self emotion-focused supportive DC* subscale, which assesses how individuals respond to their partner with empathy and under-standing during times of distress, and the 2-item *partner emotion-focused supportive DC* subscale, which assesses individuals' perceptions of how their partner empathized with them during times of distress. The 2-item *self partner problem-focused supportive DC* subscale asked participants about their own behaviors to help their partner see the problem from a new perspective; on the other hand, the 2-item *partner problem-focused supportive DC* subscale assessed romantic partners' endeavors in advice giving and problem solving. Lastly, we used the *self negative DC* subscale to assess partner reported negative DC and the *partner negative DC* subscale to assess perceived partner negative DC; they each included four items describing individuals' experiences from negative attitudes and withdrawn behaviors toward and from their partner, respectively.

For both partner reported and perceived partner DC, DC behaviors were rated on a 5-point scale (1 = *very rarely* to 5 = *very often*). The mean of all subscales were calculated, with higher scores indicating more frequent DC behaviors. The DCI has evidenced good convergent and discriminant validity and measurement invariance across gender and culture (for a review, see Nussbeck & Jackson, 2016). Acceptable reliability for each subscale of DC was achieved except for the one assessing partner reported problem-focused supportive DC in the current study (see Table 11.1). This *self problem-focused supportive DC* subscale also showed low reliability in the English validation study among heterosexual committed couples (Cronbach's $\alpha_{\text{selfmales}}$ = 0.54, $\alpha_{\text{selffemales}}$ = 0.45; Randall et al., 2015). Although caution is needed in interpreting results from this subscale, we chose to retain it in analyses to provide a parallel examination with the perceived partner version of the subscale.

Control variables. Social context may influence the likelihood of members of sexual minorities to experience symptoms of psychological distress (e.g., Hatzenbuehler, Keyes, & Hasin, 2009). Therefore, we controlled for the region where participants were recruited (effects coded as Arizona = –0.5, Alabama = 0.5). On the relational level, we controlled for relationship satisfaction, as it has been closely associated with depression (e.g., Bodenmann & Randall, 2013; Whitton & Kuryluk, 2014). We measured relationship satisfaction using the 7-item *Relationship Assessment Scale* (Hendrick, 1988). Participants reported feelings about their relationship on both positive (e.g., "How good is your relationship compared to most?) and negative items (e.g., "How many problems are there in your relationship") on a 5-point scale (1 = *poor*, 3 = *average*, 5 = *excellent*, and 1 = *not much*, 3 = *average*, 5 = *very much*, respectively). This scale has demonstrated good internal consistency as well as criterion and discriminant validity (Hendrick, 1988), and presented acceptable reliability in this study (see Table 11.1). Additionally, we controlled for relationship length, given prior findings on its moderating effects on the relationship satisfaction–depression link (Whitton & Kuryluk, 2014) and the wide range of relationship lengths reported in our sample.

DATA ANALYTIC STRATEGY

We used an actor–partner interdependence model approach for moderation analysis with nondistinguishable dyads (Garcia, Kenny, & Ledermann, 2015) to account for partners' interdependence (Kashy, Donnellan, Burt, & McGue, 2008) using SAS Proc Mixed version 9.3 (SAS Institute, 2008). Because same-sex couples are nondistinguishable, one partner's actor effects are the same as the other's actor effects, which holds true for the partner effects and the moderating effects (see Figure 11.1). In these multilevel models, level-1 (individual-level) variables include individuals' reports of family reactions to stress, DC, depression, and relationship satisfaction, while level-2 (couple-level) variables include couples' reports of region, sex, and relationship length.

    Prior to running the analyses, we examined the assumptions of residual normality, linearity, homogeneity of variance, and influential outliers. Because of a positive skew of the *depression* subscale of the DASS-21 (skew $Z = 1.93$ and kurtosis $Z = 4.75$), we performed a square root transformation on the depression score. The transformed depression score showed improved distribution (skew $Z = 0.90$ and kurtosis $Z = 0.71$), and was highly correlated with the original score, $r = 0.97$; therefore, we used the transformed score in the future analyses. We effects-coded sex (females = −0.5, males = 0.5) and grand-mean centered self-reported family reactions to partner stress and DC to reduce multicollinearity of the interaction terms (Aiken & West, 1991). Lastly, data showed a missingness rate of 8.75%. To account for this, we used maximum likelihood estimation and adopted a listwise deletion approach given its appropriateness similar to multilevel multiple imputation (Medhanie, 2013).

We performed six multilevel models (one for each type of perceived partner and partner reported DC) to test our hypotheses. In each model, we included the control variables (i.e., region, relationship satisfaction, relationship length), the independent variables (i.e., actor and partner family reactions to partner stress), the moderators (i.e., the respective type of DC and sex), and the interaction terms between the independent variables and the moderators.

RESULTS

Descriptive Statistics

Descriptive statistics and results of independent-sample t-tests by sex can be found in Table 11.1, and zero-order correlations of the main variables by sex can be found in Table 11.2. Males reported marginally lower levels of family reactions to partner stress ($M = 1.90$, $SD = 1.92$) compared to females ($M = 2.56$, $SD = 2.71$), $t(187) = 2.62$, $p = 0.06$. Also, males perceived marginally less frequent partner problem-focused supportive DC behaviors ($M = 3.58$, $SD = 0.92$) compared to females ($M = 3.85$, $SD = 0.91$), $t(188) = −1.92$, $p = 0.06$. Finally, males reported significantly more frequent negative DC from their partner ($M = 2.01$, $SD = 0.87$) compared to females ($M = 1.70$, $SD = 0.71$), $t(1, 188) = 2.59$, $p = 0.01$, and toward their partner ($M = 1.96$, $SD = 0.81$) compared to females ($M = 1.70$, $SD = 0.70$), $t(1, 188) = 2.29$, $p = 0.02$. However, there was no sex difference in self-reports of depression, perceived partner and partner reported emotion-focused supportive DC, or partner reported problem-focused supportive DC.

Conditional Main Effects of Family Reactions
to Partner Stress on Depression

Results from the six multilevel models (one for each type of DC; Table 11.3) consistently indicated that relationship satisfaction was negatively associated with depression, $ps < 0.05$. When the effects of control variables were accounted for, higher levels of actor family reactions to partner stress were associated with elevated depressive symptoms ($ps < 0.05$) among individuals in same-sex relationships, consistent with our hypothesis. However,

TABLE 11.2 *Zero-order correlations of the main study variables by sex*

Depression		Zero-Order Correlations								
	1.	2.	3.	4.	5.	6.	7.	8.	9.	10.
1. Depression (Transformed)	—	0.16†	-0.03	-0.06	-0.02	-0.01	-0.04	0.18*	0.12	-0.21*
2. Family Stress (A)	0.24†	—	0.19*	0.05	0.16†	0.04	0.25*	-0.03	-0.07	0.12
3. Family Stress (P)	0.16	0.01	—	0.08	0.03	0.21*	0.003	-0.08	-0.01	0.07
4. ESDC (PR)	0.08	0.06	0.06	—	0.38*	0.21*	0.27*	-0.69*	-0.30*	0.35*
5. ESDC (PP)	-0.10	-0.21	0.11	0.44*	—	0.05	0.52*	-0.24*	-0.58*	0.42*
6. PSDC (PR)	0.20	0.22†	-0.03	0.08	-0.05	—	0.27*	-0.11	-0.08	0.13
7. PSDC (PP)	-0.08	-0.03	0.07	0.28*	0.32*	0.18	—	-0.14	-0.37*	0.45*
8. NDC (PR)	-0.05	-0.06	0.24†	-0.39	-0.28*	0.10	-0.20	—	0.29*	-0.26*
9. NDC (PP)	-0.15	0.20	-0.07	-0.41*	-0.58*	0.18	-0.26*	0.55*	—	-0.30*
10. Relationship Satisfaction	-0.30*	-0.11	0.05	0.23†	0.51*	0.06	0.42*	-0.18	-0.44*	—

Note. Correlations for males are presented below the diagonal, and correlations for females are presented above the diagonal. A = actor; P = partner; Family Stress = family reactions to partner stress; PR = partner reported; PP = perceived partner; ESDC = emotion-focused supportive DC; PSDC = problem-focused supportive DC; NDC = negative DC. †$p < 0.10$; *$p < 0.05$.

TABLE 11.3 *Effects of stress from family reactions to partner on depression moderated by dyadic coping (DC)*

Fixed Effects	Partner Reported ESDC			Perceived Partner ESDC			Partner Reported PSDC			Perceived Partner PSDC		
	$F(df)$	F	B	$F(df)$	F	B	$F(df)$	F	B	$F(df)$	F	B
Intercept			4.70*			4.51*			4.56*			4.44*
Region[a]	(1, 95)	0.11	−0.05	(1, 95)	0.06	−0.04	(1, 95)	0.10	−0.05	(1, 95)	0.05	−0.04
Relationship Satisfaction	(1, 175)	15.24	−0.11*	(1, 175)	13.47	−0.11*	(1, 171)	14.78	−0.11*	(1, 174)	12.13	−0.10*
Relationship Length	(1, 110)	0.06	0.003	(1, 113)	0.20	0.01	(1, 112)	0.02	0.002	(1, 111)	0.02	0.002
Sex[b]	(1, 93)	0.76	0.14	(1, 94)	0.47	0.11	(1, 93)	0.79	0.14	(1, 94)	0.64	0.13
Family Stress (A)	(1, 175)	5.03	0.07*	(1, 174)	7.83	0.08*	(1, 175)	5.18	0.07*	(1, 173)	6.20	0.08*
Family Stress (P)	(1, 175)	1.27	0.03	(1, 175)	1.25	0.03	(1, 175)	1.39	0.04	(1, 175)	1.54	0.04
DC	(1, 175)	0.43	0.07	(1, 176)	0.11	−0.03	(1, 169)	0.00	0.005	(1, 172)	0.14	−0.03
Family Stress (A) × DC	(1, 175)	<0.01	−0.001	(1, 169)	4.36	−0.08*	(1, 174)	0.00	−0.06	(1, 171)	0.88	−0.03

TABLE 11.3 *(continued)*

Fixed Effects	Partner Reported NDC			Perceived Partner NDC		
	$F(df)$	F	B	$F(df)$	F	B
Intercept			4.27*			4.18*
Region[a]	(1, 172)	0.03	−0.03	(1, 95)	<0.01	0.002
Relationship Satisfaction	(1, 172)	11.44	−0.10*	(1, 175)	11.21	−0.09*
Relationship Length	(1, 112)	0.09	−0.004	(1, 108)	0.21	−0.01
Sex[b]	(1, 95)	0.28	0.09	(1, 93)	0.26	0.08
Family Stress (A)	(1, 173)	5.50	0.07*	(1, 175)	6.48	0.07*
Family Stress (P)	(1, 174)	2.19	0.04	(1, 175)	1.75	0.04
DC	(1, 172)	3.15	0.18†	(1, 175)	5.49	0.23
Family Stress (A) x DC	(1, 171)	2.27	0.06	(1, 175)	2.88	0.07†

Note. [a]Region was coded as Arizona = −0.5, Alabama = 0.5. [b]Sex was coded as female = −0.5, male = 0.5. A = actor; P = partner; Family Stress = Family Reactions to Partner Stress; ESDC = emotion-focused supportive DC; PSDC = problem-focused supportive DC; NDC = negative DC. † p <0.10; * p <0.05.

significant partner effects did not emerge; *partners'* perceived family reactions to partner stress was not linked with individuals' own depressive symptoms ($ps > 0.05$), partially supporting H1.

Moderating Effects of Sex and DC

We found no sex differences in associations between family reactions to partner stress and DC with symptoms of depression (RQ1). Therefore, we removed all the interaction terms with sex from the model for parsimony, and kept it as a control variable.

Emotion-focused supportive DC. *Partner reported* emotion-focused supportive DC did not moderate the association between family reactions to partner stress and depressive symptoms. However, in support of H2, we found a significant two-way interaction effect of family reactions to partner stress by *perceived partner* emotion-focused supportive DC on depressive symptoms, F (1, 169) = 4.36, $b = -0.08$, $p = 0.04$. We performed simple slope analyses probing one standard deviation above (+1 SD) and below (−1 SD) the mean of perceived partner emotion-focused supportive DC (Aiken & West, 1991). Higher stress from family reactions to partner stress was found to be associated with greater symptoms of depression for those who perceived *low* levels of partner emotion-focused supportive DC, $b = 0.14$, $p < 0.01$. This association was nonsignificant for individuals who perceived *high* levels of partner emotion-focused supportive DC, $b = 0.02$, $p = 0.49$. Said differently, perceived partner emotion-focused supportive DC weakened the positive association between family reactions to partner stress and depressive symptoms, as expected.

Problem-focused supportive DC. Contrary to H2, problem-focused supportive DC did not moderate the association between family reactions to partner stress and symptoms of depression, either in the *partner reported* or in the *perceived partner* problem-focused supportive DC model.

Negative DC. *Partner reported* negative DC behaviors did not moderate the association between family reactions to partner stress and reported symptoms of depression. A marginally significant main effect of *partner reported* negative DC on depressive symptoms emerged, $F(1, 172) = 3.15$, $b = 0.18$, $p = 0.08$. More frequent negative DC behaviors reported by individuals' partners were marginally linked with individuals' greater depressive symptoms. Further, we found a marginally significant interaction effect of *perceived partner* negative DC with actor family reactions to partner stress on depressive symptoms (H3), $F(1, 175) = 2.88$, $b = 0.07$, $p = 0.09$. Perceived partner negative DC exacerbated the association between higher perceived family reactions to partner and greater symptoms of depression. Specifically, those who perceived *less* frequent negative DC behaviors from their partner (–1 SD) did not report elevated depressive symptoms despite experiencing higher family reactions to partner stress, b = 0.02, p = 0.52; conversely, for those who perceived more frequent negative DC behaviors from their partner (+1 SD) higher perceived family reactions to partner stress were associated with greater symptoms of depression, b = 0.12, p < 0.01. Although marginal in significance, the pattern of findings was in the direction predicted and provided additional support for H2.

DISCUSSION

Using a dyadic sample of 95 same-sex couples, we examined the actor and partner effects of family reactions to partner stress as associated with reported symptoms of depression. As expected, when individuals reported high levels of family reactions to partner stress, such as stress from their family's lack of acceptance of their partner, they reported greater depressive symptoms (actor effects); however, we did not find any association between partner reports of family reactions stress and individuals' depressive symptoms (partner effects). These findings add to the existing literature such that despite the shared experiences in romantic relationships (e.g., Kelley, 1979), individuals' reports of depressive symptoms were more influenced by their own perceived stress from their family reactions toward their same-sex partner, and less affected by their partners' perceived stress from family reactions.

The lack of significant partner effects in our study was surprising given recent dyadic research that has examined both actor and partner effects of stress on individual well-being in heterosexual couples (e.g., Johnson, Galambos, Finn, Neyer, & Horne, 2017; Neff & Karney, 2007). Although others have found partner effects of daily stress on relationship quality in same-sex couples (Totenhagen et al., 2012), these authors did not focus on forms of sexual minority stress. Further, it may be that stressors are more likely to cross over between partners in examining relational outcomes (e.g., relationship satisfaction) as opposed to individual outcomes (e.g., individual depressive symptoms). Another explanation for the nonsignificant partner effects of family reactions to partner stress may be that when one partner experiences high levels of family reactions to partner stress, the other partner may be less likely to disclose his or her relationship to his or her family (Rostosky et al., 2007), which may lessen the likelihood of impact on the individuals' depressive symptoms.

Moderating Effects of Dyadic Coping

We also examined the moderating effects of DC given the well-documented association with relationship well-being in heterosexual couples (Falconier et al., 2015). We focused on DC that the partner reports providing (*partner reported* DC) as well as the DC that the individual reports receiving (*perceived partner* DC). Results showed a negative association between reported stress and symptoms of depression for individuals who perceived less frequent emotion-focused supportive DC from their partners. When individuals perceived more frequent emotion-focused supportive DC (e.g., empathy and understanding) from their partners, this relation was weakened. That is, perceptions of emotion-focused supportive DC buffered the negative implications of family reactions to partner stress on individual depression. This pattern is congruent with prior findings on the protective factors of this type of DC behaviors in heterosexual (e.g., Landis et al., 2013; Regan et al., 2014) and same-sex couples (Randall et al., 2017a, 2017b). In contrast to our hypothesis, we did not find that partner problem-focused DC behaviors (e.g., providing new perspectives on the problem) moderated the association. Family reactions to same-sex partner stress, including stress from introducing a new partner to the family and facing reluctance of the family to accept the partner, can be emotionally arousing (Béres-Deák, 2011), and challenging for the partner to respond with a new perspective (i.e., problem-focused supportive DC). In this sense, emotion-focused responses, including empathy and understanding, may exert a more significant effect on family reactions to partner stress with the symptoms of depression link. On the other hand, problem-focused supportive DC may be less effective for weakening the negative effects of stress between individuals' family and their partner than of stress that is more distinctly unrelated to their relationships, for example, individual illness or discrimination at work (Fife, Weaver, Cook, & Stump, 2013; Randall et al., 2017b).

Moreover, we found a marginally significant moderating effect of perceived partner negative DC such that the more frequent negative DC individuals perceived from their partners, the stronger the association between family reactions to partner stress with symptoms of depression. Perceived partner negative DC may be related to more frequent aggression in communication between partners (Bodenmann, Charvoz, Widmer, & Bradbury, 2004) and lower relationship satisfaction (Falconier et al., 2013), and directly or indirectly associated with individuals' elevated symptoms of depression (Whitton & Kuryluk, 2014). Our results are consistent with existing findings on perceived partner negative DC as a risk factor for individual and relational outcomes (Regan et al., 2014). Moreover, we showed that partner reported negative DC behaviors tended to have a more direct relationship with individuals' depressive symptoms as evidenced in the marginal main effect of partner reported negative DC in comparison to the indirect effect of *perceived* partner negative DC in this study.

Despite low to moderate correlations between partner reported and perceived partner DC (except problem-focused supportive DC behaviors among men), the discrepancy between individuals' *perceptions* of DC provided by their partners, in comparison to those partners' reported attempted behaviors, may be meaningful in understanding the strengthening or weakening effects on the stress–depression link. Specifically, individuals tend to perceive their partner as more emotionally supportive (or discouraging) than their partners' intentions to engage in DC behaviors in same-sex relationships (Landis et al., 2013). It should be noted, however, that participants reported on their own and their partner's general DC behaviors rather than reporting on DC behaviors in the face of specific stressors (in this case, family reactions to partner stress). Thus, we cannot necessarily assume that reported DC behaviors were in response to experiencing stress from family reactions to the partner. Future research may examine partner DC in the face of family reactions among same-sex couples to supplement the current findings.

Considerations of Sex Differences

Finally, we examined the potential sex differences in perceived stress, depressive symptoms, DC behaviors, and the associations among them. In our sample, females reported marginally higher levels of stress from family reactions to same-sex partner than males, consistent with previous findings with a mixed sample of female members of sexual minorities with and without a partner (Lewis et al., 2001). Also, females were found to perceive marginally more frequent problem-focused supportive DC and less frequent negative DC behaviors from their partner than males, which may reflect more harmonious communication in their same-sex relationship, as evidenced in prior literature (e.g., Roisman, Clausell, Holland, Fortuna, & Elieff, 2008). Aside from these differences, we found that both males and females showed similar levels of depressive symptoms, which were similarly associated with their perceived stress from family reactions toward their partner and moderated by partner DC behaviors.

Limitations and Future Directions

Despite the contributions of this study's findings, it is important to recognize its limitations. First, although our sample appeared to be similar to the US same-sex couple population at the time of recruitment (2013), couples in our sample reported a wide range of relationship lengths. Given this, we controlled for the potential influence relationship length may have had on depressive symptoms in our analyses, yet relationship length could also contribute to the levels of family reactions to partner stress. For example, those who had been in a committed relationship for a long time may have already introduced their same-sex partner to their family, thus reporting low levels of stress in this domain. Second, because we used a convenience sample, individuals who contacted the research team and participated in the study were self-selected. For example, participants in this study tended to report few depressive symptoms. Although we performed a transformation on the depression scores, caution is needed in generalizing our findings to the larger sexual minority individual population, especially among those who are at a high risk or have been diagnosed with major depression disorder. Moreover, as mentioned previously, we examined general partner reported and perceived partner DC behaviors; prospective research may benefit from assessing DC behaviors specific to certain stressors to unravel the unique effects DC may have to help coping with stress as a couple. Drawing from a dyadic perspective, future studies may evaluate couple-level stress specifically to understand the stress proliferation process in same-sex couples (Leblanc, Frost, & Wight, 2015). Lastly, the data we used in the present study are cross-sectional, which limits our understanding of causal associations between stress and depression. Given the illustrative example of Pat and Jamie, we cannot conclude that Pat's depressive symptoms result from her perceived family reactions to partner stress and not the other way around. Researchers may move forward with our findings and consider collecting data from a more diverse sample and adopting a longitudinal design to capture the dynamics between family reactions to partner stress, symptoms of depression, and partner DC behaviors across cultures and over a period of time.

CONCLUSION

Same-sex partners can help each other cope with the stress associated with negative family reactions to their partner, which may also help to mitigate negative associations on reported symptoms of psychological distress. These results shed light on the role same-sex partners can play in the association between specific minority stressors and symptoms of depression – individuals' perceptions of DC behaviors their partners engaged in appeared to be more influential than their partner's own report of DC behaviors. Given these findings, same-sex partners may be encouraged to try to recognize their partner's empathetic and understanding responses when experiencing stress from family reactions to their partner, which could ameliorate the negative influence such stress may have on their depressive symptoms. These findings add to the general consideration of stress as a relational construct, and the proposed "we-disease" perspective of understanding psychological distress in the context of close relationships (Bodenmann & Randall, 2013), wherein both partners are considered integral to promoting their relational well-being. Romantic partners should therefore be encouraged to be involved in helping individuals cope with stress in their lives, especially in the form of partner emotion-focused supportive DC, to decrease risk for depressive symptoms.

REFERENCES

Aiken, L. S., & West, S. G. (1991). *Multiple regression: Testing and interpreting interactions*. Newbury Park, CA: SAGE.

Béres-Deák, R. (2011). "I was a dark horse in the eyes of her family": The relationship of cohabiting female couples and their families in Hungary. *Journal of Lesbian Studies*, 15, 337–355. doi: 10.1080/10894160.2011.530153

Bodenmann, G. (1995). A systemic-transactional conceptualization of stress and coping in couples. *Swiss Journal of Psychology / Schweizerische Zeitschrift für Psychologie / Revue Suisse De Psychologie*, 54(1), 34–49.

Bodenmann, G. (2000). *Stress und coping bei paaren*. Göttingen, Germany: Hogrefe.

Bodenmann, G. (2005). Dyadic coping and its significance for marital functioning. In T. Revenson, K. Kayser, & G. Bodenmann (Eds.), *Couples coping with stress: Emerging perspectives on dyadic coping* (pp. 33–50). Washington, DC: American Psychological Association.

Bodenmann, G. (2008). *Dyadisches Coping Inventar: Testmanual* [Dyadic Coping Inventory: Test manual]. Bern, Switzerland: Huber.

Bodenmann, G., Charvoz, L., Widmer, K., & Bradbury, T. N. (2004). Differences in individual and dyadic coping among low and high depressed, partially remitted, and nondepressed persons. *Journal of Psychopathology and Behavioral Assessment*, 26, 75–85. doi: 10.1023/B:JOBA.0000013655.45146.47

Bodenmann, G., & Randall, A. K. (2013). Close relationships in psychiatric disorders. *Current Opinion in Psychiatry*, 26, 464–467. doi: 10.1097/YCO.0b013e3283642de7

Bodenmann, G., Randall, A. K., & Falconier, M. K. (2016). Coping in couples: The systemic-transactional model. In M. K. Falconier, A. K. Randall, & G. Bodenmann (Eds.), *Couples coping with stress: A cross-cultural perspective* (pp. 5–22). New York, NY: Routledge.

Buck, A. A., & Neff, L. A. (2012). Stress spillover in early marriage: The role of self-regulatory depletion. *Journal of Family Psychology*, 26, 698–708. doi: 10.1037/a0029260

Butler, E. A, Young, V., & Randall, A. K. (2010). Suppressing to please, eating to cope: The effect of overweight women's emotion suppression on romantic relationships and eating. *Journal of Social and Clinical Psychology*, 29, 559–623. doi: 10.1521/jscp.2010.29.6.599

Crosbie-Burnett, M., Foster, T. L., Murray, C. L., & Bowen, G. L. (1996). Gays' and lesbians' families-of-origin: A social cognitive-behavioral model of adjustment. *Family Relations*, 45(4), 397–403. doi: 10.2307/585169

Falconier, M. K., Jackson, J. B., Hilpert, P., & Bodenmann, G. (2015). Dyadic coping and relationship satisfaction: A meta-analysis. *Clinical Psychology Review*, 42, 28–46. doi: 10.1016/j.cpr.2015.07.002

Falconier, M. K., Nussbeck, F., & Bodenmann, G. (2013). Immigration stress and relationship satisfaction in Latino couples: The role of dyadic coping. *Journal of Social and Clinical Psychology*, 32, 813–843. doi: 10.1521/jscp.2013.32.8.813

Falconier, M. K., Randall, A. K., & Bodenmann, G. (Eds.). (2016). *Couples coping with stress: A cross-cultural perspective*. New York, NY: Routledge.

Fife, B. L., Weaver, M. T., Cook, W. L., & Stump, T. T. (2013). Partner interdependence and coping with life-threatening illness: The impact on dyadic adjustment. *Journal of Family Psychology*, 27, 702–711. doi: 10.1037/a0033871

Freitas, D. F., D'Augelli, A. R., Coimbra, S., & Fontaine, A. M. (2016). Discrimination and mental health among gay, lesbian, and bisexual youths in Portugal:

The moderating role of family relationships and optimism. *Journal of GLBT Family Studies, 12*, 68–90. doi: 10.1080/1550428X.2015.1070704

Garcia, R. L., Kenny, D. A., & Ledermann, T. (2015). Moderation in the actor–partner interdependence model. *Personal Relationships, 22*, 8–29. doi: 10.1111/pere.12060

Gilman, S. E., Cochran, S. D., Mays, V. M., Hughes, M., Ostrow, D., & Kessler, R. C. (2001). Risk of psychiatric disorders among individuals reporting same-sex sexual partners in the national comorbidity survey. *American Journal of Public Health, 91*, 933–939. doi: 10.2105/AJPH.91.6.933

Graham, J. M., & Barnow, Z. B. (2013). Stress and social support in gay, lesbian, and heterosexual couples: Direct effects and buffering models. *Journal of Family Psychology, 27*, 569–578. doi: 10.1037/a0033420

Hatzenbuehler, M. L., Keyes, K. M., & Hasin, D. S. (2009). State-level policies and psychiatric morbidity in lesbian, gay, and bisexual populations. *American Journal of Public Health, 99*, 2275–2281. doi: 10.2105/AJPH.2008.153510

Heatherington, L., & Lavner, J. A. (2008). Coming to terms with coming out: Review and recommendations for family systems-focused research. *Journal of Family Psychology, 22*, 329–343. doi: 10.1037/0893-3200.22.3.329

Hendrick, S. S. (1988). A generic measure of relationship satisfaction. *Journal of Marriage and the Family, 50*, 93–98. doi: 10.2307/352430

Johnson, M. D., Galambos, N. L., Finn, C., Neyer, F. J., & Horne, R. M. (2017). Pathways between self-esteem and depression in couples. *Developmental Psychology, 53*, 787–799. doi: 10.1037/dev0000276

Karney, B. R., & Bradbury, T. N. (1995). The longitudinal course of marital quality and stability: A review of theory, methods, and research. *Psychological Bulletin, 118*, 3–34. doi: 10.1037/0033-2909.118.1.3

Kashy, D. A., Donnellan, M. B., Burt, S. A., & McGue, M. (2008). Growth curve models for indistinguishable dyads using multilevel modeling and structural equation modeling: The case of adolescent twins' conflict with their mothers. *Developmental Psychology, 44*, 316–329. doi: 10.1037/0012-1649.44.2.316

Kelley, H. H. (1979). *Personal relationships: Their structure and processes.* Hillsdale, NJ: Lawrence Erlbaum Associates.

King, M., Semlyen, J., Tai, S. S., Killaspy, H., Osborn, D., Popelyuk, D., & Nazareth, I. (2008). A systematic review of mental disorder, suicide, and deliberate self harm in lesbian, gay and bisexual people. *BMC Psychiatry, 8*, 70–86. doi: 10.1186/1471-244X-8-70

Landis, M., Peter-Wight, M., Martin, M., & Bodenmann, G. (2013). Dyadic coping and marital satisfaction of older spouses in long-term marriage. *The Journal of Gerontopsychology and Geriatric Psychiatry, 26*, 39–47. doi: 10.1024/1662-9647/a000077

LeBlanc, A. J., Frost, D. M., & Wight, R. G. (2015). Minority stress and stress proliferation among same-sex and other marginalized couples. *Journal of Marriage and Family, 77*, 40–59. doi: 10.1111/jomf.12160

Lewis, R. J., Derlega, V. J., Berndt, A., Morris, L. M., & Rose, S. (2001). An empirical analysis of stressors for gay men and lesbians. *Journal of Homosexuality, 42*, 63–88. doi: 10.1300/J082v42n01_04

Lovibond, P. F., & Lovibond, S. H. (1995). The structure of negative emotional states: Comparison of the depression anxiety stress scales (DASS) with the Beck depression and anxiety inventories. *Behaviour Research and Therapy, 33*, 335–343. doi: 10.1016/0005-7967(94)00075-U

McCabe, S. E., Bostwick, W. B., Hughes, T. L., West, B. T., & Boyd, C. J. (2010). The relationship between discrimination and substance use disorders among lesbian, gay, and bisexual adults in the United States. *American Journal of Public Health, 100*, 1946–1952. doi: 10.2105/AJPH.2009.163147

Medhanie, A. G. (2013). *The robustness of multilevel multiple imputation for handling missing data in hierarchical linear models* (Doctoral dissertation). Retrieved from PsycINFO. (1534280883; 2014-99100-510). (Order No. AAI3589097).

Mereish, E. H., & Poteat, V. P. (2015). A relational model of sexual minority mental and physical health: The negative effects of shame on relationships, loneliness, and health. *Journal of Counseling Psychology, 62*, 425–437. doi: 10.1037/cou0000088

Meyer, I. H. (1995). Minority stress and mental health in gay men. *Journal of Health and Social Behavior, 36*, 38–56. doi: 10.2307/2137286

Meyer, I. H. (2003). Prejudice, social stress, and mental health in lesbian, gay, and bisexual populations: Conceptual issues and research evidence. *Psychological Bulletin, 129*, 674–697. doi: 10.1037/0033-2909.129.5.674

Neff, L. A., & Karney, B. R. (2007). Stress crossover in newlywed marriage: A longitudinal and dyadic perspective. *Journal of Marriage and Family, 69*, 594–607. doi: 10.1111/j.1741-3737.2007.00394.x

Nussbeck, F. W., & Jackson, J. B. (2016). Measuring dyadic coping across cultures. In M. K. Falconier, A. K. Randall, & G. Bodenmann (Eds.), *Couples coping with stress: A cross-cultural perspective* (pp. 36–53). New York, NY: Routledge/Taylor & Francis Group.

Papp, L. M., Kouros, C. D., & Cummings, E. M. (2010). Emotions in marital conflict interactions: Empathic accuracy, assumed similarity, and the moderating context of depressive symptoms. *Journal of Social and Personal Relationships, 27*, 367–387. doi: 10.1177/0265407509348810

Randall, A. K., Hilpert, P., Jimenez-Arista, L., Walsh, K. J., & Bodenmann, G. (2015). Dyadic coping in the U.S.: Psychometric properties and validity for use of the English version of the dyadic coping inventory. *Current Psychology: A Journal for Diverse Perspectives on Diverse Psychological Issues, 35*, 570–582. doi: 10.1007/s12144-015-9323-0

Randall, A. K., Tao, C., Totenhagen, C. J., Walsh, K. J., & Cooper, A. N. (2017a). Associations between sexual orientation discrimination and depression among same-sex couples: Moderating effects of dyadic coping. *Journal of Couple & Relationship Therapy, 16*, 325–345. doi: 10.1080/15332691.2016.1253520

Randall, A. K., Totenhagen, C. J., Walsh, K. J., Adams, C., & Tao, C. (2017b). Coping with gay-related stress: Effects of positive dyadic coping on anxiety in lesbian couples. *Journal of Lesbian Studies, 21*, 70–87.

Regan, T. W., Lambert, S. D., Kelly, B., McElduff, P., Girgis, A., Kayser, K., & Turner, J. (2014). Cross-sectional relationships between dyadic coping and anxiety, depression, and relationship satisfaction for patients with prostate cancer and their spouses. *Patient Education and Counseling, 96*, 120–127. doi: 10.1016/j.pec.2014.04.010

Roisman, G. I., Clausell, E., Holland, A., Fortuna, K., & Elieff, C. (2008). Adult romantic relationships as contexts of human development: A multimethod comparison of same-sex couples with opposite-sex dating, engaged, and married dyads. *Developmental Psychology, 44*, 91–101. doi: 10.1037/0012-1649.44.1.91

Rostosky, S. S., Riggle, E. D. B., Gray, B. E., & Hatton, R. L. (2007). Minority stress experiences in committed same-sex couple relationships. *Professional Psychology: Research and Practice, 38*, 392–400. doi: 10.1037/0735–7028.38.4.392

SAS Institute. (2008). *SAS/STAT 9.2 user's guide* (2nd Ed). Cary, NC: SAS Institute Inc.

Schoebi, D., & Randall, A. K. (2015). Emotional dynamics in intimate relationships. *Emotion Review, 7*, 342–348. doi: 10.1177/1754073915590620

Thibaut, J. W., & Kelley, H. H. (1959). *The social psychology of groups.* Piscataway, NJ: Transaction Publishers.

Totenhagen, C. J., Butler, E. A., & Ridley, C. A. (2012). Daily stress, closeness, and satisfaction in gay and lesbian couples. *Personal Relationships, 19*, 219–233. doi: 10.1111/j.1475–6811.2011.01349.x

Totenhagen, C. J., Curran, M. A., Serido, J., & Butler, E. A. (2013). Good days, bad days: Do sacrifices improve relationship quality? *Journal of Social and Personal Relationships, 30*, 881–900. doi: 10.1177/0265407512472475

Totenhagen, C. J., Randall, A. K., Cooper, A. N., Tao, C., & Walsh, K. J. (2017). Stress spillover and crossover in same-sex couples: Concurrent and lagged daily effects. *Journal of GLBT Family Studies, 13*, 236–256. doi: 10.1080/1550428X.2016.1203273

U.S. Census Bureau. (2013). *American community survey data on same sex couples: Characteristics of same-sex couples households.* Retrieved from: www.census.gov/hhes/samesex/files/ssex-tables-2013.xlsx

Weaver, K. M. (2014). *An investigation of gay male, lesbian, and transgender dyadic coping in romantic relationships* (unpublished doctoral dissertation). Spalding University, Louisville, KY.

Whitton, S. W., & Kuryluk, A. D. (2014). Associations between relationship quality and depressive symptoms in same-sex couples. *Journal of Family Psychology, 28*, 571–576. doi: 10.1037/fam0000011

12

"I Just Want My Wife and My Life Back": Men's Experiences of Stress and Social Support during Their Partner's Postpartum Depression

KELI STEUBER-FAZIO, KEELIN MORAN, CAITLIN MCNAIR, AND ERICA COGLAND

The birth of a child is often a joyous turning point in couples' lives. Whereas most mothers experience a normal level of stress associated with the transition to parenthood, many others cope with a period of more intense feelings, such as "baby blues" or mood swings that often disappear after a short period of time (Hoseini Omam, Panaghi, Habibi Asgarabadi, & Davoodi, 2016). When these intense feelings do not dissipate, the condition can progress into a more major depressive disorder. In fact, 13% of women in America experience postpartum depression (PPD; Miller, Hogue, Knight, Stowe, & Newport, 2012). PPD can incapacitate a mother by interfering with daily activities (Hoseini Omam et al., 2016), resulting in feelings of extreme anger that are often directed at her partner, and inhibiting the mother from bonding with or even caregiving for her new baby (see Davey, Dziurawiec, & O'Brien-Malone, 2006 for a review).

Another person positioned centrally to this experience is the partner of the woman coping with PPD. The father is managing a series of transitions, from taking on the role of a new parent, adjusting to the presence of a young baby, to ultimately helping in the wake of his partner's depression. Despite the prominent role they play, very little research has explored and documented men's experiences as their partner copes with PPD. The limited research on the topic found that men in this situation often feel depressed themselves, have uncertainty about the future of their family, and have confusion about the medical aspects and severity of PPD in general (Davey et al., 2006). Research also suggests that in couples in which wives are managing PPD, husbands and wives very rarely interpret the situation similarly, which impedes their ability to communicate effectively about it (Everingham, Heading, & Connor, 2006).

In light of the limited research and the magnitude of the implications of PPD on the family as a unit, this study examines the perspective of men as their partner copes with PPD. Utilizing data from an online support forum for fathers supporting a woman coping with PPD, this chapter describes the results of a thematic analysis of the major stressors described by male partners of mothers with PPD, as well as the types of social support desired by the father. The results are discussed in terms of their implications for future research and practice regarding the interdependent experiences of partners in the face of PPD.

TRANSITIONING TO PARENTHOOD AND DEPRESSION

Having a child is one of the happiest, and most stressful life transitions a couple might experience (Cowan & Cowan, 2000). Along with the joy of a new baby comes increased financial burden, reduced intimacy, decreased companionate activities, and unfamiliar caregiving tasks (Cowan & Cowan, 2000). In addition to these stressors, the chronic fatigue of new parents often amplifies issues. The normal stress that coincides with new parenthood is taxing in itself on couples; however, simultaneously coping with depression can further exacerbate an already trying time.

Although PPD is largely labeled and treated as a mental health condition afflicting a new mother, the effects of the disease have a much farther reach. For every mother coping with depression, there is a partner, sibling, parent, or friend experiencing the harrowing residual effects. PPD has the capacity to stress marriages, strain friendships, and isolate the mother in ways that can perpetuate the negative effects associated with the condition. Given their daily interaction with the mother and baby, it is not surprising that fathers are adversely affected by this major depression (Davey et al., 2006). Whereas some couples have experienced PPD as a heightened form of prior depression in the mother, about half of the women diagnosed with PPD are struggling with their first depressive episode (Stowe, Landry, & Porter, 1995). Although both scenarios are difficult, partners in the latter situation do not have prior experiences or skillsets for how to best manage the disease. Further complicating matters, 10.4% of new fathers are coping with prenatal or postpartum depression themselves (Paulson & Bazemore, 2010). In any of these cases, fathers are managing the normal stressors associated with the birth of their child, the debilitating depression of their wife, and all the residual – and serious – effects that come along with managing PPD as both a parent and a partner.

Despite the detrimental effects that PPD can have on men's lives, there is limited research on the social and emotional needs of men as they cope with it (Paulson & Bazemore, 2010). The qualitative research that does exist highlights the depth of the stress and frustration that fathers experience as their partner manages PPD (see Davey et al., 2006 for a review). In light of the primary role fathers play in caregiving for the baby and mother during postnatal depressive episodes, it is imperative to begin understanding their experiences during this time. Recognizing ways to help educate and support men during PPD might limit the negative implications of the disease for the family. We know very little about the emotional experiences of men as they contend with this disease, and even fewer studies within this already small group illuminate the major social and emotional stressors fathers cope with as they manage PPD within their families. To address this goal, we advance the following research question:

RQ1: What types of stressors are experienced by male partners of women with PPD?

SOCIAL SUPPORT

One of the theoretical lenses for examining men's experiences with PPD is to consider the social support they need as they contend with it. Considerable research has documented the psychological benefits of receiving social support during stressful experiences (Sarason, Sarason, & Gurung, 1997). Social support, defined as verbal or nonverbal communication intended to provide assistance to others perceived to need aid (Burleson & MacGeorge, 2002), coincides with greater perceptions of control, self-efficacy, esteem, and life satisfaction (Goodwin & Plaza, 2000; Shaw, Krause, Chatters, Connell, & Ingersoll-Dayton, 2004; Symister & Friend, 2003; Uchino, 2009). Receipt of social support is also linked to positive behavior changes (Reblin & Uchino, 2008; DiMatteo, 2004) and positive relational outcomes (Conger, Rueter, & Elder, 1999; Verhofstadt, Buysse, & Ickes, 2007). Social support has been found to be a crucial resource in helping distressed people cope with trauma, manage their emotional upset, reframe stressors, and generally feel better about who they are as individuals (Burleson, 2003; Burleson & MacGeorge, 2002).

People can provide support in a variety of ways (Xu & Burleson, 2001). Informational support provides factual information or advice, such as sharing information about medicines that treat PPD or giving websites that offer resources for managing it. Emotional support involves expressing interpersonal solidarity. This support can usually be communicated by showing love or care for a person through listening, showing compassion, and being "on their side." Network support involves connecting people both socially and through other forms of resources. Helping people find others going through a similar experience is one way to extend network support, as it helps to integrate them into a community that is empathic to their situation. Esteem support works to enhance the perceived self-worth a person has. Reminding the person of their successes or positive characteristics are ways to offer esteem support. Tangible support is a form of practical help. A person can offer financial assistance, logistical help such as organizing transportation or meal trains, or any other support that can make day-to-day life easier. Social support that meets people's needs has been found to promote enhanced coping ability, affect, reappraisal of a traumatic situation, and physiological health (Bodie, Burleson, & Jones, 2012).

In light of the various benefits of social support during times of stress, it is important to explore the type of social support that men whose partners are coping with PPD might desire. Unfortunately, both women and men seem to be hiding their struggles. In one study, many women reported they feared disclosing about their PPD because they felt others would deem them a bad mother or they might lose their children (Chew-Graham, Sharp, Chamberlain, Folkes, & Turner, 2009). Similarly, a study of Australian men whose wives had PPD reported that they felt reluctance to reach out for help so that they could maintain the appearance that things were fine (Davey et al., 2006). Once they did reach out, they felt as though people attempted to share the burden. Taken together, the potential for the receipt of social support during a health stressor is well documented; however, the hesitation to disclose about the stressor impedes those benefits (Steuber & High, 2015). A first step in helping men communicate their emotional and logistical needs during this time is to identify the type of comfort and help they desire, especially in light of both partners working to conceal PPD. Therefore, in an effort to better understand men's perspectives, we advance our second research question:

RQ2: What is the role of social support in men's experiences of their partner's PPD?

METHOD

To investigate the issues relevant to fathers of babies whose birth mothers are coping with PPD, this study examined an online forum dedicated to this population. The design of the forum involved fathers being invited to share their experiences with PPD, and then other people were able to comment and dialogue about their own experiences in relation to that story. This data source was selected because, in contrast to more traditional surveys or interviews, these online venues showcase discourse that is salient to the fathers as they help their child's mother cope with the disease rather than issues that are guided by the researcher's agenda (see Steuber & Solomon, 2008 for a similar format). This approach is especially important for this particular demographic, as the father might work to protect his partner, and the anonymous nature of the internet might enable him to share his needs in a safe and anonymous environment. In addition, of the little research that is available, much of the data are from a subset of the population in which the mother is being medically treated, leaving a large portion of PPD families that are without clinical help noticeably missing. The clinical versus nonclinical population distinction is important, as often fathers are not aware of signs or symptoms of PPD, further limiting their ability to manage it (Everingham et al., 2006). Therefore, having a venue that slowly builds data across time as individuals check in and start new strings of dialogue is beneficial not just because of the content they privilege, but also because it allows for many perspectives to be represented in an otherwise difficult sample to collect. The following sections further explain the procedures and analysis.

SAMPLE

The online forum on which the data are listed is public domain and requires no password for accessing it; however, the listing of the exact website and usernames are masked to protect any identifying details. The website was found by utilizing search engines to locate online support forums for fathers and, on arriving at this site, the decision was made to utilize data solely from this venue because both the initial contributors and the commenters were predominately men. Other sites had both men and women offering insight, with many women discussing the experience of their husband on his behalf. The goal was to gather the perspective of the father, exclusively, in this study, and this forum best served that purpose. The design of this forum included fathers being invited by one of the website administrators to submit their story, and then the administrator would follow up at various (nonstandard) points of time with the fathers to get updates. At the time the data were archived for this study, the forum included 24 invited narratives, with a large number of comments following some and none after others. The data from all the stories and all the comments were included in this analysis and divided into units such that each story was one unit, and each comment following it was one unit. The data resulted in 107 pages of single-spaced text and 163 units of analysis ($N = 163$).

ANALYTIC PROCEDURES

This study mirrored the analysis utilized by Steuber and Solomon (2008), in which they first conducted a general theme analysis of online health forums so that no assumptions were made about the stressors related to the health condition, and then followed with a secondary theme analysis that was conducted with an eye toward identifying categories related to concepts identified by a relevant theory. This two-step process offers a holistic view of the stressors and desired support strategies, and it allows the data to speak from the perspective of the father, as well as organizes those ideas in theoretically and practically beneficial ways.

The first step in the analysis involved identifying general sources of stress for the husbands whose partners had PPD. The data were read through four times, and on the fifth read researchers began to take note of reoccurring themes. Themes were identified based on their frequency, intensity, and extensiveness (Krueger, 1998; Rabiee, 2004). Themes were considered frequent if they appeared readily in the data. Intense themes were marked based on the depth of feeling with which the view was expressed. If the theme was represented across units broadly, they were marked as extensive. Following Strauss and Corbin's (1998) framework for coding, open coding was utilized to identify central concepts and their dimensions within the data. Then axial coding was conducted to map out the connections within and across the most prominent themes. This enabled collapsing and assimilating themes to streamline the analysis. Once the stressors that were more prominently represented in the data were organized into themes, the data were read again through a social support lens. The same process was followed as outlined in the first step for the identification of themes.

RESULTS

This study explored two research questions related to the stressors and social support experiences of men whose partner copes with PPD. The general stressors of PPD are well documented. What are far less explored are the experiences of men who are caregiving for both the baby and the mother during PPD. A theme analysis of desired social support of those partners is warranted, but it would best serve to first provide some insight into the stressors that manifest in the text of, in this case, partners of women coping with PPD. Accordingly, the following section showcases the most prominent themes related to stress that emerged in response to RQ1. The data are presented verbatim from the message boards and therefore retain all spelling and typographical errors to retain authenticity.

The Turning Point: "I will never forget that morning for as long as I live"

One of the most prominent experiences of fathers whose partner was coping with PPD was the moment they realized the severity of their situation. Whether it involved an alarming display of behavior by the mother, or resulted from the culmination of a series of events, that point exemplified a defining moment in their PPD journey. Some men recalled a memory that stands still to them, such as seeing their wife in a new light for the first time:

I found her curled up in the fetal position on our bed, shaking uncontrollably and crying into the bed. She told me that she felt like she was dying . . . She jumped off the bed and told me that she couldn't hold him (the baby), rushing out of the room and leaving me wondering just what was happening to my wife (#1).

Similarly, another new dad recalls disturbing dialogue that indicated something was seriously awry. The following example details a conversation one man had with his wife:

"I don't want to do this anymore" . . . "Do what?" . . . "Keep living." Nothing in my life has come close to causing as much worry, anger, frustration, despair, and fear as dealing with PPD . . . Nothing in my life prepared me to hear those words for the woman I loved so much. Nothing had prepared me to deal with how quickly our wonderful life with our new baby had spiraled down into thoughts of suicide . . . I felt like the life we had built together was falling apart (#4).

The serious nature of these pivotal moments was engraved in these men's minds as the beginning of a long journey. For example, one man stated, "When I found her she was almost catatonic with Andrew on her lap . . . My heart sank and I knew we were in for the fight of our lives" (#19). Similarly, another man recalls his wife changing the foundation of their marriage, "My spouse even told me I could sleep with other women . . . which I have not done" (#7). Some men experienced this realization in a less climactic way. Instead, it was the culmination of a series of events that forced them to realize their new normal. One man stated, "I almost feel like all hope is gone, like Im losing my relationship, my new son, and myself, like life just wont let me live it." (#23). Regardless of how the epiphany emerged, these turning points represented a pivotal moment that redefined their lives as they knew it. This theme represents the turning point from ambiguity to clarity – the defining moments when the severity of their situation crystallized, and when the pieces of their lives shifted in ways they had not anticipated on their journey to parenthood.

Concerns over Rebuilding the Relationship: "I just want my life and wife back"

Easily the most frequent, intense, and extensive theme was the concern men had over whether they could regain the lives they had prior to PPD. These quotes exemplify the loss men felt about their normal day-to-day functions, as well as missing their partner. Some men described how they felt in their daily lives, which involved becoming the primary caretaker for their family. The following quote illuminates one experience:

Suddenly I was caring for not just myself, but also my wife and baby. My view of how my life was going to go was shaken. I had to confront my fears, my frustrations, and my disappointments and carry on (#4).

Another man echoes the magnitude of the disruption and exhaustion of the situation:

I am worn down, broken, and tired . . . I am literally 100% committed between my work, and my kids. I have no time to myself. I pray to God every day that my wife will find some peace and that we can have a "normal" family and a "normal" life together. I look forward to the day when my wife and I can enjoy our family together and count our blessings instead of our misery. I've got to keep the faith, and be the rock for my family (#10).

In addition to taking on the primary caregiving role for their family, many men missed the partnership they had with their wife. Extensively throughout the text, the point about desiring the relationship they had with their wife prior to PPD trumped most other issues. This was the most extensive subset of the theme, with the majority of submissions touching on it in some capacity. Some men were short and to the point, such as, "She is less and less the person that I once knew. I feel like I'm living with a stranger at times . . . I just want my wife and my life back" (#12), and, "I pray daily that I will one day get my wife back" (#31). Others, such as the two that follow, gave a more nuanced view of their concerns over losing their wife and the life they created together:

I began to feel helpless, lost, and alone; I had no idea what happened to my wife and began to wonder if she would ever come back to me. It was easily the hardest and most trying time of my life and I began to feel depressed (#1).

Similarly, the next quote shows the despair one man feels as he tries to wait out the depression:

I pray for the same thing every day to have her back the way she was. I can't move on because my heart lies with my family. This is probably the hardest thing that I will ever have to go through because there just seems to be no end in sight. I feel bad for my son. This was not the life I wanted for him (#62).

Unfortunately, some men worried that there was no way to regain their life prior to PPD because of their inability to shake the negative memories and feelings associated with their experience. One man stated:

After all the bad things finally starts to get better for her but I now feel hate and anger towards her and I don't know how to turn those feeling off because I do care for her and love her, but I don't feel in love with her anymore and I feel like I despise her. It's like I gave her my heart just to crush me and now she wants me to love her but I don't know how anymore (#63).

Similarly, another husband laments about the woman he married:

I swear me and you are on the same boat only I don't think my wife will ever change back to who I fell in love with. Like seriously I feel like I'm getting treated like a child. I honestly don't know what to do anymore or what to believe . . . So if anyone has the same situation or can give me any tips that would be great (#111).

This theme highlights the loss the men feel as they struggle to maintain some normalcy in their life. Not only are they missing their day-to-day functions prior to PPD, they feel as though their partner is temporarily or permanently lost to them. The depth of their desire to return to "normal" is tangible.

Critiques: "She makes me feel like a crappy husband"

Another theme identified by its frequency and extensiveness was having to cope and process critiques received from their wife. It is important to state that these men indicated, repeatedly, that they love their wife and they do not believe these behaviors are indicative of her character; however, they believe part of coping with the disease is finding healthy communicative and internal ways of dealing with the critiques they receive from the mothers. For example, one man noted that "We can no longer joke around with one another. And to be honest I do not know if I love her anymore and just there cause I am used to her" (#13). One man stated, in response to the critiques his wife makes about him, "Sometimes I even question myself if she isn't right about the things she says about me ... she makes me feel like a crappy husband, which I'm pretty sure I am not" (#54). Another father noticed the stark difference between before and after the birth of their child:

Before we had our daughter, my wife loved me and cared about me. Now, I feel that she thinks I'm in the way. My wife says mean things to me. A lot. When I tell her that it hurts my feelings, she argues that she's sick of being the bad guy. I just have to sit there and take it ... There's constant digs about my parenting (#59).

Another man talked about the struggle he had experienced during PPD, saying his wife used to, "love and hate me at the same time. Insult me, belittle me, tell me I'm less of a man, threaten me ... sometimes she made me feel like if she had others in her life that would have been there for her, she wouldn't need me, actually she would tell me that" (#63). This example illuminates the extent to which the critiques challenged both the behavior and, at times, character of the men. This theme was not intense in elaboration, which limits the variety and length of the quotes used to exemplify it, but they were frequent and extended throughout the units of data.

The general stressors highlighted in this section offer a glimpse of the main worries or stressors that permeated the discourse. Men identifying the turning point moments, concerns over rebuilding their relationships, and struggling with critiques from the mothers as the prominent sources of stress during this time. With these themes as a foundation, the following section shares the results of an analysis of the themes related to social support of fathers whose partner was coping with PPD.

SUPPORT FOR STRESS

Now that the sources of stress are identified, attention can be turned to the type of social support men enacted or desired in the forums related to those issues (RQ2). Three themes emerged with regard to social support. The first theme, consultation, represented the problem-solving features of the interactions the men were having on the forum. The second theme featured the way that men considered fellow PPD fathers as almost comrades, having to "fight the good fight" together in honor of their families and wives. Finally, a theme of community emerged with regard to people and systems that supported them during the stressful time. The following sections expand on these themes in detail and connect them to the types of social support intertwined within them.

Consultation. Easily the most logical and serious theme, men worked to offer informational and emotional support by sharing their own experiences with readers. In sharing their thoughts, men offered a combination of practical support addressing the pragmatics of coping with PPD in the family as well as emotional support that discussed ways to manage feelings commonly associated with the stressor. For example, one man laid out his advice in terms of a game plan for fathers:

> If you make failure an option when dealing with PPD, you will fail. She will make you furious, she will make you scared, she will make you want to cut your losses and take your children away from her. You must remember this is not her talking. She is sick, and you might be the only thing in the world that can keep her from killing herself, killing your child, or both. You need, and must, take any and all support you can. You will need it, but when the rubber hits the road the responsibility may lie completely on your shoulders (#20).

Another man advised fathers against being secretive about their PPD experiences, both for the sake of helping others through sharing, as well as by addressing the PPD directly as a family:

> While parts of this story may be quite scary at times, I think it's important to share what happened to us, for it may help you be more prepared. And, know this, you and your family can and will get through whatever happens. Just don't ignore it. And believe me it will get better, for you have to BELIEVE; it's the most important part!!! (#17)

Whereas some men responded to submitters' questions directly in a chain of responses, others offered more global advice. Not all of the suggestions were positive, however. Some consultations acted as warnings for what was to come:

> I learned that if you just leave them alone, you're neglecting them and if you show you care you're smothering. It's almost an unattainable matter to make your wife happy

enough. Then you have to deal with the rejection, lack of intimacy. My spouse even told me that I could sleep with other women . . . which I have not done (#7).

Unlike the prior quote, which showed a major shift in the marriage, many others focused more exclusively on advising about issues of rebuilding trust. As one man stated, "As I look back, one major challenge was building trust up again. It can be hard to be afraid of leaving your child with her Mom, but over time the trust can be built" (#17). Yet another said, "My biggest worry is her coming home and trusting her again" (#2). Many of the men who submitted to the forum discussed trust in terms of comfort with leaving the child in her care, that she would seek help if needed in the future, and some men offered advice as to how to respond if their wives committed infidelity while suffering from PPD. As these quotes illuminate, much of the informational support came in the form of caregiving or, as exemplified above, warnings of difficulties they will face as they emerge out of the PPD episode.

The most poignant types of consultations came with specific, logical suggestions for the men, but they were also riddled with emotional support. The quote below exemplifies this type of advice:

I wish I could tell you the magic solution. I didn't find it myself. Learn all you can, be as loving as you can and find support from knowledgeable people . . . Know that what you and she experiences is not your fault, not your wife's fault, and that it will get better. Help her to feel secure in her home, secure with you, that you care immensely for her and your daughter. Know that it gets very difficult for husbands too, don't take it personally . . . you are in a "storm". Yes. Learn and love" (#47).

Similarly, many men offered practical support and emotional support in the form of advising others in effective ways to proceed. The advisement was presented in the text in a consultation manner, as many times the chain of comments were a slowly built dialogue that resulted in a collectively constructed offering of support. The advice given would sometimes be in response to questions asked, or it would be offered as a parallel to another submitter's response. This theme was extensive and intense, and had moderate frequency in the data.

Camaraderie. The most frequent and extensive support theme that permeated the data was that of a brotherhood. Especially when there were strings of comments following a story, the men would clearly state their relief in learning that other men were experiencing the same hardship. In this demonstration of weak-tie support, the men provide emotional support simply by informing others that they are not alone. For example, one man said, "Finished reading this in utter disbelief that you just described much of what I've been going through with my wife for the last 12 years!!" (#49) and, "Hey guys, first of all I wish I could have a beer or two with all of you" (#83). These men would often start their post with a statement addressing the comment prior to theirs, and others would directly link up to another person's story at the end of their statement. For example, "The story sounds exactly like mine . . . congrats on your reconciliation with your wife. I can only hope that mine has the same result" (#23), and, "Wow, verbatim what I'm going through . . . I hope my story has an upswing as yours does" (#25).

The text of the comments suggest that men were combing through others' examples, looking for a light at the end of the tunnel:

I concur with all three of these stories, and mine is similar. Two years removed from my son being born, wife still in a heavy depressive state. Two long years, I've read so many times that you have to be patient it takes time. If it's like Michael above, 7 years?!? I don't think I can last that long (#10).

This quote shows perceived commonality across others' stories and the sharing of one's own story. Some men directly addressed one another as individuals, "[Name Withheld], are you there? Tell me how it went. Is there any end to this because I am going through the same identical situation . . . this is hell, did not know my life can turn into this . . ." (#45), and others addressed the group more collectively, "I am in the boat guys! PLEASE tell me I am not nuts!" (#43). Regardless of how they go about this camaraderie, these men created a cohesive identity that is supportive for other members of the group.

Taken together, this theme beautifully showcased how men personalized the discourse in thoughtful and unique ways. By directly addressing individuals or the group as a collective, they enhanced their ability to provide emotional support to one another. The camaraderie displayed, and the commitment by so many of the commentators to foster it, was one of the most powerful themes of the study.

COMMUNITY

The theme of community emerged by the frequent and extensive representations of it in the text. A unit was labeled as representing the community category if it spoke about other individuals in their social network as playing a salient role in their PPD narratives. Emotional and informational support were the two forms most represented in this theme. The stories varied in valence concerning community, with some comments representing positive effects of the people to whom they had turned for support, and other units indicating the heavy implications of a nonsupportive community. One man's comments showed his relief in finding someone in his health care network that seemed to understand the precarious nature of his experience:

When we walked into his office there was a totally different attitude toward us than at the hospital. The doctored just listened. He allowed us, mostly myself, to explain our whole ordeal. He allowed me to express a lot of the anger and frustration I had about the situation. He then patiently explained the nature of depression and how Serotonin levels in the brain affect mood. He continually reassured us that Pam would get better.

He explained what medications he was prescribing and what the effects would be of each. He allowed us to ask a lot of questions. He was compassion and caring. Suddenly I felt like we had someone on our side helping us to heal Pam, rather than a system treating her like a criminal. It was a huge turning point for us (#4).

Another man documented the features of his social network that helped sustain him as he and his family struggled with PPD:

There have been many things that have helped me through this, but I think the key is the insight that I have been able to gain with the help of my wife, her doctors, the staff at the mother– baby units, pop psychology books, and my own experiences with psychotherapy (#3).

It is important to note that not all network comments indicated a positive impact, as many of these men discussed the helpful community components because of their relief of finding them after a hard or negative experience.

Beyond the health care component, men discussed the role that family can play when it comes to community issues. One dad noticed how his wife's mother struggled seeing her daughter cope with PPD and being hospitalized for it:

What makes this newsworthy is that when I told this news to her mother, she said, 'Well if I visit her I visit her. She chose to stay there.' I mentioned this, not to criticize her mother, but to point out that even those closest to the women going through postpartum depression can reach their limit (#20).

This man discussed how much her mother helped him care for his wife, but how she began to struggle with why her daughter could not emerge from the depressive episode over time.

Finally, men directly addressed the feeling of community that the power of the Internet provided them. Similar to the camaraderie theme in nature, this subset of the theme highlighted how the Internet has given them access to a community that proved to be an incredible form of support for them. To exemplify this point, one man wrote:

I know the power of that the internet provides. Putting useful info like PPD resources and descriptions of other people's experiences really shows what good the internet can do in actually helping people. It seems to me that awareness is the key. The more a thing is talked about, the less mysterious and frightening it seems (#3).

These three themes highlight the role of social support in men's experiences with their partner's PPD. Fathers used emotional, practical, and network support in effective ways to help one another, and men visibly desired emotional support to help them keep feelings of hope. The following section discusses the implications of these results.

DISCUSSION

The goal of this study was to examine the perspective of men whose partner was coping with PPD. An analysis of online forums for discussing this perspective revealed three themes outlining sources of stress for the fathers, followed by a second theme analysis that highlighted forms of social support the men desired or received. The first research goal addressed the general stressors, and it was found that men were stressed by the memory or turning point of when they knew something "wasn't right" with their partner. They also listed the criticism that was commonly distributed by their partner as a major source of stress, as well as their concern that they would never be able to rebuild their relationship or get back the person their partner was prior to PPD. The second analysis identified the presence of social support in three formats. The first was a sense of camaraderie with other men experiencing the same PPD life. The second was a genuine desire for advice, or consultation, in which men both very literally asked for advice via direct questions and were willing to share pieces of information that helped them survive the ordeal. Finally, themes of community support permeated the discourse. Men would note how family and health care professionals either helped or hindered their process of caring for their family, oftentimes citing how men should allow the community to help and embrace them as they coped with PPD.

Practical Implications

One of the most intense and frequent themes we found was the experience of criticism husbands perceived from their wives. Within the parameters of a relationship in which one partner is not coping with depression, chronic criticism is often treated as a downfall of the partnership (Shapiro & Gottman, 2004). When considering the presence of depression, however, criticism might be functioning as a feature of the situation rather than representative of the culture of the relationship. In our data, men would comment that it was unlike their wife to be so negative or insulting to them. In these cases, when negativity and criticism is not normative of the partnership, husbands could work to reframe how they respond to the criticism directed to them by their wife. One practice that might aid in distinguishing between situational criticism and chronic criticism is what therapists call relationship awareness (Acitelli, 2002). Being relationally aware entails recognizing and adjusting one's own behaviors to view the relationship as a unit, which in large part is associated with adopting dual perspectives and considering the current experiences of the partner. Some specific ways of enacting these relational lenses are to encourage fathers, when possible, to recognize that the criticism directed toward them is a function of the depression rather than how their wife actually views their partnership or the father's capabilities. In our data, men were understandably hurt by what they perceived to be lack of belief in their abilities to father, or in comments that made them feel less appreciated or desired. If these behaviors are not indicative of those that happen prior to the PPD, it might be a useful exercise to help fathers dismiss them as fleeting and recognize they are likely not personal, but situational.

A second feature of the data was that men were concerned with getting their wife and partnership back to "normal." One important feature in terms of helping husbands prepare for parenthood and PPD is that having a child is a turning point that brings with it a "new normal." Kleiman and Wenzel (2014) suggest that individuals work to recalibrate their expectations when confronted with parenthood more broadly, and PPD specifically. Helping fathers recognize that "good" marriages come in various forms, or that PPD can be a part of their story of strength rather than their marital downfall, might be important components of framing their relationship during this stressful time. Most families cope with PPD for a limited amount of time, and recovering or managing from postnatal anxieties and depressions can be accelerated by proper health care. Reminding fathers that there will be ebbs and flows, and teaching them to expect these obstacles, might help when confronting them. In a similar vein, many men reached out for a sliver of hope as they struggled during this time. Encouraging fathers that the depression is serious, but can be temporary if properly addressed, might help in them visualizing this intense time as a chapter in their partnership, rather than the defining moment of their marriage.

The data from this study suggest that men are coping with loneliness, hurt, and uncertainty. Unfortunately, men will need to rely heavily on coping skills during this stressful experience. Research on posttraumatic growth suggests that social support coincides with problem-focused coping, as well as the ability to manage self-depression and perceive positive opportunities during adversity (Tedeschi, Park, & Calhoun, 1998). Our data also point toward social support as a mechanism for managing the stressors associated with PPD. Often, emotional support is the facet that is less attended to in male support circles (Steuber & Solomon, 2008), but the outward appreciation of it in our data was obvious. Whereas women often cite their partner as the main form of desired emotional support, they also lean on other female counterparts for additional support resources when it comes to discussing feelings and emotions surrounding their experiences (Negron, Martin, Almog, Balbierz, & Howell, 2013). The results from this study suggest that men might function similarly within this context when it comes to reaching out to other men for emotional support, which is a deviation from research in other contexts. Future examinations should consider the pragmatics and accessibility of these online forums when it comes to the provision of support, as well as inquire about other helpful sources and how men can access them.

Directions for Future Research

Although this research project highlighted common stressors for and social support of men coping with a partner's PPD, our findings provide only a glimpse into this perspective. Future research needs to use a theoretical lens to begin connecting the dots in ways that can lead to effective interventions and means for helping men, individually, and the family, as a unit, during PPD. Some theoretical perspectives that could shed light on this experience are ones that consider stigma and disclosure (i.e., the disclosure decision-making model; Greene, 2009), and other theoretically driven work that links disclosure to social support (see Steuber & High, 2015 as an example). Both of these areas of work consider how perceptions of judgment or concerns about being treated differently inhibit the revelation of one's health condition. Because social support can be obtained only if a person is aware of a stressor, and considering PPD is often stigmatizing and therefore hidden, exploring these variables together is important.

The relational turbulence theory is another theory that could offer insight into the relational stressors that men face as they cope with PPD in their family (RTT; Solomon, Knobloch, Theiss, & McLaren, 2016). RTT considers the relational uncertainty and perceived interference that are inherent during relational transitions, and this theory has been used to explore other stressful health conditions such as infertility (Steuber & Solomon, 2008) and breast cancer (Weber & Solomon, 2008), as well as the transition to parenthood more broadly (Theiss, Estlein, & Weber, 2013). Because men articulated uncertainty about the future of their relationship, extending our focus beyond general well-being and exploring relational well-being is an important facet of helping these families return to a satisfied state as they emerge from the PPD experience.

Finally, extending research into the area of marital support might be a fruitful direction for improving PPD experiences for couples. We know that there are support gaps in terms of desired and received support between spouses (Xu & Burleson, 2001), but we know far less about the efficacy partners have in their abilities to provide appropriate and meaningful support for each other. Put differently, helping fathers feel confident in their executions of support behaviors could increase their own and their marital well-being during the postpartum time. Part of this could be explored by education about PPD, and others could be connected back to relational awareness (Acitelli, 2002) so that fathers can increase their chances of knowing the desired support their wife wants so they can increase the chances of their wife perceiving support during the stressor.

Strengths and Limitations

Extracting data from online support forums contributed both strengths and weaknesses to this study. The primary benefit was that the text provided narratives from men actively coping with a partner suffering from PPD that were unsolicited by the researchers. A weakness of this approach is that the sample is restricted in terms of generalizability to men with consistent Internet access, which might exclude lower socioeconomic groups (Calvert, Rideout, Woolard, Barr, & Strouse, 2005). The anonymous nature of the online forum also made it difficult to discern demographic information about the contributors. The two-step analysis provided a holistic perspective of both stressors and the role of social support in PPD experiences of men, but it was only an initial examination of the interplay of support and PPD.

Future studies should move to probe these issues more thoroughly in men, and directly ask them what types of support they would find valuable at different points in their PPD experience. For example, men might find that practical support in the form of help caring for their child, staying with the mother so they can attend work without concern over leaving the mother and child unattended, and having health care providers that listen and are knowledgeable in the variations in intensity and symptoms of the disease, might be what they initially desire in the early weeks or months. As time passes, they might want help nurturing their relationship back to a strong foundation or continued care when and if they have a new baby. Both future research and interventions should consider not just the immediate and crisis-driven care that is needed, but should also help establish satisfactory individual and relational well-being.

CONCLUSION

This chapter began by situating the male perspective of PPD as an under-studied, yet imperative, point of view during this health crisis. Although this study represents only a first step in the goal of illuminating fathers' needs during PPD, the data highlighted common sources of stress and the representation of support presented in online forums. Namely, men recalled the turning points that represented their realization of the severity of their situations, the concerns they had over whether they could reclaim their prior relationship, and the criticisms they oftentimes faced from their wife as she coped with PPD. In terms of social support, the presence of informational and emotional support was evident, as men offered advice and consultation to one another. They also exhibited a strong desire for and provision of emotional support by way of fostering camaraderie for one another. Finally, men discussed how tangible, informational, and network support can be provided, both positively and negatively, by the community of people around them. This study lays the foundation for future work on social support and other theoretically driven research on fathers' experiences of stress and social support during their partner's PPD.

REFERENCES

Acitelli, L. (2002). Relationship awareness: Crossing the bridge between cognition and communication. *Communication Theory, 12*, 92–112. doi: 10.1111/j.1468–2885.2002. tb00261

Bodie, G. D., Burleson, B. R., & Jones, S. M. (2012). Explaining the relationships among supportive message quality, evaluations, and outcomes: A dual-process approach. *Communication Monographs, 79*, 1–22. doi: 10.1080/03637751.2011.646491

Burleson, B. R. (2003). The experience and effects of emotional support: What the study of cultural and gender differences can tell us about close relationships, emotion and interpersonal connection. *Personal Relationships, 10*, 1–23. doi: 10.1111/pere.12150

Burleson, B. R., & MacGeorge, E. L. (2002). Supportive communication. In M. L. Knapp & J. A. Daly (Eds.), *Handbook of interpersonal communication* (3rd ed., pp. 374–424). Thousand Oaks, CA: SAGE.

Calvert, S. L., Rideout, V. J., Woolard, J. L., Barr, R.F., & Strouse, G. A. (2005). Age, ethnicity, and socioeconomic patterns in early computer use: A national survey. *American Behavior Scientist, 48*, 590–607. doi: 10.1177/0002764204271508

Chew-Graham, C., Sharp, D., Chamberlain, E., Folkes, L., & Turner, K. (2009). Disclosure of symptoms of postnatal depression, the perspectives of health professionals and women: A qualitative study. *Family Practice, 10*, 1–9. doi: 10.1186/1471–2296-10–7

Conger, R. D., Rueter, M. A., & Elder, G. H. (1999). Couple resilience to economic pressure. *Journal of Personality and Social Psychology, 76*, 54–71. doi: 10.1037/0022–3514.76.1.54

Cowan, C. P., & Cowan, P. A. (2000). *When partners become parents: The big life change for couples.* Mahwah, NJ: Lawrence Erlbaum Associates.

Davey, S. J., Dziurawiec, S., & O'Brien-Malone, A. (2006). Men's voices: Postnatal depression from the perspective of male partners. *Qualitative Health Research, 16*, 206–220. doi: 10.1177/1049732305281950

DiMatteo, M. R. (2004). Social support and patient adherence to medical treatment: A meta-analysis. *Health Psychology, 23*, 207–218. doi: 10.1037/0278–6133.23.2.207

Everingham, C. R., Heading, G., & Connor, L. (2006). Couples' experiences of postnatal depression: A framing analysis of cultural identity, gender, and communication. *Social Science and Medicine, 62*, 1745–1756. doi: 10.1016/j.socsimed.2005.08.039.

Goodwin, R., & Plaza S. H. (2000). Perceived and received social support in two cultures: Collectivism and support among British and Spanish students. *Journal of Social Personal Relationships, 17*, 282–291. doi: 10.1177/0265407500172007

Greene, K. (2009). An integrated model of health disclosure decision-making. In T. D. Afifi & W. A. Afifi (Eds.), *Uncertainty, information management, and disclosure decisions* (pp. 226–254). New York, NY: Routledge.

Hoseini Omam, S. S., Panaghi, L., Habibi Asgarabadi, M., & Davoodi, J. (2016). The relation between social support and marital satisfaction & couples' depression after the birth of the first child. *European Psychiatry, 33*, S779. doi: 10.1016/j.europsy.2016.01.2336

Kleiman, K., & Wenzel, A. (2014). *Tokens of affection: Reclaiming your marriage after postpartum depression.* New York, NY: Routledge.

Krueger, J. (1998). Enhancement bias in descriptions of self and others. *Personality and Social Psychology Bulletin, 24*, 505–516. doi: 10.1177/0146167298245006

Miller, A., Hogue, C., Knight, B., Stowe, Z., & Newport, D. J. (2012). Maternal expectations of postpartum social support: Validation of the postpartum social support questionnaire during pregnancy. *Archives of Women's Mental Health, 15*, 307–311. doi: 10.1007/s00737-012-0287-x

Negron, R., Martin, A., Almog, M., Balbierz, A., & Howell, E. (2013). Social support during the postpartum period: Mothers' views on needs, expectations, and mobilization of support. *Maternal Children Health Journal, 17*, 616–623. doi: 10.1007/s10995-012-1037-4

Paulson, J. F., & Bazemore, S. D. (2010). Prenatal and postpartum depression in fathers and its association with maternal depression: A meta-analysis. *Journal of the American Medical Association, 303*, 1961–1969. doi: 10.1001/jama/2010.605.

Rabiee, F. (2004). Focus group interview and data analysis. *Proceedings of the Nutrition Society, 63*, 655–660. doi: 10.1079/PNS2004399

Reblin, M. A., & Uchino, B. N. (2008). Social and emotional support and links to physical health. *Current Opinions in Psychiatry, 21*, 201–205. doi: 10.1097/yco.0b013e3282f3ad89

Sarason, B. R., Sarason, I. G., & Gurung, R. A. R. (1997). Close personal relationships and health outcomes: A key to the role of social support. In S. Duck (Ed.), *Handbook of personal relationships* (2nd ed., pp. 547–573). Chichester, England: Wiley.

Shapiro, A. F., & Gottman, J. M. (2004). The Specific Affect Coding System. In P. K. Kerig & D. H. Baucom (Eds.), *Couple observational coding systems* (pp. 191–208). Mahwah, NJ: Lawrence Erlbaum.

Shaw, B. A., Krause, N., Chatters, L. M., Connell, C. N., & Ingersoll-Dayton, B. (2004). Emotional support from parents early in life, aging, and health. *Psychology and Aging, 12*, 458–472. doi: 10.1037/0882-7974.19.1.4

Solomon, D. H., Knobloch, L. K., Theiss, J. A., & McLaren, R. M. (2016). Relational turbulence theory: Explaining variation in subjective experiences and communication within romantic relationships. *Human Communication Research, 42*, 507–532. doi: 10.1111/hcre.12091

Steuber, K. R., & High, A. C. (2015). Disclosure strategies, social support, and quality of life in infertile women. *Human Reproduction, 30*, 1635–1642. doi: 10.1093/humrep/devo93

Steuber, K. R., & Solomon, D. H. (2008). Relational uncertainty, partner interference, and infertility: A qualitative study of discourse within online forums. *Journal of Social and Personal Relationships, 25*, 831–855. doi: 10.1177/0265407508096698.

Symister, P., & Friend, R. (2003). The influence of social support and problematic support on optimism and depressions in chronic illness: A prospective study evaluating self-esteem as a mediator. *Health Psychology, 22*, 123–129. doi: 10.1037/0278-6133.22.2.123

Stowe, Z. N., Landry, J. C., & Porter, M. R. (1995). The use of depression rating scales in women with postnatal depression. In A. F. Schatzberg & C. B. Nemeroff (Eds.), *New research program and abstracts of the 148th annual meeting of the American Psychiatric Association* (pp. 17–57). Miami, FL: American Psychiatric Press.

Strauss, A., & Corbin, J. (1998). *Basics of qualitative research.* Thousand Oaks, CA: SAGE.

Tedeschi, R. G., Park, G. L., & Calhoun, L. G. (1998). *Posttraumatic growth: Positive changes in the aftermath of crisis.* Mahwah, NJ: Lawrence Erlbaum Associates.

Theiss, J. A., Estlein, R., & Weber, K. M. (2013). A longitudinal assessment of relationship characteristics that predict new parents' relationship satisfaction. *Personal Relationships, 20*, 216–235. doi: 10.1111/j.1475-6811.2012.01406.x

Uchino, B. N. (2009). Understanding the links between social support and physical health: A life-span perspective with emphasis on the separability of perceived and received support. *Perspectives on Psychological Science, 4*, 236–255. doi: 10.1111/j.1745-6924.2009.01122.x

Verhofstadt, L. L., Buysse, A., & Ickes, W. (2007). Social support in couples: An examination of gender differences using self-report and observational methods. *Sex Roles, 57*, 267–282. doi: 10.1007/s11199-007-9257-6

Weber, K. M., & Solomon, D. H. (2008). Locating relationship and communication issues among stressors associated with breast cancer. *Health Communication, 23*, 548–559. doi: 10.1080/10410230802465233

Xu, Y., & Burleson, B. R. (2001). Effects of sex, culture, and support type on perceptions of spousal social support: An assessment of the "support gap" hypothesis in early marriage. *Human Communication Research, 24*, 535–566. doi: 10.1093/hcr/27.4.535

13

Communication Skills (Comskil) Training for Oncology Nurses to Improve Patient-Centered Care

SMITA C. BANERJEE, RUTH MANNA, AND PATRICIA A. PARKER

Nurses play a key role on the oncology health care team. They tend to spend the most time with patients, and patients report being more comfortable communicating with nurses than with their physicians (McCarthy, 2014). Nurses are information and communication facilitators and provide support to patients and families (Farrington & Townsend, 2014; McLennon et al., 2013). Nurses typically report learning how to communicate with patients by watching others or through their experience (Mishelmovich, Arber, & Odelius, 2016). However, few of their mentors and colleagues received communication skills training and likely did not have systematic strategies for handling communication challenges. Communication skills are not innate and experience alone does not generally improve nurses' skills (Happ et al., 2011; Wright, 2012). Further, few nurses have formal training in difficult communication tasks such as discussing end-of-life (EOL) issues and responding to challenging family interactions (Sullivan, Lakoma, & Block, 2003). Several surveys of nurses at all experience levels have demonstrated that many feel unprepared to address these complicated and emotionally laden communication tasks and do not have a systematic plan for discussing difficult news (e.g., Baer & Weinstein, 2013; Chen & Raingruber, 2014; Peterson et al., 2010; Sivesind et al., 2003). Oncology nurses have expressed a considerable need for training in areas such as working with family challenges and EOL communication (Jors et al., 2016).

Effective communication is central to optimal patient-centered care in oncology (Epstein & Street, 2007; Institute of Medicine, 2013). In fact, in some studies, health care practitioner–patient communication has been identified as one of the most essential facets of patient care (Fuszard, Slocum & Wiggers, 1990). Oncology patients' view of good communication with nurses is that it is patient-centered, sensitive, and empathic; provides information in simple language; and offers opportunities to ask questions and express emotions and concerns (e.g., Newell & Jordan, 2015; Skea, Maclennan, Entwistle, &

N'Dow, 2014; Thorne et al., 2010). Researchers have shown that poor communication is prevalent within oncology settings and aspects of communication by nurses may be associated with increased risk of burnout, negatively impact patient well-being, and hinder optimal patient-centered care (Finke, Light, & Kitko, 2008; Gomez-Urquiza et al., 2016; McCabe, 2004; Thorne et al., 2005; Wittenberg-Lyles, Goldsmith, & Ferrell, 2013). Two research reviews found that nurses who were genuine, competent, knew how to facilitate patient disclosure, and had effective communication skills were more likely to promote better communication (Tay, Hegney, & Ang, 2011; Uitterhoeve et al., 2009). Conversely, nurses who were task-oriented or who had low self-awareness of their own verbal behaviors were found to inhibit communication (Tay et al., 2011). Thus, research clearly indicates a need for systematic training to help nurses learn communication skills to provide better patient care. This was also highlighted in the Institute of Medicine recommendations on promoting high quality cancer care, whereby the recommendations emphasized the importance of providing communication skills training to empower nurses to take a leadership role in modeling effective collaboration with patients and families (Ferrell, McCabe, & Levit, 2013).

NURSES AS "RELATIONAL PARTNERS"

Role of oncology nurses as informational partners, relational bridges, coordinators, advocates, educators, and facilitators has been described by many (e.g., Bridges et al., 2013; Havens, Vasey, Gittell, & Lin, 2010; Tariman & Szubski, 2015; Zaider et al., 2016). However, we describe the role of oncology nurses as "relational partners," as nurses are an integral part of the oncology team and are uniquely positioned to not only initiate and model supportive care to the patient and family, but also be an advocate for the patient and family unit when negotiating their wishes to the other members of the oncology team. Nurses have frequent contact with the patients and families and often assume partnership roles as they translate the perspectives of health care providers to the family and vice versa (Hamric, 2001; Koutsopoulou, Papathanassoglou, Katapodi, & Patiraki, 2010).

However, assuming the role of relational partner is fraught with communication stressors and challenges. A study that explored communication barriers reported by seven nurse managers to better identify communication skills needed for oncology nurses to practice patient-centered care revealed an imminent need for nurses to learn how to manage their intermediary role between patients, families, and physicians. Nurse managers reported that oncology nurses face communication challenges when they are caught in the middle between patients, families, and physicians (Wittenberg-Lyles et al., 2013), therefore underscoring the need for communication skills training for oncology nurses.

THEORETICAL FOUNDATIONS FOR COMMUNICATION SKILLS TRAINING: A BRIEF REVIEW

Advancements in the field of communication skills training have emphasized the need for theoretically sound training programs while acknowledging that the current theoretical basis of the communication trainings is generally weak (Brown & Bylund, 2008; Cegala & Broz, 2002; Hulsman, 2009). Coyne and Racioppo (2000) reaffirm the need for the development and testing of interventions or training programs explicitly designed from theoretical frameworks that can help explain why intervention or training components have been selected and how those components should be expected to improve outcomes. Cegala and Broz (2002) suggest that literature from research into provider–patient communication, communication theory, and educational psychology may help clarify the theoretical basis of communication skills training. Published reports on communication skills training have relied on a handful of theories to help support the development of their specific communication skills training module. Brown and Bylund (2008) describe (1) goals, plans, and action (GPA) theories and (2) sociolinguistic theory as foundations of Memorial Sloan Kettering's (MSK's) Communication Skills Training and Research (Comskil) Model, while Donovan and Ward (2001) discuss Leventhal's common-sense model (CSM) as foundations for their "representational approach to patient education." In this section, we present a brief review (see Kissane et al., 2012) of the aforementioned theories that may be well suited for formulating theoretical foundations of communication skills training.

Goals, plans, and action (GPA) theories. This theoretical framework is based on the assumption that when communicating, people rely on goals and plans to guide their communication (Berger, 1997). *Goals* are defined as future states of affairs that an individual is committed to achieving or maintaining. *Plans* are more concrete than goals and are cognitive representations of the behaviors that are intended to help enable goal attainment. *Actions*, even more concrete, are the behaviors that are carried out or enacted in an effort to realize the goal (Berger, 1997; Wilson & Morgan, 2006). Given that the GPA model proposes connecting goals to actions through plans, it seems to have utility for application in communication skills training. It is important to emphasize that to attain a single goal, multiple plans and actions may be proposed. For instance, in order to teach "responding empathically to patients, i.e., to recognize or elicit and respond to patients' empathic opportunities in order to communicate understanding, alleviate distress and provide support" (goal), the strategy of "recognize or elicit a patient's empathic opportunity" (plan) may be accomplished through acknowledgment, or encouragement of expression of feelings (actions). As well, "responding empathically to patients" (goal) could be attained using the strategy of "work toward a shared understanding of a patient's emotions or experience" (plan), which may be accomplished through asking open questions, clarifying, or restating (actions; see Pehrson et al., 2016).

Sociolinguistic theory. Sociolinguistic theory describes the process of communication from two orientations: the position-centered approach and the person-centered approach. The position-centered approach takes into account the communicator's reliance on a restricted code of communication, following the rules and norms of a communication situation. The role-based characteristics of the participants (e.g., physician to patient) are maintained during the process of communication. The person-centered approach, on the other hand, explains that communicators adapt their communication in response to the perspectives, feelings, and intentions of others (Miller, 2002). For instance, consider the scenario whereby an inpatient oncology nurse walks in to a room and mentions something about changing the intravenous (IV) infusion bag. Patient makes (sad) eye contact with the nurse and states, "I'm just so scared of what the future holds." In response to this interaction, the nurse from a position-centered approach may respond with, "The doctor will be here shortly and you can discuss all your problems with him. I will change the IV bag and will be back with your next medication shortly." Conversely, a nurse from a person-centered approach may pause whatever he or she is doing, pull a chair, sit next to the patient, and ask, "I am sure this is a very stressful time for you. But I am here for you . . . please talk to me. What's making you scared?" The second example clearly demonstrates providing social support and comfort in order to encourage the patient to share concerns and fears. Empathy and warmth overlap the relational facet of person-centered communication. Application of sociolinguistic theory to communication skills training could help health care practitioners identify and adapt to a variety of communication contexts (see Brown & Bylund, 2008).

Leventhal's common-sense model (CSM). Leventhal's common-sense model (CSM) is a self-regulation model that builds a comprehensive explanatory model of illness shared by the physician–patient dyad with reciprocal cross-checking and updating to ensure mutual accomplishment of this shared representation as a prototype of illness and health (McAndrew et al., 2008). CSM focuses on two sets of factors that describe the relationship between care seeking and patient management of chronic illness: (1) patients' representations of illnesses and treatments and (2) how patients appraise somatic changes (i.e., symptoms and function; Cameron, Leventhal, & Leventhal, 1993; Horne, 2003; Skelton & Croyle, 1991). In other words, patients hold a series of attitudes and beliefs (which may be medically sound or unsubstantiated) as their representations of illness. Patients also develop representations of treatment, perceived causal routes of action, expectations regarding efficacy, timeframes for action, and consequences (side effects). These representations of illness and treatment are interpreted and continually modified as new information is presented (from health care practitioners, friends, family, and mass media) and adjusted to (Leventhal, 2005).

Research has consistently established that these representations have five key domains: identity, cause, timeline, consequences, and control/ cure (Baumann, 2003; Leventhal, Leventhal, & Cameron, 2001). Action plans, as well as specific times and places for implementing treatment, link both the representations of illness and treatments to performance. From a physician–patient interaction perspective, it is important for clinicians to appreciate the multiple levels at which these representations operate and how they guide patients' preferences for treatment and the behaviors in which they engage over time (Hale, Treharne, & Kitas, 2007).

Thus, the three aforementioned theories (i.e., the GPA theory, patient-centered sociolinguistic theory, and the CSM of illness representation) become integrated in the communication skills training program, with the utmost objective of optimizing patient care.

CURRENT STATE OF COMMUNICATION SKILLS TRAINING PROGRAMS FOR ONCOLOGY NURSES

Many different types of communication skills training programs have been designed and delivered to oncology nurses (e.g., Delvaux et al., 2004; Heaven, Clegg, & Maguire, 2006; Kruijver et al., 2001; van Weert, Jansen, Spreeuwenberg, van Dulmen, & Bensing, 2011; Wilkinson, Perry, Blanchard, & Linsell, 2008), with varying outcomes (Moore, Rivera Mercado, Grez Artigues, & Lawrie, 2013). A Cochrane review of communication skills training for health care professionals working in oncology included 15 randomized controlled trials, with six trials focused on nurses. The review concluded that communication skills training for oncology health care providers can result in improvements of some communication skills, particularly gathering information skills and empathy. However, given the variation in study design, duration, and presence/absence of consolidation (or additional booster) training, the review concluded with a call for further research on effectiveness of communication skills training, both for the health care provider and patients (Moore et al., 2013)

MEMORIAL SLOAN KETTERING'S COMSKIL TRAINING FOR ONCOLOGY NURSES

The Communication Skills Training and Research Laboratory at Memorial Sloan Kettering (MSK) was created to train oncology providers in communication skills to improve communication with cancer patients and their families and enhance their overall adaptation to the illness. Traditionally, through its inception in 2005, the Communication Skills Training and Research Laboratory focused on developing communication training modules to support oncology physicians in communicating with oncology patients and their families throughout the cancer trajectory (Bylund et al., 2011). Following the development and successful implementation of the physician training program, our research and training group was approached by nursing leadership at MSK requesting support in developing Comskil training for the nurses. In meetings with the nursing leadership, we identified a list of three topics where nurses reported communication challenges: challenges in communicating empathically, challenges in having end-of-life (EOL) conversations, and challenges with conflicting families. However, we needed more data to help develop the Comskil training program for nurses.

To identify unmet communication needs of nurses, our team conducted a qualitative survey of 121 oncology nurses that focused on understanding specific forms of communication challenges they faced in the three aforementioned areas: challenges in communicating empathically, challenges in having EOL conversations, and challenges with conflicting families. Thematic analyses revealed six themes that described the challenges in communicating empathically with patients: dialectical tensions, burden of carrying bad news, lack of skills for providing empathy, perceived institutional barriers, challenging situations, and perceived dissimilarities between the nurse and the patient. The findings for challenges in having EOL conversations revealed five themes: dialectical tensions, discussing specific topics related to EOL, lack of skills for providing empathy, patient/family characteristics, and perceived institutional barriers (Banerjee et al., 2016). Finally, results for challenges with conflicting families revealed two themes: family interactions inhibiting quality care (demanding, controlling, and angry families) and differing viewpoints regarding patient care (disagreements between patient and family, disagreements between family members, and disagreements between family and health care team; Zaider et al., 2016). Overall, our study emphasized the need for institutions to provide communication skills training to their oncology nurses for navigating through challenging patient and family interactions.

In response to the needs survey described earlier, we developed a one-day Comskil training for nurses that offered three 2-hour long modules: (1) *Responding Empathically to Patients*: The goal of this module is to recognize or elicit and respond to patients' empathic opportunities in order to communicate understanding, alleviate distress, and provide support (Pehrson et al., 2016); (2) *Discussing Death, Dying, and EOL Goals of Care*: The goal of this module is to support the patient/family during their discussions and the decision-making process regarding EOL care (Coyle et al., 2015); and (3) *Challenging Interactions with Families*: The goal of this module is to use a collaborative and supportive approach to navigate difficult interactions with caregiving families (Zaider et al., 2016).

The curriculum for these modules was based on best practices in the literature (Brown & Bylund, 2008), a qualitative needs assessment survey of inpatient nurses' communication challenges (Banerjee et al., 2016), and was modeled after MSK's prior Comskil training program for oncologists (Bylund et al., 2011). Three booklets were developed for the training program (one for each module respectively). These booklets were sent to participants before their scheduled training and can serve as a resource for trainees after they come to training (Bylund et al., 2010). Participants are asked to review the material prior to attending training. Next, we will present preliminary results of the training for both inpatient and outpatient oncology nurses.

METHODS

Participants

A total of 410 nurses ($N = 410$; 342 inpatient nurses, 68 outpatient nurses) working in the oncology setting at MSK participated in a one-day nursing Comskil training program from January 2012 to November 2014. These nurses were from a number of settings across the hospital, including acute care, pediatrics, critical care, and urgent care, and were nominated by their nurse leaders to attend the Comskil training. A total of 37 Comskil trainings were offered between January 2012 and November 2014, with approximately 12 nurses participating in each training.

Nursing Comskil Training

Oncology nurses attended a 1-day, 3-module nursing Comskil training, comprising an introductory lecture (*Introduction to the Comskil Conceptual Model*) followed by three 2-hour modules (a total of 6.15 hours of communication skills training). The three modules included in the training were: *Responding Empathically to Patients, Discussing Death, Dying, and End-of-Life Goals of Care*, and *Responding to Challenging Interactions with Families*. Each module is comprised of two parts: (1) a 30-minute presentation that provides a rationale for the module's topic, reviews current literature on the topic, presents our recommended communication approach to address the challenges highlighted in the module, and shows demonstration videos that illustrate MSK nurses using our recommended communication approach with a simulated patient (each participant is also provided a printed booklet on the module); and (2) a 90-minute small group role play session that allows the participants to take turns and practice during an encounter with simulated patients (SPs).

The didactic presents our recommended blueprint for the module [the blueprint is a map that contains the communication goal (i.e., the desired outcome of the consultation)], and a recommended sequence of communication strategies (i.e., a priori plans that direct communication behavior toward the successful realization of the communication goal), skills (i.e., a standalone utterance by which a clinician can further the clinical dialogue, and thus achieve a strategy), and process tasks (i.e., sets of dialogues or nonverbal behaviors that create an environment for effective communication that are key to achieving a strategy) that are key to goal attainment. The majority of time in each training module was devoted to small groups of three learners, each working through role play scenarios, tailored to the discipline of the nurse participants. These role play sessions are co-facilitator-led sessions, wherein participants reflect on their interaction with the SP immediately following their role play, receive critical feedback from their peers/group members and facilitators, and review their performance on video playback. The SPs also provide feedback on the communication interaction, focusing on what aspects of the communication worked/did not work and why. The role plays for the first two modules, i.e., *Responding Empathically to Patients* and *Discussing Death, Dying, and End-of-Life Goals of Care* were presented in a small group format and the role play for the third module *Responding to Challenging Interactions with Families* was presented in a large group format (and referred to as a fishbowl).

Evaluation

The foundation for the evaluation of Comskil training program for nurses was based on the Kirkpatrick model, which is widely used in program evaluation (Kirkpatrick, 1967). The Kirkpatrick model includes assessment at four levels that measure (1) the reaction of the learners/participants, (2) their learning, (3) their behavior, and (4) the overall results on patient outcomes. With prior experience in the use of Kirkpatrick model in evaluation of Comskil training program for oncologists (Bylund et al., 2011), we modeled the operationalization of each of the four levels in the following ways: (1) nurse participant's self-reported perception of the Comskil training, both overall and for each module; (2) nurse participants' self-reported and demonstrated communication skills learning using self-efficacy measures and standardized patient assessments (SPAs; simulated patients using standardized scripts), respectively; (3) nurse participants' use of communication skills with real patients in their respective work setting; and (4) patient-reported outcomes. For the early phase of the Comskil training program for nurses, our focus was on determining the acceptability and preliminary efficacy of the program, and we focused on the first two levels of assessments that measure the reactions of the participants, and their learning (Banerjee et al., 2017).

Level 1: Participants' reactions. Nurse participants completed a paper-and-pencil evaluation survey after completion of each of the three modules (Banerjee et al., 2017). The evaluation survey contained six statements assessing post-training perceptions regarding the skills learned and application of skills in nursing clinical practice, measured on a 5-point Likert scale (1 = *strongly disagree* to 5 = *strongly agree*). For example, "The skills I learned in this module will allow me to provide better patient care," "The module prompted me to critically evaluate my own communication skills," and "I feel confident that I will use the skills I learned in this module." In addition, nurses were asked to rate the effectiveness of the four curricular activities, including the didactic teaching, exemplary videos, role play experiences, and booklet, on a 3-point Likert scale (1 = *Did not aid in my learning at all* to 3 = *Aided in my learning a lot*).

Level 2: Participant learning. Participant learning was operationalized in two different ways: a self-reported self-efficacy measure, and demonstration of skills uptake used in pre- and post-training SPAs. First, nurse participants' self-efficacy was assessed by a self-reported retrospective pre–post measure for self-efficacy (Hill & Betz, 2005), in which nurse participants respond to the following two questions post-training (the questions were tailored to match the module): (1) "Before this module, I felt confident responding empathically to patients/discussing death, dying, and end-of-life goals of care/ responding to challenging interactions with families," and (2) "Now that I have attended this module, I feel confident responding empathically to patients/discussing death, dying, and end-of-life goals of care/responding to challenging interactions with families."

Second, nurse participant learning was assessed through demonstration of skills uptake in SPAs in pre- and post-training. A SPA constitutes an 8-minute video recorded interaction between the nurse and the simulated patient (SP; a trained actor) on a given clinical scenario, using standardized scripts by the SP. SPAs were completed both pre- and post-training, and two trained coders coded all the SPA videos using the Comskil Coding System adapted to nurse clinical scenarios (Bylund et al., 2010).

Comskil Coding

We used the Comskil Coding System (CCS; Brown & Bylund, 2008; Bylund et al., 2010) to code all the video recorded SPAs. The CCS codes verbal utterances (frequency of skills) that are present in the nurse-standardized patient interaction, but does not code nonverbal behaviors (see Table 13.3 for a list of skills that were coded). Two research assistants were trained to code

TABLE 13.1 *Participant-rated perception of nurse communication skills training* (n = 410)

Item from Program Evaluation	Inpatient Nurses (*n* = 342) Agree or Strongly Agree (%)				Outpatient Nurses (*n* = 68) Agree or Strongly Agree (%)			
	Module 1	Module 2	Module 3	Overall	Module 1	Module 2	Module 3	Overall
1. I feel confident that I will use the skills I learned today.	97.4	96.4	91.1	95.0	97.1	95.4	98.6	97.0
2. The skills I learned today will allow me to provide better patient care.	97.4	98.2	91.5	95.7	94.1	97.0	98.6	96.5
3. The workshop prompted me to critically evaluate my own communication skills.	97.5	96.8	90.5	95.0	98.5	98.5	95.6	97.6
4. The experience of video feedback/large group role play was helpful to the development of my skills.	82.3	38.6	77.2	82.7	89.7	87.6	88	88.5
5. The skills I learned were reinforced through the feedback I received in the small group.	97.4	97.0	—	97.2	98.5	98.4	—	98.4
6. The small group/fishbowl facilitator was effective.	97.6	98.5	89.3	95.2	98.5	96.9	95.5	97.0

Note. Module 1 = responding empathically to patients; Module 2 = discussing death, dying, and EOL goals of care; Module 3 = responding to challenging interactions with families.

the video recorded SPAs, and were blind to the pre- or post-status of SPAs. The coding process was divided into two blocks. In the first block, both coders started with coding the same designated subset of videos (10% of the video recordings), which were assessed for intercoder agreement. On establishment of adequate reliability (minimum 75% agreement between coders), the two coders independently coded 20% of the dataset. Similar procedures were carried out in the second block of coding, with 10% of the data coded by both coders (and assessed for intercoder reliability), followed by both coders independently coding 20% of the SPAs (see Banerjee et al., 2017).

Data Analysis

For Level 1: participants' reaction, a rating of *agree* or *strongly agree* was considered to be an indicator of satisfaction with the module, and was analyzed descriptively. For Level 2: participant learning, paired *t*-tests were used to assess significant improvements in self-efficacy pre- and post-training. Finally, for assessing skill uptake, paired *t*-tests were used to assess changes in frequency of skills from pre- to post-training. Given that we conducted paired *t*-tests on 20 individual skills, 5 skill categories, and 1 overall skill index, we applied Bonferroni correction ($0.05/26 = 0.002$), and considered only *t* values that were significant at the $p < 0.01$ level (see Banerjee et al., 2017).

RESULTS

Results for Level 1: Participants' Reaction

Nurse participants rated the Comskil training program very favorably, as evidenced by high endorsement ($\geq 80\%$ participants choosing *agree* or *strongly agree*) of the statements evaluating the Comskil training (See Table 13.1). More than 90% of nurse participants, both from inpatient and outpatient settings, indicated high endorsement (agreed or strongly agreed) of five of the six evaluation items (with one item, "The experience of video feedback/large group role play was helpful to the development of my skills," receiving endorsement by more than 80% but less than 90% of participants; see Table 13.1). In addition, a large majority of nurse participants (>90%) rated each individual module component as aiding in learning (as indicated by ratings of "somewhat aided my learning" and "aided my learning a lot"; see Table 13.2).

TABLE 13.2 *Participant-rated perception of training components for nurse communication skills training*

Item from Program Evaluation	Inpatient Nurses (*n* = 342) Somewhat Aided My Learning or Aided My Learning a Lot (%)				Outpatient Nurses (*n* = 68) Somewhat Aided My Learning or Aided My Learning a Lot (%)			
	Module 1	Module 2	Module 3	Overall	Module 1	Module 2	Module 3	Overall
1. Didactic teaching	96.1	97.8	95.6	96.6	98.6	100.0	98.5	99.0
2. Exemplary video	96.1	99.1	96.9	97.4	98.5	98.5	96.9	98.0
3. Role play/ Fishbowl experience	99.4	98.8	98.2	98.8	100.0	100.0	100.0	100.0
4. Booklet	95.8	94.6	92.9	94.6	94.8	98.2	94.5	95.8

Note. Module 1 = responding empathically to patients; Module 2 = discussing death, dying, and EOL goals of care; Module 3 = responding to challenging interactions with families.

Results for Level 2: Participant Learning

Results for Level 2 will be presented in the two different ways in which learning was operationalized: a self-reported self-efficacy measure and demonstration of skills uptake used in pre- and post-training SPAs.

Self-efficacy. Paired sample *t*-tests were performed to assess overall changes in self-efficacy and self-efficacy for each of the specific modules. Overall for inpatient nurses, nurses' self-efficacy significantly improved [*t*(1016) = 31.17, *p* < 0.001] from pre- (*M* = 3.31, *SD* = 0.88) to post-training (*M* = 4.05, *SD* = 0.65). In particular, inpatient nurse participants' self-efficacy in responding empathically to patients significantly increased [*t*(340) = 18.59, *p* < 0.001] from pre- (*M* = 3.59, *SD* = 0.69) to post-training (*M* = 4.22, *SD* = 0.56). Similarly, inpatient nurse participants' self-efficacy in discussing death, dying, and EOL goals of care significantly increased [*t*(338) = 21.52, *p* < 0.001] from pre- (*M* = 3.03, *SD* = 1.02) to post-training (*M* = 3.99, *SD* = 0.70). Finally, inpatient nurse participants' self-efficacy in responding to challenging family interactions significantly increased [*t*(336) = 15.11, *p* < 0.001] from pre- (*M* = 3.30, *SD* = 0.79) to post-training (*M* = 3.93, *SD* = 0.64). A similar pattern of results was evident in the outpatient nurse cohort, with improved self-efficacy, overall, and for each of the three modules (see Table 13.3).

Skills uptake. Significant increases in overall skill use from pre- to post-training was evident for inpatient nurses, but not for outpatient nurses [*t*(333)

TABLE 13.3 *Self-efficacy in ability to complete task performance*

Self-Efficacy Items	Inpatient Nurses (n = 342)			Outpatient Nurses (n = 68)		
	M	SD	Paired Sample t-test	M	SD	Paired Sample t-test
Overall						
Before this module I felt confident about task.	3.31	0.88		3.30	0.85	
Now that I have attended this module I feel confident in my ability to perform task.	4.05	0.65	$t(1,016) = 31.17$**	4.00	0.69	$t(201) = 12.35$**
Responding empathically to patients						
Before this module I felt confident responding empathically to patients.	3.59	0.69		3.61	0.70	
Now that I have attended this workshop, I feel confident responding empathically to patients.	4.22	0.56	$t(340) = 18.59$**	4.16	0.59	$t(66) = 6.64$**
Discussing death, dying, and end-of-life goals of care						
Before this module, I felt confident discussing death, dying and end-of-life goals of care.	3.03	1.02		2.91	0.95	
Now that I have attended this workshop, I feel confident discussing death, dying and end-of-life goals of care.	3.99	0.70	$t(338) = 21.52$**	3.93	0.75	$t(66) = 9.45$**
Responding to challenging interactions with families						
Before this module, I felt confident responding to challenging interactions with families.	3.30	0.79		3.39	0.73	
Now that I have attended this workshop, I feel confident responding to challenging interactions with families.	3.93	0.64	$t(336) = 15.11$**	3.90	0.69	$t(67) = 5.81$**

**$p < 0.001$.

= 4.27, $p < 0.001$ vs. $t(67) = 1.01$, $p = 0.32$]. For inpatient nurses, the biggest gain was observed in empathic skills, while other skill categories failed to demonstrate clear significance. In particular, four out of five empathic skills (encourage expression of feelings, acknowledge, normalize, and praise patient efforts) significantly increased from pre- to post-training. Additionally, a significant increase was observed in one out of five questioning skills (clarify). No significant gains from pre- to post-training were observed in any of the agenda setting skills, information organization skills, or checking skills. However, for outpatient nurses, none of the skill categories demonstrated significant improvements. One out of five empathic skills (normalize) significantly increased from pre- to post-training (see Table 13.4).

DISCUSSION

Results from our inpatient and outpatient nurse trainings demonstrate a successful implementation of a communication skills training program for nurses at a major cancer center. The results for inpatient nurses provide evidence through favorable program evaluation, significant gains in self-efficacy regarding communicating with patients in various contexts, and significant improvement in several empathic skills, as well as in clarifying skills (see Banerjee et al., 2017). The results for outpatient nurses provide evidence through favorable program evaluation, significant gains in self-efficacy regarding communicating with patients in various contexts, and significant improvement in one empathic skill. We believe the unique contribution of the Comskil training program is to demonstrate that communication training in oncology can be integrated into a busy institution's regular practice, and offered to inpatient and outpatient nurses. Our ultimate objective is to encourage self-critique and foster self-reflection in clinicians that will help them provide optimal patient care.

We learned multiple lessons from the implementation of this training program. First, we learned that Comskil training was evaluated positively by the learners. The results from both inpatient and outpatient cohorts clearly indicated that Comskil training was received favorably by the nurses. The experience of video feedback was less favored as compared to other training components, possibly due to learner anxiety and self-consciousness of seeing oneself on screen. However, the endorsement of video feedback was not too low to raise concern about altering that aspect of training.

Second, it was clear that the nurses reported improved self-efficacy (i.e., improved beliefs about their capabilities to perform the key patient care tasks), such as responding to emotions and discussing EOL goals. We believe that the strong sense of improved self-efficacy is achieved through the role play sessions, where the learners are asked to identify challenging aspects of communication and, relatedly, craft their own learning objective.

TABLE 13.4 *Nurse training SPA (skills coding) results*

Skills	Inpatient Nurses (n = 342)			Outpatient Nurses (n = 68)		
	Pre-training M (SD)	Post-training M (SD)	t (df = 333)	Pre-training M (SD)	Post-training M (SD)	t (df = 67)
Agenda setting	0.08 (0.30)	0.08 (0.27)	−0.30	0.12 (0.33)	0.19 (0.43)	1.22
Declare agenda	0.07 (0.26)	0.07 (0.25)	−0.17	0.12 (0.33)	0.15 (0.36)	0.53
Invite agenda	0.01 (0.08)	0.01 (0.09)	0.45	0.00 (0.00)	0.03 (0.17)	1.43
Negotiate agenda	0.00 (0.00)	0.00 (0.00)	—	0.00 (0.00)	0.01 (0.12)	1.00
Take stock	0.01 (0.08)	0.00 (0.00)	−1.42	—	—	
Checking	0.61 (0.95)	0.70 (0.92)	1.65†	0.82 (0.95)	1.03 (1.05)	1.51
Check understanding	0.58 (0.91)	0.66 (0.86)	1.40	0.79 (0.89)	0.96 (0.95)	1.23
Check preference	0.02 (0.17)	0.04 (0.32)	1.04	0.03 (0.17)	0.07 (0.40)	1.35
Questioning	4.63 (2.10)	4.85 (2.21)	1.50	4.10 (2.00)	3.93 (2.17)	−0.55
Ask open questions	3.39 (1.76)	3.33 (1.77)	−0.54	2.10 (1.79)	2.19 (1.40)	0.39
Clarify	0.19 (0.52)	0.38 (0.77)	3.85***	0.22 (0.67)	0.19 (0.47)	−0.31
Restate	0.14 (0.43)	0.19 (0.45)	1.35	0.21 (0.48)	0.25 (0.53)	0.54
Endorse question asking	0.13 (0.37)	0.19 (0.43)	1.77†	0.31 (0.55)	0.40 (0.65)	1.14
Invite questions	0.78 (0.92)	0.75 (0.85)	−0.50	1.26 (1.05)	0.90 (1.01)	−2.56*
Information organization	0.35 (0.58)	0.37 (0.58)	0.58	0.31 (0.58)	0.27 (0.54)	−0.54
Preview	0.02 (0.13)	0.01 (0.09)	−1.00	0.06 (0.24)	0.01 (0.12)	−1.35
Summarize	0.01 (0.11)	0.04 (0.19)	2.34*	0.01 (0.12)	0.04 (0.21)	1.00
Transition	0.09 (0.33)	0.06 (0.29)	−1.42	0.15 (0.36)	0.09 (0.29)	−1.27

Review next steps	0.22 (0.45)	0.26 (0.44)	1.20	0.09 (0.29)	0.12 (0.33)	0.70
Empathic communication	2.31 (2.16)	2.91 (2.29)	4.03***	3.03 (2.11)	3.46 (1.93)	1.29
Encourage expression of feelings	0.36 (0.73)	0.56 (0.79)	3.87***	0.85 (1.23)	0.91 (1.09)	0.31
Acknowledge	0.46 (0.81)	0.60 (0.80)	2.47**	1.07 (1.06)	1.16 (1.17)	0.52
Validate	1.28 (1.57)	1.26 (1.42)	-0.22	0.96 (1.23)	0.91 (1.06)	-0.25
Normalize	0.07 (0.28)	0.17 (0.42)	3.88***	0.15 (0.40)	0.43 (0.68)	2.99**
Praise patient efforts	0.13 (0.40)	0.31 (0.67)	4.37***	0.00 (0.00)	0.04 (0.21)	1.76†
All skills	7.96 (3.57)	8.90 (3.40)	4.27***	8.38 (3.28)	8.87 (3.10)	1.01

†$p < 0.10$; *$p < 0.05$; **$p < 0.01$; ***$p < 0.001$.

The role plays are then tailored to the challenges identified by the learners themselves. Engaging in such an interaction with an SP gives them an opportunity to use communication skills and to observe meaningful differences in patients' verbal and nonverbal behaviors. In addition, critical feedback from their peers, facilitators, and, at the end, the SP, helps the learner understand helpful (and unhelpful) communication skill utilization.

Third, the results from SPAs demonstrated marginal improvements in skill uptake, particularly in empathic skills. This is an important outcome of our training, as nurses had identified their struggles in communicating empathically with patients (Banerjee et al., 2016). In addition, the results showing skills uptake for inpatient nurses were stronger than the results for outpatient nurses. Despite the fact that both nursing cohorts received the same training (with the exemplary videos and role plays tailored to the respective scenarios), we did not observe similar demonstrable skills uptake in the outpatient cohort. The reason for this could be attributed to the smaller number of outpatient nurses who participated in the Comskil training program. The low numbers were due to a lack in funding for the outpatient nurses to attend regular Comskil trainings. However, the trend observed in the training does indicate the possibility of significant improvements in the use of empathic skills in the outpatient cohort, as well.

Fourth, our results did not show improvements across all skill categories. In particular, nurses from both inpatient and outpatient cohorts did not demonstrate significant uptake in the other four skill categories (i.e., agenda setting, checking, questioning, and information organization). The different roles of nurses, from inpatient bedside nurses, to outpatient nurses who work as part of a disease management team, to outpatient nurses who function in nurse-run clinics, may have been a confounding factor, as not all skills categories may be relevant for all nurses. A future extension of this study will be to examine skills uptake in specific nursing disciplines to understand relevance of different skills in varied clinical setups.

Limitations

This study was not without limitations. This study was carried out at one cancer center in the northeast United States, and results may not be generalizable to other cancer hospital settings. Second, we evaluated the Comskil training program only up to the second level of the Kirkpatrick model (Kirkpatrick, 1967). Future work should assess more broad applications of training, particularly the transference of communication skills from a lab setting to the real world (with real oncology patients) and patient-reported outcomes. Third, we did not assess nurse participants' prior experience with communication skills training and years of oncology experience. Future research could assess moderators of program effectiveness, including prior communication skills training, years of experience, and attitude toward communication skills training (Banerjee et al., 2017). Finally, we did not assess effects of the Comskil training on nurse-level outcomes. Research informs us that ineffective communication with patients and families may negatively affect the nurses by increasing their levels of stress, lack of job satisfaction, and emotional burnout (Emold, Schneider, Meller, & Yagil, 2011; Potter et al., 2010). Providing a communication skills training can be considered as an institutional resource to invest in uplifting the morale of its nurses and should be assessed in future research.

CONCLUSION

Communication skills training (specifically MSK's Comskil training) is feasible and a useful model of training to improve clinician–patient communication. Our experience of implementation, both with inpatient and outpatient oncology nurses, suggests that nurses not only rated the program favorably, but also reported improved self-efficacy in their capabilities to perform the key patient care tasks and demonstrated skills uptake in use of empathic skills. Future research on transference of learning to real nurse–patient interactions and patient-reported outcomes will help us define the parameters of training reach and establish outcomes that are in concordance with the Institute of Medicine core elements of high-quality health care, defined as "providing care that is respectful of and responsive to individual preferences, needs, and values and ensuring that patient values guide all clinical decisions" (Institute of Medicine, 2001, p. 6).

REFERENCES

Baer, L., & Weinstein, E. (2013). Improving oncology nurses' communication skills for difficult conversations. *Clinical Journal of Oncology Nursing, 17*, E45–E51. doi: 10.1188/13.CJON.E45-E51

Banerjee, S. C., Manna, R., Coyle, N., Hammonds, S., Gallegos, T. E., Zaider, T., . . . Parker, P. A. (2017). The implementation and evaluation of a communication skills training program for oncology nurses. *Translational Behavioral Medicine, 7*, 615–623. doi: 10.1007/s13142-017-0473-5.

Banerjee, S. C., Manna, R., Coyle, N., Shen, M. J., Pehrson, C., Zaider, T., . . . Bylund, C. L. (2016). Oncology nurses' communication challenges with patients and families: A qualitative study. *Nurse Education in Practice, 16*, 193–201. doi: 10.1016/j.nepr.2015.07.007

Baumann, L. C. (2003). Culture and illness representation. In L. D. Cameron & H. Leventhal (Eds.), *The self-regulation of health and illness behavior* (pp. 242–254). New York, NY: Routledge.

Berger, C. R. (1997). *Planning strategic interaction: Attaining goals through communicative action*. Mahwah, NJ: Lawrence Erlbaum Associates.

Bridges, J., Nicholson, C., Maben, J., Pope, C., Flatley, M., Wilkinson, C., … Tziggili, M. (2013). Capacity for care: Meta-ethnography of acute care nurses' experiences of the nurse–patient relationship. *Journal of Advanced Nursing*, 69, 760–772. doi: 10.1111/jan.12050

Brown, R.F., & Bylund, C. L. (2008). Communication skills training: Describing a new conceptual model. *Academic Medicine*, 83, 37–44. doi: 10.1097/ACM.0b013e31815c631e

Bylund, C. L., Brown, R. F., Bialer, P. A., Levin, T. T., Lubrano di Ciccone, B., & Kissane, D. W. (2011). Developing and implementing an advanced communication training program in oncology at a comprehensive cancer center. *Journal of Cancer Education*, 26, 604–611. doi: 10.1007/s13187-011-0226-y

Bylund, C. L., Brown, R., Gueguen, J. A., Diamond, C., Bianculli, J., & Kissane, D. W. (2010). The implementation and assessment of a comprehensive communication skills training curriculum for oncologists. *Psycho-Oncology*, 19, 583–593. doi: 10.1002/pon.1585

Cameron, L., Leventhal, E. A., & Leventhal, H. (1993). Symptom representations and affect as determinants of care seeking in a community-dwelling, adult sample population. *Health Psychology*, 12, 171–179. doi: 10.1037/0278-6133.12.3.171

Cegala, D. J., & Broz, S. L. (2002). Physician communication skills training: A review of the theoretical backgrounds, objectives and skills. *Medical Education*, 36, 1004–1016. doi: 10.1046/j.1365-2923.2002.01331.x

Chen, C. H., & Raingruber, B. (2014). Educational needs of inpatient oncology nurses in providing psychosocial care. *Clinical Journal of Oncology Nursing*, 18, E1–E5. doi: 10.1188/14.CJON.E1-E5

Coyle, N., Manna, R., Shen, M. J., Banerjee, S. C., Penn, S., Pehrson, C., … Bylund, C. L. (2015). Discussing death, dying, and end-of-life goals of care: Adaptation and initial evaluation of a communication skills training module for oncology nurses. *Clinical Journal of Oncology Nursing*, 19, 697–702. doi: 10.1188/15.CJON.697-702

Coyne, J. C., & Racioppo, M. W. (2000). Never the twain shall meet? Closing the gap between coping research and clinical intervention research. *The American Psychologist*, 55, 655–664. doi: 10.1037/0003-066X.55.6.655

Delvaux, N., Razavi, D., Marchal, S., Bredart, A., Farvacques, C., & Slachmuylder, J. L. (2004). Effects of a 105 hours psychological training program on attitudes, communication skills and occupational stress in oncology: A randomized study. *British Journal of Cancer*, 90, 106–114. doi: 10.1038/sj.bjc.6601459

Donovan, H. S., & Ward, S. (2001). A representational approach to patient education. *Journal of Nursing Scholarship*, 33, 211–216. doi: 10.1111/j.1547-5069.2001.00211.x

Emold, C., Schneider, N., Meller, I., & Yagil, Y. (2011). Communication skills, working environment and burnout among oncology nurses. *European Journal of Oncology Nursing*, 15, 358–363. doi: 10.1016/j.ejon.2010.08.001.

Epstein, R. M., & Street, R. L. (2007). *Patient-centered communication in cancer care: Promoting healing and reducing suffering*. Bethesda, MD: National Cancer Institute.

Farrington, N., & Townsend, K. (2014). Enhancing nurse-patient communication: A critical reflection. *British Journal of Nursing*, 23, 771–775. doi: 10.12968/bjon.2014.23.14.771

Ferrell, B., McCabe, M. S., & Levit, L. (2013). The Institute of Medicine report on high-quality cancer care: Implications for oncology nursing. *Oncology Nursing Forum*, 40, 603–609. doi: 10.1188/13.ONF.603-609.

Finke, E., Light, J., & Kitko, L. (2008). A systematic review of the effectiveness of nurse communication with patients with complex communication needs with a focus on the use of augmentative and alternative communication. *Journal of Clinical Nursing, 17*, 2012–2015. doi: 10.1111/j.1365–2702.2008.02373.x

Fuszard, B., Slocum, L. I., & Wiggers, D. E. (1990). Rural nurses. Part II, Surviving the nurse shortage. *The Journal of Nursing Administration, 20*(5), 41–46. Retrieved from: http://journals.lww.com/jonajournal/Citation/1990/05000/Rural_Nurses__Part_II,_Surviving_the_Nurse.10.aspx

Gomez-Urquiza, J., Aneas-Lopez, A., Fuente-Solana, E., Albendin-Garcia, L., Diaz-Rodriquez, L., & Fuente, G. (2016). Prevalence, risk factors and levels of burnout among oncology nurses: A systematic review. *Oncology Nursing Forum, 43*, E104-E120. doi: 10.1188/16.ONF.E104-E120

Hale, E. D., Treharne, G. J., & Kitas, G. D. (2007). The common-sense model of self-regulation of health and illness: How can we use it to understand and respond to our patients' needs? *Rheumatology, 46*, 904–906. doi: 10.1093/rheumatology/kem060

Hamric, A. B. (2001). Reflections on being in the middle. *Nursing Outlook, 49*, 254–257. doi: 10.1067/mno.2001.120247

Happ, M. B., Garrett, K., Thomas, D. D., Tate, J., George, E., Houze M, . . . Sereika, S. (2011). Nurse-patient communication interactions in the intensive care unit. *American Journal of Critical Care, 20*, e28–e40. doi: 10.4037/ajcc2011433

Havens, D. S., Vasey, J., Gittell, J. H., & Lin, W. T. (2010). Relational coordination among nurses and other providers: Impact on the quality of patient care. *Journal of Nursing Management, 18*, 926–937. doi: 10.1111/j.1365–2834.2010.01138.x

Heaven, C., Clegg, J., & Maguire, P. (2006). Transfer of communication skills training from workshop to workplace: The impact of clinical supervision. *Patient Education & Counseling, 60*, 313–325. doi: 10.1016/j.pec.2005.08.008

Hill, L. G., & Betz, D. L. (2005). Revisiting the retrospective pretest. *American Journal of Evaluation, 26*, 501–517. doi: 10.1177/1098214005281356

Horne, R. (2003). Treatment perceptions and self-regulation. In L. D. Cameron & H. Leventhal (Eds.), *The self-regulation of health and illness behavior* (pp. 138–153). London: Routledge.

Hulsman, R. L. (2009). Shifting goals in medical communication. Determinants of goal detection and response formation. *Patient Education & Counseling, 74*, 302–308. doi: 10.1016/j.pec.2008.12.001

Institute of Medicine. (2013). *Delivering high-quality cancer care: Charting a new course for a system in crisis*. Washington, DC: National Academies Press.

Institute of Medicine; Committee on Quality of Health Care in America. (2001). *Crossing the quality chasm: A new health system for the 21st century*. Washington, DC: National Academies Press.

Jors, K., Seibel, K., Bardenheuer, H., Buchheidt, D., Mayer-Steinacker, R., Viehrig, M., . . . Becker, G. (2016). Education in end-of-life care: What do experienced professionals find important? *Journal of Cancer Education, 31*, 272–278. doi: 10.1007/s13187-015-0811-6

Kirkpatrick, D. L. (1967). Evaluation of training. In R. Craig & I. Bittel (Eds.), *Training and development handbook*. New York, NY: McGraw-Hill.

Kissane, D. W., Bylund, C. L., Banerjee, S. C., Bialer, P., Levin, T., Maloney, E. K., & D'Agostino, T. (2012). Special series (Whole patient): Communication skills training for oncology professionals. *Journal of Clinical Oncology, 30*, 1242–1247. doi: 10.1200/JCO.2011.39.6184

Koutsopoulou, S., Papathanassoglou, E. D. E., Katapodi, M. C., & Patiraki, E. I. (2010). A critical review of the evidence for nurses as information providers to cancer patients. *Journal of Clinical Nursing*, *19*, 749–765. doi: 10.1111/j. 1365–2702.2009.02954.x

Kruijver, I. P. M., Kerkstra, A., Kerssens, J. J., Holtkamp, C. C. M., Bensing, J. M., & van de Wiel, H. B. M. (2001). Communication between nurses and simulated patients with cancer: Evaluation of a communication training program. *European Journal of Oncology Nursing*, *5*, 140–153. doi: 10.1054/ejon.2001.0139

Leventhal, H. (2005). Health psychology: Past, present, and future. *The European Health Psychologist*, *1*, 3–5.

Leventhal, H., Leventhal, E., & Cameron, L. D. (2001). Representations, procedures, and affect in illness self-regulation: A perceptual-cognitive approach. In A. Baum, T. Revenson, & J. Singer (Eds.), *Handbook of health psychology* (pp. 19–48). New York, NY: Lawrence Erlbaum Associates.

McAndrew, L. M., Musumeci-Szabo, T. J., Mora, P. A., Vileikyte, L., Burns, E., Halm, E. A., ... Leventhal, H. (2008). Using the common sense model to design interventions for the prevention and management of chronic illness threats: From description to process. *British Journal of Health Psychology*, *13*, 195–204. doi: 10.1348/ 135910708X295604.

McCabe, C. (2004). Nurse-patient communication: An exploration of patients' experiences. *Journal of Clinical Nursing*, *13*, 41–49. doi: 10.1111/j. 1365–2702.2004.00817.x

McCarthy, B. (2014). Patients' perceptions of how healthcare providers communicate with them and their families following a diagnosis of colorectal cancer and under-going chemotherapy treatment. *European Journal of Oncology Nursing*, *18*, 452–458. doi: 10.1016/j.ejon.2014.05.004

McLennon, S. M., Lasiter, S., Miller, W. R., Amlin, K., Chamness, A. R., & Helft, P. R. (2013). Oncology nurses' experiences with prognosis-related communication with patients who have advanced cancer. *Nursing Outlook*, *61*, 427–436. doi: 10.1016/j. outlook.2012.12.001

Miller, K. (2002). *Communication theories: Perspectives, processes, and contexts.* Boston, MA: McGraw-Hill.

Mishelmovich, N., Arber, A., & Odelius, A. (2016). Breaking significant news: The experience of clinical nurse specialists in cancer and palliative care. *European Journal of Oncology Nursing*, *21*, 153–159. doi: 10.1016/j.ejon.2015.09.006

Moore, P. M., Rivera Mercado, S., Grez Artigues, M., & Lawrie, T. A. (2013). Communication skills training for healthcare professionals working with people who have cancer. *Cochrane Database of Systematic Reviews*, *3*, CD003751. doi: 10.1002/14651858.CD003751.pub3

Newell, S., & Jordan, Z. (2015). The patient experience of patient-centered communication with nurses in the hospital setting: A qualitative systematic review protocol. *JBI Database of Systematic Reviews and Implementation Reports*, *13*, 76–87. doi: 10.11124/jbisrir-2015-1072.

Pehrson, C., Banerjee, S. C., Manna, R., Shen, M. J., Hammonds, S., Coyle, N., ... Bylund, C. L. (2016). Responding empathically to patients: Development, implementation, and evaluation of a communication skills training module for oncology nurses. *Patient Education & Counseling*, *99*, 610–616. doi: 10.1016/j.pec.2015.11.021

Peterson, J., Johnson, M. A., Halvorsen, B., Apmann, L., Chang, P. C., Kershek, S., ... Pincon, D. (2010). What is it so stressful about caring for a dying patient?

A qualitative study of nurses' experiences. *International Journal of Palliative Nursing, 16*, 181–187. doi: 10.12968/ijpn.2010.16.4.47784

Potter, P., Deshields, T., Divanbeigi, J., Berger, J., Cipriano, D., Norris, L., & Olsen, S. (2010). Compassion fatigue and burnout: Prevalence among oncology nurses. *Clinical Journal of Oncology Nursing, 14*, E56–E62. doi: 10.1188/10.CJON.E56-E62

Sivesind, D., Parker, P. A., Cohen, L., Demoor, C., Bumbaugh, M., Throckmorton, T., . . . Baile, W. F. (2003). Communicating with patients in cancer care: What areas do nurses find most challenging? *Journal of Cancer Education, 18*, 202–209. doi: 10.1207/s15430154jce1804_7

Skea, Z. C., Maclennan, S. J., Entwistle, V. A., & N'Dow, J. (2014). Communicating good care: A qualitative study of what people with urological cancer value in interactions with health care providers. *European Journal of Oncology Nursing, 18*, 35–40. doi: 10.1016/j.ejon.2013.09.009

Skelton, J. A., & Croyle, R. T. (1991). *Mental representation in health and illness.* New York, NY: Springer-Verlag.

Sullivan, A. M., Lakoma, M. D., & Block, S. D. (2003). The status of medical education in end-of-life care: A national report. *Journal of General Internal Medicine, 18*, 685–695. doi: 10.1046/j.1525-1497.2003.21215.x

Tariman, J. D., & Szubski, K. L. (2015). The evolving role of the nurse during the cancer treatment decision-making process: A literature review. *Clinical Journal of Oncology Nursing, 19*, 548–556. doi: 10.1188/15.CJON.548-556

Tay, L. H., Hegney, D., & Ang, E. (2011). Factors affecting effective communication between registered nurses and adult cancer patients in an inpatient setting: A systematic review. *International Journal of Evidence-Based Healthcare, 9*, 151–164. doi: 10.1111/j.1744-1609.2011.00212.x.

Thorne, S. E., Bultz, B. D., Baile, W. F., & SCRN Communication Team. (2005). Is there a cost to poor communication in cancer care? A critical review of the literature. *Psycho-Oncology, 14*, 875–884. doi: 10.1002/pon.947

Thorne, S., Oliffe, J., Kim-Sing, C., Hislop, T. G., Stajduhar, K., Harris, S. R., . . . Oglov, V. (2010). Helpful communications during the diagnostic period: An interpretive description of patient preferences. *European Journal of Cancer Care, 19*, 746–754. doi: 10.1111/j.1365-2354.2009.01125.x

Uitterhoeve, R., Bensing, J., Dilven, E., Donders, R., deMulder, P., & van Achterberg, T. (2009). Nurse-patient communication in cancer care: Does responding to patient's cues predict patient satisfaction with communication? *Psycho-Oncology, 18*, 1060–1068. doi: 10.1002/pon.1434

van Weert, J. C., Jansen, J., Spreeuwenberg, P. M., van Dulmen, S., & Bensing, J. M. (2011). Effects of communication skills training and a Question Prompt Sheet to improve communication with older cancer patients: A randomized controlled trial. *Critical Reviews in Oncology-Hematology, 80*, 145–159. doi: 10.1016/j.critrevonc.2010.10.010

Wilkinson, S., Perry, R., Blanchard, K., & Linsell, L. (2008). Effectiveness of a three-day communication skills course in changing nurses' communication skills with cancer/palliative care patients: A randomized controlled trial. *Palliative Medicine, 22*, 365–375. doi: 10.1177/0269216308090770

Wilson, S. R., & Morgan, W. M. (2006). *Goals–Plans–Action Theories: Theories of goals, plans and planning processes in families.* Thousand Oaks, CA: SAGE.

Wittenberg-Lyles, E., Goldsmith, J., & Ferrell, B. (2013). Oncology nurse communication barriers to patient-centered care. *Clinical Journal of Oncology Nursing, 17*, 152–158. doi: 10.1188/13.CJON.152-158

Wright, R. (2012). Communication skills for the "caring" nurse. Pearson Education. Retrieved from: www.pearsonlongman.com/tertiaryplace/pdf/ros_wright_effecti ve_comm_skills_for_the_caring_nurse_aug2012.pdf.

Zaider, T. I., Banerjee, S. C., Manna, R., Coyle, N., Pehrson, C., Hammonds, S., ... Bylund, C. L. (2016). Responding to challenging interactions with families: A training module for inpatient oncology nurses. *Families, Systems and Health, 34,* 204–212. doi: 10.1037/fsh0000159

PART V

COMMUNICATION PATTERNS IN HEALTH AND
RELATIONSHIPS

14

Alcoholic and Nonalcoholic Parents' Orientations toward Conformity and Conversation as Predictors of Attachment and Psychological Well-Being for Adult Children of Alcoholics

MARIE C. HAVERFIELD AND JENNIFER A. THEISS

Alcoholism is a family illness that has implications for the physical, emotional, and psychological well-being of the spouse and children of individuals with alcoholism (Johnson & Stone, 2009). One in four families in the United States is affected by alcoholism (Grant, 2000), with approximately 26.8 million children growing up with a parent with alcoholism (Alcohol and Drug Programs [ADP], 2007). Children of parents with alcoholism tend to experience more frequent depression and struggle to develop healthy intimate relationships when compared to children of parents without alcoholism (Drejer, Theikjaard, Teasedale, Schulsinger, & Goodwin, 1985). Adult children of alcoholics (ACoA) who had a distressed relationship with a parent report feelings of alienation, poor communication ability, difficulty trusting others, increased emotional longing, negative attitudes toward the parent, and increased anxiety (Kelley et al., 2011; Straussner & Fewell, 2011). Taken together, these findings suggest that the interpersonal conditions in families coping with alcoholism can have a lasting effect on the well-being of ACoA. Thus, the goal of this study is to examine how communication patterns in families coping with a parent's alcoholism are associated with psychological outcomes for ACoA in adulthood.

We draw on family communication patterns theory (Koerner & Fitzpatrick, 2002a; Ritchie & Fitzpatrick, 1990) as the theoretical foundation for this study. The theory identifies two dimensions of communication in the family system: conformity orientation and conversation orientation (Ritchie & Fitzpatrick, 1990). A family's conformity and conversation orientations can be influential in shaping children's information processing ability, behavioral outcomes, and psychosocial outcomes (Schrodt, Witt, & Messersmith, 2008). Applications of family communication patterns theory have assumed that all family members share a similar co-orientation with regard to communication behavior within the family (Koerner & Fitzpatrick, 2002b). Although some families may enact uniform communication patterns that allow for a universally shared communication orientation in the family, this approach tends to overlook circumstances in which each parent may enact different patterns of conformity and conversation (e.g., Miller-Day & Marks, 2006). In families coping with a parent's alcoholism, for example, the parent with and without alcoholism may enact different communication patterns with their children, such that each parent would create distinct expectations for conformity and conversation (Rangarajan & Kelly, 2006). Accordingly, this study examines the extent to which ACoA perceive that the parent with and without alcoholism enact similar or different communication orientations and the associations that each parent's communication patterns share with ACoA's psychological well-being in adulthood.

This study has theoretical and practical implications for understanding communication patterns in families coping with a parent's alcoholism. Theoretically, we extend family communication patterns theory by (a) applying it to the context of distressed families and (b) examining ACoA perceptions of the degree to which the parent with and without alcoholism enact similar communication patterns with similar effects. In doing so, we challenge the assumption that all family members adopt a singular co-orientation with regard to family communication patterns, and explore the possibility for divergent communication patterns with different family members. Pragmatically, this study is important for understanding how perceptions of communication in families coping with a parent with alcoholism can have lasting effects on attachment and well-being. In practice, this study can inform interventions with families coping with a parent's alcoholism by helping to identify the ways in which family communication patterns are linked with various outcomes for children in this context. In this chapter, we summarize the assumptions of family communication patterns theory as they relate to psychological outcomes for ACoA, and we report the results of a study designed to explore these associations.

FAMILY COMMUNICATION PATTERNS THEORY

The interactions that take place within families are influential for the socialization of family members and the transference of shared values and beliefs (Burleson, Delia, & Applegate, 1995; Ritchie & Fitzpatrick, 1990). Family members establish norms for behavior and co-construct their family culture through interpersonal interaction (Reiss, 1981). Family communication patterns theory provides a framework for characterizing communication behavior within families (Fitzpatrick & Ritchie, 1994; Koerner & Fitzpatrick, 2002a). The theory identifies two dimensions that define family communication: conformity orientation and conversation orientation. *Conformity orientation* reflects the degree to which all family members are expected to share the same attitudes, values, and beliefs. Families that have a high conformity orientation promote traditional family hierarchies, interdependence between family members, conflict avoidance, and family harmony. Families that have a low conformity orientation encourage individuality and equality for all family members and expect less cohesion in the family. *Conversation orientation* reflects the degree to which family members communicate openly and share information about a variety of topics. Families with a high conversation orientation engage in frequent conversations and they value spontaneous interaction characterized by openness and honesty. Low conversation oriented families engage in less frequent and less open interactions between family members and they do not view communication as an essential aspect of family functioning.

Communication patterns in the family are associated with an array of psychological outcomes for children. For example, families that enact open and constructive communication have children who demonstrate better social competence and the ability to regulate emotion (Carle & Chassin, 2004; Farrell, Barnes, & Banerjee, 1995). Children from conversation-oriented families demonstrate increased self-efficacy, stronger academic ability, and fewer adjustment problems (Rueter & Koerner, 2008; Tajalli & Ardalan, 2010). In addition, children from conversation-oriented families engage in more relational maintenance behaviors and have closer friendships than children in low conversation-oriented families (Ledbetter, 2009). Families that emphasize high conformity are known to produce more regulatory behavior, less empathy, and less perspective-taking than those low in conformity (Koerner & Cvancara, 2002). Conformity orientation has been found to be both positively (Hamon & Schrodt, 2012) and negatively (Koerner & Fitzpatrick, 1997) associated with depression, and it is negatively associated with self-esteem (Hamon & Schrodt, 2012). Taken together, this evidence suggests that conformity orientation and conversation orientation are influential factors in children's psychological adjustment.

Family communication patterns in families coping with alcoholism are not well-documented. Early research on the topic indicated that children of parents with alcoholism are often discouraged from communicating about various topics in the family to prevent upset for the parent with alcoholism (Black, 1982). Families coping with a parent's alcoholism tend to express fewer feelings and have lower regard for other family members (Jones & Houts, 1992). More recent studies continue to show that family members struggle to manage conflicts or express positive feelings in the homes of families coping with a parent's alcoholism (Johnson, 2001). Some recent work has shown that a father's alcoholism is more influential to family communication patterns than is a mother's alcoholism, such that the severity of paternal alcoholism is positively associated with higher conformity orientation and is negatively associated with conversation orientation, but severity of maternal alcoholism does not predict either orientation (Rangarajan & Kelly, 2006). These findings present the possibility of different communication styles between mothers and fathers with alcoholism. Along these lines, within families coping with alcoholism, the parent with and without alcoholism may each adopt different communication orientations. Although research utilizing family communication patterns theory typically applies one communication orientation to the entire family unit, there are a variety of family circumstances that may promote different communication patterns with each parent. For example, divorced parents may each enact different communication behaviors when they have custody of their children, stepparents may encourage a different communication environment than biological parents, and parents who are chronically ill or absent may promote communication behaviors that the healthy or present partner does not promote. Along these lines, we wonder if ACoA may perceive their parent with and without alcoholism differently in terms of their orientations toward conformity and conversation. Accordingly, we advance the following research question:

RQ1: To what extent do ACoA perceive parents with and without alcoholism to be similar or different in their conformity orientation and conversation orientation?

ATTACHMENT STYLES ASSOCIATED WITH FAMILY COMMUNICATION PATTERNS

According to attachment theory (Bowlby, 1969), a primary caregiver's availability and sensitivity during infancy and early childhood shapes children's internal representations of the self. Thus, caregivers who are available and respond sensitively to their children's distress influence their children's evaluation of the self as worthy of attention and affection, but parents who fail to provide sensitive and responsive care could promote a model of self as unworthy and undeserving of attention and love. Two dimensions serve as the foundations for people's attachment style (Bartholomew, 1990; Fraley, Waller, & Brennan, 2000): anxiety and avoidance. The *anxiety dimension* reflects the degree to which individuals have internalized a sense of their own self-worth and expect others to respond to them positively or negatively. The *avoidance dimension* reflects the degree to which individuals expect others to be generally available and supportive. Thus, the dimensions of anxiety and avoidance represent general expectations about the worthiness of self and the reliability of others (Griffin & Bartholomew, 1994).

Within the context of a family coping with a parent's alcoholism, caregiving quality may be compromised by parents' preoccupation with their own or their partner's alcoholism. When parents' attention to their children is impaired by these factors, children may react in disorganized, detached, and disruptive ways, and they may also develop an insecure attachment style

(Erdman, 1998). In families coping with a parent's alcoholism, one or both parents may be prone to periodic, if not chronic, distancing from their children. Thus, children growing up with a parent with alcoholism are at risk for the development of an insecure attachment style, particularly to the alcoholic parent. Prior research has shown that parents with alcoholism have a high conformity orientation and a low conversation orientation (Rangarajan & Kelly, 2006). Moreover, family communication patterns have been found to moderate associations between family stressors and attachment styles in families coping with a parent's alcoholism (Rangarajan, 2008). In general, conformity orientation should predict increased anxiety and avoidance because individuals may have difficulty establishing their own self-worth and trusting others in a context where their input is not valued. In contrast, conversation orientation should predict decreased anxiety and avoidance because it reflects the degree of parental involvement and responsiveness that are required for a secure attachment style. Thus, we advance the following hypotheses:

H1: Perceptions of the conformity orientation of the parent (a) with alcoholism and (b) without alcoholism are positively associated with ACoA self-reported attachment anxiety and avoidance.

H2: Perceptions of the conversation orientation of the parent (a) with alcoholism and (b) without alcoholism are negatively associated with ACoA self-reported attachment anxiety and avoidance.

One important consideration is whether parents with and without alcoholism exert the same degree of influence on their children's attachment outcomes. On one hand, parents with alcoholism may be absent in the parenting process, which suggests that the communication patterns of the parent without alcoholism would be more salient in shaping attachment outcomes than those of the parent with alcoholism. On the other hand, parents with alcoholism may behave in ways that are more dysfunctional due to their disease, which may have a more significant impact on children's development. For example, individuals with alcoholism, as a consequence of their disease, tend to prioritize alcohol over family, neglect family and work obligations, become verbally and physically abusive, and withdraw from loved ones (Straussner & Fewell, 2011). Moreover, during bouts of heavy alcohol abuse, parents with alcoholism often render themselves emotionally and physically unavailable to their spouse and children (Eiden, Edwards, & Leonard, 2002). Thus, we wonder whether the relative absence of and inconsistent nurturing from a parent with alcoholism is more or less influential to a child's attachment style than a potentially more consistent and engaged caregiving style of a parent without alcoholism. To investigate this, we pose another research question:

RQ2: To what extent do parents with and without alcoholism have similar degrees of influence on their children's attachment anxiety and avoidance?

ATTACHMENT ORIENTATION AS A PREDICTOR OF PSYCHOLOGICAL WELL-BEING FOR ACOA

The dimensions of attachment are associated with a variety of psychological and relational outcomes in adulthood. In this study, we highlight three psychological outcomes that are relevant to ACoA and are likely to be predicted by attachment style: (a) depression, (b) resilience, and (c) self-esteem.

Depression is one psychological outcome that is predicted by attachment orientation and particularly germane to the experiences of ACoA. *Depression*, as a clinical disorder, refers to feelings of sadness, anger, and loss that impact healthy functioning (Fava & Cassano, 2008). Factors that can lead to depression include stressful life events, difficulty coping, and interpersonal struggles (Compas, Connor-Smith, Saltzman, Thomsen, & Wadsworth, 2001; Grant, Compas, Thurm, McMahon, & Gipson, 2004; Sullivan, Neale, & Kendler, 2000). Research on attachment has found that insecure attachment styles are associated with increased levels of anxiety and depression (Muris, Mayer, & Meesters, 2000). ACoA are especially susceptible to depression due to the many risk factors to which they are exposed during childhood (Hall & Webster, 2007; Harter & Taylor, 2000). For example, ACoA report high levels of stress, difficulty adjusting to life events, and an increase in negative self-perception (Hall & Webster, 2007; Hall & Webster, 2002; Hall, Webster, & Powell, 2003). Taken together, these findings suggest that attachment anxiety and avoidance may predict depressive symptoms for ACoA. Thus, we advance the following hypothesis:

H3: Attachment anxiety and avoidance are positively associated with symptoms of depression for ACoA.

Resilience is another outcome for ACoA that is also predicted by attachment style. *Resilience* is broadly defined as an individual's ability to positively overcome adverse circumstances (Palmer, 1997). Children growing up in the home of a family coping with a parent's alcoholism are highly susceptible to risk factors that inhibit resilience, such as over-responsibility, high levels of conflict, and parental neglect (Hall & Webster, 2007). Secure, dismissing, and fearful attachment styles are associated with increased resilience, whereas the preoccupied attachment style is negatively associated with resilience (Karreman & Vingerhoets, 2012). Thus, we expect that increased attachment anxiety and avoidance may hamper resilience for ACoA. Accordingly, we advance the following hypothesis:

H4: Attachment anxiety and avoidance are negatively associated with resilience for ACoA.

Finally, self-esteem is an outcome that has been linked with both attachment style and experiences of children of parents with alcoholism. *Self-esteem* refers to an individual's perception of self-worth, with high self-esteem relating to higher levels of confidence and low self-esteem reflecting feelings of inadequacy (Baumeister, 1993). Various studies have shown that children of parents with alcoholism have lower self-esteem than their peers who are raised in a home with a family not coping with a parent's alcoholism (Beesley & Stoltenberg, 2002; Berkowitz & Perkins, 1988; Bush, Ballard, & Fremouw, 1995; Drake & Vaillant, 1988; Beaudoin, Murray, Bond, & Barnes, 1997). In addition, research has consistently found support for the relationship between secure attachment and positive representations of the self, including high levels of self-esteem and self-efficacy (Thompson, 1999). Similarly, individuals who are high on the anxiety dimension experience greater fluctuation in self-esteem based on negative interpersonal feedback and individuals who are high on the avoidance dimension have fewer fluctuations in self-esteem based on positive feedback (Hepper & Carnelley, 2012). These findings suggest that attachment orientation is a significant predictor of self-esteem. Thus, we propose the following hypothesis:

H5: Attachment anxiety and avoidance are negatively associated withself-esteem in ACoA.

The model in Figure 14.1 summarizes our hypotheses. Specifically, we predicted that ACoA's perceptions of the conformity orientation of parents with and without alcoholism is positively associated with attachment anxiety and avoidance (H1), and conversation orientation is negatively associated with the attachment dimensions (H2). Next, we predicted that ACoA's attachment anxiety and avoidance are positively associated with depressive symptoms (H3) and negatively associated with resilience (H4) and self-esteem (H5). In addition to our hypothesized paths, we included paths between several variables in the model that are known to share significant correlations.

METHOD

To test our hypotheses, we recruited ACoA to complete an online survey about their family communication patterns in their family of origin, attachment orientation, and experiences of depression, resilience, and self-esteem in adulthood. Participants were recruited by responding to announcements posted in online listservs of support groups for family and friends of individuals with alcoholism (e.g., www.ncadd.org; www.al-anon.alateen.org; www.breining.edu). The criteria for selecting these platforms included active member participation, number of members, and the likeliness of reaching a large population of ACoA. To be eligible to participate in the study, individuals had to (1) be 18 years of age or

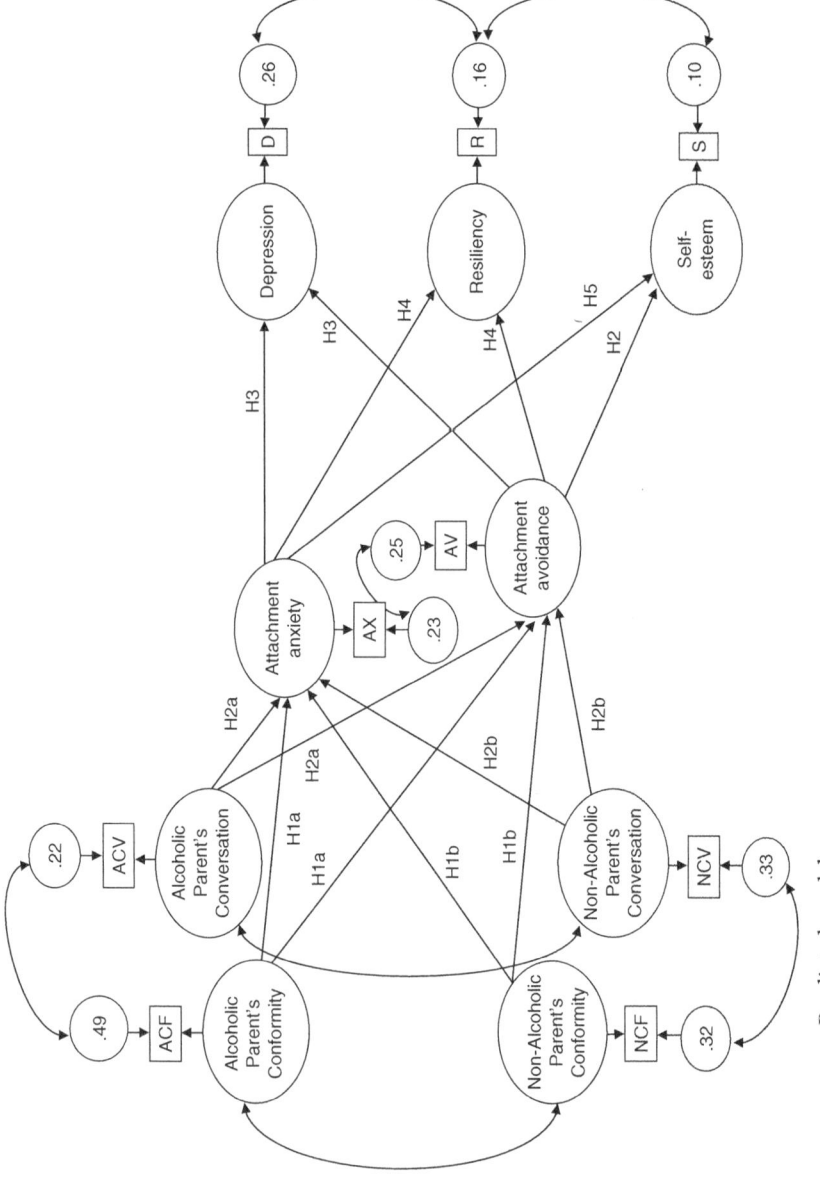

FIGURE 14.1 Predicted model.

older, (2) be a self-proclaimed child of a parent with alcoholism, and (3) have Internet access. The first 200 people to complete the survey received a $15 gift card.

Sample

The initial sample included 968 participants, but individuals who indicated that both of their parents had alcoholism ($N = 345$) were eliminated prior to analysis so that we could compare effects for parents with and without alcoholism. The final sample included 623 ACoA (537 female, 85 male, 1 missing). Participants ranged in age from 18 to 87, with a mean age of 47.96 ($SD = 14.41$). The majority of respondents were white/Caucasian (91.5%), with others identifying as Hispanic/Latino (4.3%), African American (2.2%), Native American (2.2%), Asian-Pacific Islander (1.4%), Middle Eastern (0.2%), and 1.4% other. Respondents reported living in 48 different states, as well as Canada and the Virgin Islands. The majority of participants had a father with alcoholism (76.6%), with fewer individuals reporting a mother with alcoholism (23.4%).

Measures

We conducted confirmatory factor analyses on all multi-item scales to ensure that they were unidimensional and externally valid (Hunter & Gerbing, 1982). The criteria for a good fitting factor structure were $\chi^2/df < 3.0$, Comparative Fit Index (CFI) > 0.95, and Root Mean Squared Error of Approximation (RMSEA) < 0.06. After confirming satisfactory fit, composite scores were constructed by averaging the responses to scale items.

Family communication patterns. We asked respondents to report on the conformity orientation and the conversation orientation for their mother and father separately. Then, based on their indication of whether it was their mother or their father with alcoholism, we recoded the variables into alcoholic's and nonalcoholic's conformity orientation and conversation orientation. We assessed conformity orientation and conversation orientation using a condensed version of the 26-item Revised Family Communication Patterns Instrument (Fitzpatrick & Ritchie, 1994), removing items involving politics and hypothetical statements. Respondents indicated their agreement with items on a 6-point scale (1 = *strongly disagree* to 6 = *strongly agree*). Four items were used to evaluate the conformity orientation of each parent (e.g., "When anything really important was involved, my [mother/father] expected me to obey without question"; "In our home, my [mother/father] usually had the last word"; Alcoholic Parent: $\alpha = 0.82$, $M = 4.35$, $SD = 1.65$; Nonalcoholic Parent: $\alpha = 0.82$, $M = 3.98$, $SD = 1.33$). Four items that measured the conversation orientation for each parent (e.g., "My [mother/father] often asked my opinion when the family was talking about something"; "I talked to my [mother/father] about feelings and emotions"; Alcoholic Parent: α = 0.86, M = 2.18, SD = 1.28; Nonalcoholic Parent: α = 0.86, M = 2.99, SD = 1.53).

Attachment dimensions. We used a shortened version of the 36-item revised Experiences in Close Relationships Scale (ECR-R; Fraley et al., 2000). Individuals indicated their agreement on a 6-point scale (1 = *strongly disagree* to 6 = *strongly agree*). Four items measured attachment anxiety (e.g., "I worry a lot about my relationships"; "I often worry that my partner doesn't really love me"; α = 0.92, M = 3.51, SD = 1.68), and six items measured attachment avoidance (e.g., "I'm afraid that I will lose my partner's love"; "I get uncomfortable when a romantic partner wants to be very close"; α = 0.86, M = 3.29, SD = 1.35).

Depressive symptoms. We measured depressive symptoms using the Center for Epidemiologic Studies Depression Scale (CES-D; Wood, Taylor, & Joseph, 2010). Prior to data collection, three items were removed due to redundancy. Respondents used a 6-point scale (1 = *strongly disagree* to 6 = *strongly agree*) to indicate their agreement with statements characterizing their feelings in the past week. Six items were included as depressive symptoms (e.g., "I felt depressed"; "I thought my life had been a failure"; α = 0.84, M = 3.04, SD = 1.28).

Self-esteem. Self-esteem was assessed by the degree to which the participant is confident in his or her personal value or maintains a positive self-image (Blascovich & Tomaka, 1991). Participants reported their agreement with items on a 5-point scale (1 = *strongly disagree* to 5 = *strongly agree*). Five items were used to measure self-esteem (e.g., "I feel that I am a person of worth, at least on an equal plane with others"; "I feel that I have a number of good qualities"; α = 0.88, M = 3.86, SD = 0.91).

Resilience. Resilience was operationalized through a composite measure of survey items assessing the degree to which the participant believes he or she has the ability to cope with adversity, maintain life balance, and maintain an optimistic perspective (Wagnild & Young, 1993). Participants reported their agreement with items on a 6-point scale (1 = *strongly disagree* to 6 = *strongly agree*). Five items measured resilience (e.g., "Keeping interested in things is important to me"; "My belief in myself gets me through hard times"; α = 0.82, M = 4.58, SD = 0.93).

RESULTS

Preliminary Analyses

As a starting point, we conducted independent samples *t*-tests to evaluate all of our variables for sex differences. Results revealed no significant differences between males and females on any of the variables. We then examined the bivariate correlations among all of our variables (see Table 14.1). A final preliminary test was conducted to address RQ1, which inquired about the extent to which parents with and without alcoholism were similar or different in their conformity and conversation orientations. We conducted paired samples *t*-tests to check for mean differences between ACoA's perceptions of the parent with and without alcoholism on the conformity orientation and the conversation orientation. Results revealed that parents with and without alcoholism were significantly different on the conformity orientation (t (612) = 3.86, $p < 0.001$), such that parents with alcoholism ($M = 4.35$, $SD = 1.65$) were perceived as having a higher conformity orientation than parents without alcoholism ($M = 3.98$, $SD = 1.33$). In addition, parents with and without alcoholism were significantly different on the conversation orientation (t (612) = –10.56, $p < 0.001$), such that parents with alcoholism ($M = 2.18$, $SD = 1.28$) were perceived as having a lower conversation orientation than parents without alcoholism ($M = 3.00$, $SD = 1.53$). These results suggest that ACoA perceive their parents differently in terms of their conformity and

TABLE 14.1 *Bivariate correlations among all variables*

	1	2	3	4	5	6	7	8
1. Alcoholic's Conversation								
2. Alcoholic's Conformity	–0.22 ***							
3. Nonalcoholic's Conversation	0.03	–0.00						
4. Nonalcoholic's Conformity	–0.05	0.29 ***	–0.16 ***					
5. Attachment Avoidance	0.05	–0.09 *	0.05	–0.16 ***				
6. Attachment Anxiety	0.02	0.01	0.12 **	–0.15 ***	0.63 ***			
7. Depression	0.02	0.02	0.07	–0.06	0.36 ***	0.44 ***		
8. Resiliency	–0.02	0.09 *	0.07	0.18 ***	–0.22 ***	–0.28 ***	–0.51 ***	
9. Self-Esteem	–0.05	0.08	–0.02	0.18 ***	–0.40 ***	–0.43 ***	–0.53 ***	0.62 ***

$^*p < 0.05$; $^{**}p < 0.01$; $^{***}p < 0.001$.

conversation orientation such that parents with alcoholism expect their children to be agreeable and obedient, whereas parents without alcoholism shoulder more of the burden in terms of engaging children in open conversations and encouraging disclosure and sharing. Taken together, these findings are significant because they imply that family communication patterns may not be consistently enacted across different family relationships.

Test of Hypothesized Model

To test our hypotheses, we conducted a structural equation model (SEM) using Amos 20. We used parcels as single-item indicators of the latent variable, with the error variance of each parcel set to $(1 - \alpha)(\sigma)$ to account for measurement error in our scales (Bollen, 1989). Again, our criteria for a good fitting model were $\chi^2/df < 3.0$, CFI > 0.95, and RMSEA < 0.06. The data indicated that the initial model did not provide an adequate fit to the data (χ^2 (15) = 3.11, CFI = 0.97, RMSEA = 0.07). We reviewed the modification indices for the model and identified paths with the largest modification index to be added to the model one at a time until we achieved a satisfactory model fit. We added one direct path from the nonalcoholic parent's conversation orientation to resilience, which resulted in a model that adequately fit the data (χ^2 (14) = 2.46, CFI = 0.98, RMSEA = 0.06).

Results indicated that ACoA's perceptions of the alcoholic parent's conformity orientation and conversation orientation were not significantly associated with either attachment avoidance or anxiety (see Figure 14.2); thus, H1a and H2a were unsupported. In contrast, ACoA's perception of the nonalcoholic parent's conformity orientation was positively associated with attachment anxiety and ACoA's perception of the nonalcoholic parent's conversation orientation was negatively associated with both anxiety and avoidance. Thus, H1b was partially supported and H2b was fully supported. In addition, ACoA's self-reported attachment avoidance and anxiety were both positively associated with depression (H3) and negatively associated with resilience (H4) and self-esteem (H5). Thus, H3, H4, and H5 were all fully supported. Finally, the added path in the model indicates that ACoA's perception of the nonalcoholic parents' conversation orientation is positively associated with resilience.

Recall that RQ2 inquired about whether parents with and without alcoholism have similar degrees of influence over their children's attachment orientation. The results indicated that perceptions of alcoholic parents' conformity orientation and conversation orientation are not significantly associated with self-reported attachment style, but perceptions of nonalcoholic parents' conformity orientation predicts attachment anxiety and perceptions of conversation orientation predicts both attachment anxiety and avoidance. A path was also added between the reports for nonalcoholic parents'

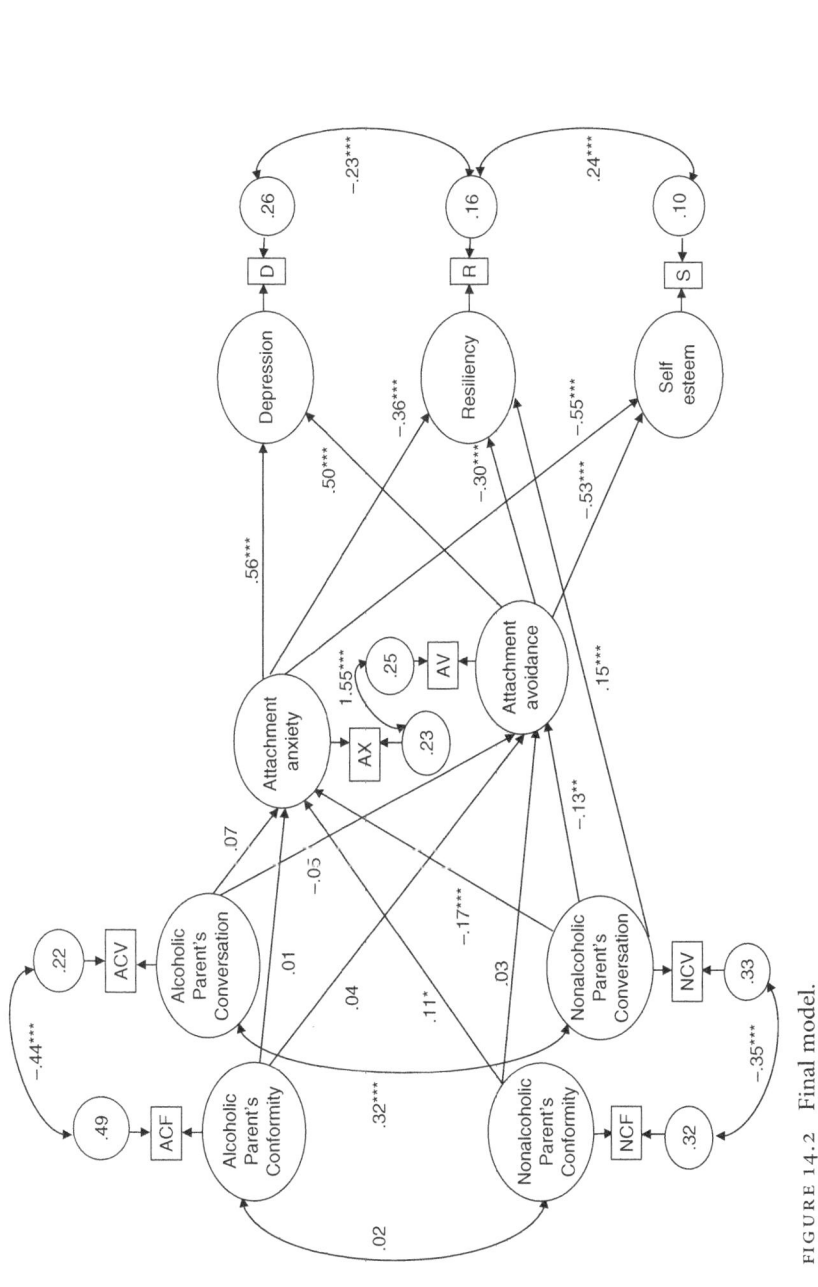

FIGURE 14.2 Final model.

conversation orientation and resilience. Thus, the results suggest that the family communication patterns of the parent without alcoholism are more influential for children's development and adjustment than those of the parent with alcoholism.

DISCUSSION

This study challenged the assumptions of family communication patterns theory (Fitzpatrick & Ritchie, 1994; Koerner & Fitzpatrick, 2002a) by exploring the ways in which communication dynamics of parents with and without alcoholism differentially contribute to attachment style and psychological outcomes for ACoA. The results indicate that ACoA's perceptions of the conformity orientation and conversation orientation of the nonalcoholic parent predict dimensions of attachment anxiety and avoidance for ACoA, which in turn predict increased levels of depression and decreased resiliency and self-esteem. Surprisingly, ACoA's perceptions of the conformity orientation and conversation orientation of the parent with alcoholism were not significant predictors of ACoA attachment. In this section, we discuss the results in terms of implications for extending theory and for helping families that are coping with a parent's alcoholism.

Implications for Advancing Family Communication Patterns Theory

As a starting point, this study examined the degree to which ACoA perceive similar orientations toward conformity and conversation in their parent with versus without alcoholism in an effort to determine whether a dominant communication style was present. Results of a paired samples *t*-test revealed that ACoA perceive their parent with alcoholism as higher in conformity orientation and lower in conversation orientation than their parent without alcoholism. Common characteristics of individuals with alcoholism include low frustration tolerance, desire for perfection, anxiety, poor self-image, and a sense of loneliness (NIAAA, 2010). In addition, parents with alcoholism are often inconsistent with their affection, vacillating between demonstrations of love and warmth at certain times and rejection at others (Woititz, 1989). In contrast, the parent without alcoholism must often overcompensate for the erratic behavior of their spouse to ensure that their children's needs are being met. Thus, it is not surprising that ACoA would have different perceptions of the communication patterns of their parent with and without alcoholism.

This result has important implications for the development of family communication patterns theory because it suggests that parents may not always promote the same communication patterns in the family and, even if they do, it does not mean that is how other members of the family perceive those patterns. Although most applications of family communication patterns theory assess perceptions of the conformity orientation and conversation orientation for the family as a whole, our results suggest that there is utility in evaluating perceptions of family communication patterns from a variety of vantage points. We can envision a variety of family circumstances in which each parent may enact different communication patterns with their children, such as in divorced families, stepfamilies, military families that are separated during deployment, or families in which one parent is suffering from illness. The results of this study indicate that distressed families, in particular, are likely to perceive different communication patterns enacted by each parent. Similarly, Rangarajan and Kelly (2006) found that parents with and without alcoholism have different orientations toward family communication. In addition, Miller-Day and Marks (2006) found that fathers' conformity orientation and conversation orientation predicted disordered eating behavior in children, but mothers' communication patterns did not. So what does this mean for family communication patterns theory? We believe this provides an opportunity to examine the implications and perceptions of dueling communication orientations in the family. The theory tends to assume that parents co-construct a social reality in the family in which they both communicate with children in the same way and to the same effect. Our results suggest that this may not be the case, and calls for further theorizing about the complexity of balancing communication patterns across parents. Family communication patterns theory may need to evolve to account for each parent's unique influence in the family as well as the corresponding perceptions of parent's communication orientations.

The results of this study also revealed that ACoA's perceptions of the communication patterns of parents without alcoholism predicted attachment anxiety and avoidance, but perceptions of the communication patterns of parents with alcoholism did not. This finding was surprising given that individuals with alcoholism tend to provide relatively inconsistent nurturing for their children (e.g., Woititz, 1989), which should be influential in shaping attachment outcomes. Why would the parent without alcoholism have more influence on attachment style than the parent with alcoholism? We have identified two possible explanations for this finding. First, a methodological explanation has to do with the distribution of fathers and mothers with alcoholism in our sample. Three-quarters of our sample reported that their father was the parent with alcoholism, so there were very few mothers with alcoholism in this sample. Given that mothers are typically the primary source for pair-bonding in the formation of attachment style (Bowlby, 1969), it is possible that our results reflect the fact that fathers, in general, are less influential in the development of attachment styles, and most of the parents with alcoholism in this sample were fathers. Second, a contextual explanation has to do with the way children of parents with alcoholism may relate to their parent with alcoholism. As a coping mechanism, many children of parents with alcoholism distance themselves from their parent with alcoholism and become more independent (Masten et al., 1995). Thus, children may buffer themselves from the negative influence of a parent with alcoholism by limiting interaction. Notably, this may be especially true for daughters with fathers with alcoholism, who were heavily represented in our sample.

The results of this study point to two important considerations for extending family communication patterns theory. First, our findings call into question the utility of family communication patterns theory for at-risk families. Prior research has tended to test the theory within intact families and measure only one communication orientation for the entire family (e.g., Schrodt et al., 2008). The results of this study suggest that some tenets of family communication patterns theory may not translate to families with nontraditional structures and relationships. Given the rich diversity that characterizes modern families, a theory that is broader in scope and applicable to more diverse family experiences would be ideal. Second, our findings call into question the idea of a co-orientation around communication behavior in the family (Koerner & Fitzpatrick, 2002a). We found that ACoA perceive different conversation orientations and conformity orientations for their parent with and without alcoholism. At the very least, this finding suggests that families characterized by separated or absentee parents may not conform to a single communication orientation in the family; however, given that the majority of the parents with alcoholism in this study were fathers, we wonder if the differing communication orientations observed in this study are less a reflection of a parent's alcoholism and more a reflection of each parent's gender. To the extent that mothers and fathers enact different communication behaviors based on traditional gender roles, children may perceive separate communication climates around each parent rather than a single communication orientation for the whole family. In other words, a lack of co-orientation in the family may not be isolated to at-risk families, it may be possible in any family where each parent enforces different expectations for communication behavior. Future research on family communication patterns theory should explore this possibility.

Implications for Families Coping with a Parent's Alcoholism

The results of this study provide important insight for children of parents with alcoholism, primary caregivers in a home of a family coping with alcoholism, and practitioners working with these families. Research on the family members of individuals with alcoholism is limited, and what is available focuses primarily on descriptions of the emotional and psychological outcomes for children of parents with alcoholism, with little attention to the dynamics of the family coping with alcoholism that may contribute to such outcomes. We believe that family communication patterns theory was a useful tool for examining the dynamics of communication in families coping with alcoholism that contribute to various outcomes for children as they become adults.

Our results suggest that the conversation orientation in the family, particularly the conversation orientation of the parent with alcoholism, is more influential in shaping outcomes for ACoA than the conformity orientation. The conversation orientation of the parent without alcoholism was negatively associated with attachment anxiety and avoidance. Moreover, the direct path that was added to the model revealed a positive association between ACoA perceptions of the conversation orientation of the parent without alcoholism and ACoA's resilience. Thus, families coping with a parent's alcoholism should be encouraged to engage in open communication about a variety of topics. Internalizing traumatic experiences can increase contemplation, anxiety, and mood turbulence (Larson & Chastain, 1990; Roemer & Borkovec, 1994), amplify psychological issues (Gross & Levenson, 1993), and intensify rates of illness (Larson & Chastain, 1990). An open communication environment allows ACoA to talk through concerns or triumphs, which can potentially mitigate emotional or psychological issues stemming from their family situation (Pennebaker, 1985). Discussing the negative experiences affecting ACoA can also be an important part of the coping process (Bareket-Bojmel & Shahar, 2011). Children of Alcoholics (CoA) and ACoA may struggle to talk about their experiences given that many families affected by alcoholism attempt to stifle communication about the illness (Black, 1982). In these instances, CoA and ACoA may benefit from seeking external support from a professional such as a counselor or therapist. Although increased communication may not be beneficial in all situations, our results suggest that CoA may benefit from talking about their feelings, either with their parent(s) or with a third party.

In contrast, the conformity orientation of parents with and without alcoholism is somewhat less influential for shaping ACoA's attachment styles. Perceptions of the conformity orientation of parents without alcoholism was positively associated with attachment anxiety, but it was the only communication orientation that was significant. On one hand, it is encouraging that few of the family communication patterns were significantly associated with attachment anxiety. On the other hand, parents should be aware that creating a family climate that is high in conformity orientation prevents children from forming their own ideas and opinions, which can encourage feelings of low self-worth. Particularly in families with a parent with alcoholism, pressuring children to adopt homogeneous opinions about the situation can lead to frustration and discourage dialogue. Thus, families coping with a parent's alcoholism should make an effort to encourage conversation and to allow family members to express their differing feelings about their family experiences.

The outcomes we investigated in this study included depression, resilience, and self-esteem. Although a number of previous studies have shown that ACoA struggle with these psychological outcomes in adulthood, few investigations have considered how perceptions of communication might contribute to them. In our study, these variables were most strongly and directly predicted by the ACoA's dimensions of attachment anxiety and avoidance. These results provide a bit of bad news for ACoA who are trying to cope with the effects of having a parent with alcoholism. Given that attachment styles are developed at a very young age and tend to be persistent across the lifespan (Ainsworth, Blehar, Waters, & Wall, 1978; Bowlby, 1969), ACoA with insecure attachment styles may continually struggle to bolster self-esteem, combat depression, and be resilient in the face of hardship. Finding attachment relationships in adulthood that can contribute to more positive working models of the self and others may be an important step in adopting more positive psychological outcomes in adulthood.

Strengths, Limitations, and Future Directions

This study has several strengths. First, we were able to recruit a rather large sample, which included participants from nearly every state and multiple countries. Thus, our sample is representative of ACoA from a variety of different communities. Second, we measured ACoA's perceptions of conformity orientation and conversation orientation for parent with and without alcoholism separately, which allowed us to examine how parents may diverge in their family communication patterns and whether each parent had equal influence on children's outcomes. Although this is in contrast to the tradition of family communication patterns theory, we believe our findings demonstrate the importance of testing theory in diverse contexts, and present an opportunity for extending the scope of the theory. Finally, whereas much of the literature on ACoA is descriptive in nature, our investigation was informed by theory. By applying family communication patterns theory to explain the dynamics of families coping with a parent's alcoholism, we were able to extend the literatures on both ACoA and families coping with alcoholism.

There were also some limitations in this study. First, the sample was heavily skewed with females, which limits our ability to generalize to the experiences of male ACoA. The distribution of males and females in the sample is representative of the groups from which they were recruited, which report that 86% of members are female. More research is needed to better understand the experiences of male ACoA and to determine if daughters and sons are similarly affected by a parent's alcoholism. Second, the majority of participants identified their father as the parent with alcoholism, so the results of this study may not successfully generalize to families with mothers with alcoholism. Moreover, the large number of fathers with alcoholism calls into question whether high conformity orientations and low conversation orientations are typical of parents with alcoholism or fathers more generally. Additional research is needed to verify differences in communication patterns for fathers versus mothers with alcoholism. Third, the average age of participants suggests that we recruited a more mature sample who may have already found successful ways to cope with their parent's alcoholism as they became further removed from their family of origin. A younger sample may have reported more significant barriers to their psychological well-being. Fourth, we recruited our sample through support groups for ACoA, which suggests that participants were already seeking treatment and support to help them cope with their parent's alcoholism; thus, we were unlikely to recruit individuals who are particularly distressed by their experiences with a parent with alcoholism. Finally, the fact that our sample was predominantly white/Caucasian may obscure any cultural factors that are enmeshed with families affected by alcoholism.

Future research can expand on this study in a number of ways. First, whereas the vast majority of research on family communication patterns has relied on self-reports of individuals' perceptions of the interaction patterns within their family, we believe that an important next step is to observe how conformity and conversation orientations are manifest in communication behavior within the family. Particularly in the context of families coping with alcoholism, it is important to understand how family members interact with and around a parent with alcoholism and the impact that those interactions can have for the well-being of spouses and children in the future. Second, rather than focusing on ACoA's retrospective accounts of their family dynamics, we encourage researchers to observe features of family communication at various stages of the life span for families coping with alcoholism and to obtain data from various perspectives in the family. A more holistic view of the dynamics in families coping with a parent's alcoholism is necessary for developing effective communication-based interventions for children and parents who are struggling directly or indirectly with this disease.

REFERENCES

Ainsworth, M. D. S., Blehar, M. C., Waters, E., & Wall, S. (1978). *Patterns of attachment: A psychological study of the strange situation.* Hillsdale, NJ: Lawrence Erlbaum Associates.

Alcohol and Drug Programs (ADP) Resource Center. (2007). *Children of alcoholics: Important facts* (99–2567). Publication No. 99–2567. Retrieved from: www.google .com/url?sa=t&rct=j&q=&esrc=s&source=web&cd=10&ved=0CHYQFjAJurl=http:// www.adp.cahwnet.gov/rc/pdf/2567.pdf&ei=AqdwUIKRHoXyogH J10DADw&usg=FQjCNHrshvqVl_5f1CWTil_TxqSKWz7VQ&sig2=22n4wBYWLW6 O-hXYDiVREA

Bareket-Bojmel, L., & Shahar, G. (2011). Emotional and interpersonal consequences of self-disclosure in a lived, online interaction. *Journal of Social and Clinical Psychology, 30*, 732–759. doi: 10.1521/jscp.2011.30.7.732

Bartholomew, K. (1990). Avoidance of intimacy: An attachment perspective. *Journal of Social and Personal Relationships, 7*, 147–178. doi: 10.1177/0265407590072001

Baumeister, R. (1993). *Self-esteem: The puzzle of low self-regard.* New York, NY: Plenum. doi: 10.1007/978-1-4684-8956-9

Beaudoin, C. M., Murray, R. P., Bond, J. Jr., & Barnes, G. E. (1997). Personality characteristics of depressed or alcoholic adult children of alcoholics. *Personality & Individual Differences, 23*, 559–567. doi: 10.1016/S0191-8869(97)00080-9

Beesley, D., & Stoltenberg, C. D. (2002). Control, attachment style, and relationship satisfaction among adult children alcoholics. *Journal of Mental Health Counseling, 24*, 281–298.

Berkowitz, A., & Perkins, H. W. (1988). Personality characteristics of children of alcoholics. *Journal of Consulting and Clinical Psychology, 56*, 206–209. doi: 10.1037/0022-006X.56.2.206

Black, C. (1982). *It will never happen to me.* Denver, CO: MAC Printing and Publications Division.

Blascovich, J., & Tomaka, J. (1991). Measures of self-esteem. In J. P. Robinson, P. R. Shaver, & L. S. Wrightsman (Eds.), *Measures of personality and psychological attitudes* (pp. 115–155). New York, NY: Academic Press. doi: 10.1016/B978-0-12-590241-0.50008-3

Bollen, K. A. (1989). *Structural equations with latent variables.* New York, NY: John Wiley & Sons. doi: 10.1002/9781118619179

Bowlby, C. (1969). *Attachment and loss (Vol. 1).* New York, NY: Basic Books.

Burleson, B. R., Delia, J. G., & Applegate, J. L. (1995). The socialization of person-centered communication skills: Parental contributions to the social-cognitive and communication skills of their children. In M. A. Fitzpatrick & A. L. Vangelisti (Eds.), *Explaining family interactions* (pp. 34–76). Thousand Oaks, CA: SAGE. doi: 10.4135/9781483326368.n2

Bush, S., Ballard, M. E., & Fremouw, W. (1995). Attributional style, depression, and self-esteem: Adult children of alcoholic and non-alcoholic parents. *Journal of Youth and Adolescence, 24*, 177–185. doi: 10.1007/BF01537148

Carle, A. C., & Chassin, L. (2004). Resilience in a community sample of children of alcoholics: Its prevalence and relation to internalizing symptomatology and positive affect. *Applied Developmental Psychology, 25*, 577–595. doi: 10.1016/j.appdev.2004.08.005

Compas, B. E., Connor-Smith, J. K., Saltzman, H., Thomsen, A. H., & Wadsworth, M. E. (2001). Coping during childhood and adolescence: Problems, progress, and potential. *Psychological Bulletin, 127,* 87–127. doi: 10.1037/0033-2909.127.1.87

Drake, R. E., & Vaillant, G. E. (1988). Predicting alcoholism and personality disorder in a 33-year longitudinal study of children of alcoholics. *British Journal of Addiction, 83,* 799–807. doi: 10.1111/j.1360-0443.1988.tb00515.x

Drejer, K., Theikjaard, A., Teasedale, T. W., Schulsinger, F., & Goodwin, D. W. (1985). A prospective study of young men at high risk for alcoholism: Neuropsychological assessment. *Alcoholism: Clinical and Experimental Research, 9,* 498–502. doi: 10.1111/j.1530-0277.1985.tb05590.x

Eiden, R. D., Edwards, E. P., & Leonard, K. E. (2002). Mother-infant and father-infant attachment among alcoholic families. *Development and Psychopathology, 14,* 253–278. doi: 10.1017/S0954579402002043

Erdman P. (1998) Conceptualizing ADHD as a contextual response to parental attachment. *American Journal of Family Therapy, 26,* 177–185. doi: 10.1080/01926189808251097

Farrell, M. P., Barnes, G. M., & Banerjee, S. (1995). Family cohesion as a buffer against the effects of problem-drinking fathers on psychological distress, deviant behavior, and heavy drinking in adolescents. *Journal of Health and Social Behavior, 36,* 377–385. doi: 10.2307/2137326

Fava, M., & Cassano, P. (2008). Mood disorders: Major depressive disorder and dysthymic disorder. In T. A. Stern, J. F. Rosenbaum, M. Fava, J. Biederman, & S. L. Rauch (Eds.), *Massachusetts General Hospital comprehensive clinical psychiatry* (1st ed.). Philadelphia, PA: Mosby Elsevier. doi: 10.1016/B978-0-323-04743-2.50031-7

Fitzpatrick, M. A., & Ritchie, L. D. (1994). Communication schemata within the family: Multiple perspectives on family interaction. *Human Communication Research, 20,* 275–301. doi: 10.1111/j.1468-2958.1994.tb00324.x

Fraley, R. C., Waller, N. G., & Brennan, K. A. (2000). An item response theory analysis of self-report measures of adult attachment. *Journal of Personality and Social Psychology, 78,* 350–365. doi: 10.1037/0022-3514.78.2.350

Grant, B. F. (2000). Estimates of U.S. children exposed to alcohol abuse and dependence in the family. *American Journal of Public Health, 90,* 112–116. doi: 10.2105/AJPH.90.1.112

Grant, K. E., Compas, B. E., Thurm, A. E., McMahon, S. D., & Gipson, P. Y. (2004). Stressors and child and adolescent psychopathology: Measurement issues and prospective effects. *Journal of Clinical Child and Adolescent Psychology, 33,* 412–425. doi: 10.1207/s15374424jccp3302_23

Griffin, D. W., & Bartholomew, K. (1994). Models of the self and other: Fundamental dimensions underlying measures of adult attachment. *Journal of Personality and Social Psychology, 67,* 430–445. doi: 10.1037/0022-3514.67.3.430

Gross, J. J., & Levenson, R. W. (1993). Emotional suppression: Physiology, self-report, and expressive behavior. *Journal of Personality and Social Psychology, 64,* 968–970. doi: 10.1037/0022-3514.64.6.970

Hall, C. W., & Webster, R. E. (2002). Traumatic symptomatology characteristics of adult children of alcoholics. *Journal of Drug Education, 32,* 195–211. doi: 10.2190/U29W-LF3W-748L-A48 M

Hall, C. W., & Webster, R. E. (2007). Risk factors among adult children of alcoholics. *International Journal of Behavioral Consultation Therapy, 3,* 494–511. doi: 10.1037/h0100819

Hall, C. W., Webster, R. E., & Powell, E. J. (2003). Personal alcohol use in adult children of alcoholics. *Alcohol Research, 8,* 157–162.

Hamon, J. D., & Schrodt, P. (2012). Do parenting styles moderate the association between family conformity orientation and young adults' mental well-being? *Journal of Family Communication*, *12*, 151–166. doi: 10.1080/15267431.2011.561149

Harter, S. L., & Taylor, T. L. (2000). Parental alcoholism, child abuse, and adult adjustment. *Journal of Substance Abuse*, *11*, 31–44. doi: 10.1016/S0899-3289(99)00018-8

Hepper, E. G., & Carnelley, K. B. (2012). The self-esteem roller coaster: Adult attachment moderates the impact of daily feedback. *Personal Relationships*, *19*, 504–520. doi: 10.1111/j.1475–6811.2011.01375.x

Hunter, J. E., & Gerbing, D. W. (1982). Unidimensional measurement, second-order factor analysis, and causal models. In B. M. Straw & L. L. Cummings (Eds.), *Research in organizational behavior 4* (pp. 267–299). Greenwich, CT: JAI Press.

Johnson, P. (2001). Dimensions of functioning in alcoholic and nonalcoholic families. *Journal of Mental Health Counseling*, *23*, 127–136.

Johnson, P., & Stone, R. (2009). Parental alcoholism and family functioning: Effects on differentiation levels of young adults. *Alcoholism Treatment Quarterly*, *27*, 3–18. doi: 10.1080/07347320802586601

Jones, D. C., & Houts, R. (1992). Parental drinking, parent/child communication, and the social skills of young adults. *Journal of Studies on Alcohol*, *53*, 48–56. doi: 10.15288/jsa.1992.53.48

Karreman, A., & Vingerhoets, J. J. M. (2012). Attachment and well-being: The mediating role of emotion regulation and resilience. *Personality and Individual Differences*, *53*, 821–826. doi: 10.1016/j.paid.2012.06.014

Kelley, M. L., Braitman, A., Henson, J. M., Schroeder, V., Ladage, J., & Gumienny, L. (2011). Relationships among depressive mood symptoms and parent and peer relations in collegiate children of alcoholics. *American Journal of Orthopsychiatry*, *80*, 204–212. doi: 10.1111/j.1939–0025.2010.01024.x

Koerner, A. F., & Cvancara, K. E. (2002). The influence of conformity orientation on communication patterns in family conversations. *Journal of Family Communication*, *2*, 133–152. doi: 10.1207/S15327698JFC0203_2

Koerner, A. F., & Fitzpatrick, M. A. (1997). Family type and conflict: The impact of conversation orientation and conformity orientation on conflict in the family. *Communication Studies*, *48*, 59–78. doi: 10.1080/10510979709368491

Koerner, A. F., & Fitzpatrick, M. A. (2002a). Toward a theory of family communication. *Communication Theory*, *12*, 70–91. doi: 10.1111/j.1468–2885.2002.tb00260.x

Koerner, A. F., & Fitzpatrick, M. A. (2002b). Understanding family communication patterns and family functioning: The roles of conversation orientation and conformity orientation. In W. B. Gudykunst (Ed.), *Communication yearbook 26* (pp. 36–68). Mahwah, NJ: Lawrence Erlbaum Associates. doi: 10.1080/23808985.2002.11679010

Larson, D., & Chastain, R. (1990). Self-concealment: Conceptualization, measurement, and health implications. *Journal of Social and Clinical Psychology*, *9*, 439–455. doi: 10.1521/jscp.1990.9.4.439

Ledbetter, A. M. (2009). Family communication patterns and relational maintenance behavior: Direct and mediated associations with friendship closeness. *Human Communication Research*, *35*, 130–147. doi: 10.1111/j.1468–2958.2008.01341.x

Masten, A. S., Coatsworth, J. D., Neemann, J., Gest, S. D., Tellegen, A., & Garmezy, N. (1995). The structure and coherence of competence from childhood through adolescence. *Child Development*, *66*, 1635–1659. doi: 10.2307/1131901

Miller-Day, M., & Marks, J. D. (2006). Perceptions of parental communication orientation, perfectionism, and disordered eating behaviors of sons and daughters. *Health Communication*, 19, 153–163. doi: 10.1207/s15327027hc1902_7

Muris, P., Mayer, B., & Meesters, C. (2000). Self-reported attachment style, anxiety, and depression in children. *Social Behavior and Personality*, 28, 157–162. doi: 10.2224/sbp.2000.28.2.157

National Institute on Alcohol Abuse and Alcoholism. (2010). Rethinking drinking: Alcohol and your health. NIH Publication No. 13–3770. Retrieved from: http://pubs.niaaa.nih.gov/publications/RethinkingDrinking/Rethinking_Drinking.pdf

Palmer, N. (1997). Resilience in adult children of alcoholics: A nonpathological approach to social work practice. *Health & Social Work*, 22, 201–209. doi: 10.1093/hsw/22.3.201

Pennebaker, J. W. (1985). Traumatic experience and psychosomatic disease: Exploring the roles of behavioural inhibition, obsession, and confiding. *Canadian Psychology*, 26, 82–95. doi: 10.1037/h0080025

Rangarajan, S. (2008). Mediators and moderators of parental alcoholism effects on offspring self-esteem. *Alcohol and Alcoholism*, 43, 481–491. doi: 10.1093/alcalc/agn034

Rangarajan, S., & Kelly, L. (2006). Family communication patterns, family environment, and the impact of parental alcoholism on offspring self-esteem. *Journal of Social and Personal Relationships*, 23, 655–671. doi: 10.1177/0265407506065990

Reiss, D. (1981). *The family's construction of reality*. Cambridge, MA: Harvard University Press.

Ritchie, D. L., & Fitzpatrick, M. A. (1990). Family communication patterns: Measuring intrapersonal perceptions of interpersonal relationships. *Communication Research*, 17, 523–544. doi: 10.1177/009365090017004007

Roemer, L., & Borkovec, T. D. (1994). Effects of suppressing thoughts about emotional material. *Journal of Abnormal Psychology*, 103, 467–474. doi: 10.1037/0021-843X.103.3.467

Rueter, M. A., & Koerner, A. F. (2008). The effect of family communication patterns on adopted adolescent adjustment. *Journal of Marriage and Family*, 70, 715–727. doi: 10.1111/j.1741-3737.2008.00516.x

Schrodt, P., Witt, P. L., & Messersmith, A. S. (2008). A meta-analytical review of family communication patterns and their associations with information processing, behavioral, and psychosocial outcomes. *Communication Monographs*, 75, 248–269. doi: 10.1080/03637750802256318

Straussner, S. A., & Fewell, C. H. (Eds.). (2011). *Children of substance-abusing parents: Dynamics and treatment*. New York, NY: Springer Publishing Company.

Sullivan, P. F., Neale, M. C., & Kendler, K. S. (2000). Genetic epidemiology of major depression: Review and meta-analysis. *American Journal of Psychiatry*, 157, 1552–1562. doi: 10.1176/appi.ajp.157.10.1552

Tajalli, F., & Ardalan, E. (2010). Relation of family communication patterns with self-efficacy and academic adjustment. *Journal of Psychology*, 14, 62–78.

Thompson, R. (1999). Early attachment and later behavior. In J. Cassidy & P. R. Shaver (Eds.), *Handbook of attachment: Research, theory, & clinical applications* (pp. 265–286). New York, NY: Guilford Press.

Wagnild, G. M., & Young, H. M. (1993). Development and psychometric evaluation of the resilience scale. *Journal of Nursing Measurement*, 1, 165–178.

Woititz, J. G. (1989). *The self-sabotage syndrome: Adult children in the workplace*. Deerfield Beach, FL: Health Communications.

Wood, A. M., Taylor, P. J., & Joseph, S. (2010). Does the CES-D measure a continuum from depression to happiness? Comparing substantive and artifactual models. *Psychiatry Research, 177*, 120–123. doi: 10.1016/j.psychres.2010.02.003

15

Alzheimer's Caregiver Distress in Adulthood: The Role of Time Invested in Caregiving and Family Verbal Aggression in Childhood

LINDSAY SUSAN ALOIA AND ANNE M. STONE

An estimated 5.3 million individuals in the United States suffer from Alzheimer's disease (Centers for Disease Control and Prevention, 2016). Alzheimer's disease is a chronic, progressive neurodegenerative illness characterized by impaired cognitive abilities and behavior disturbances, including memory loss, attention deficits, disorientation, the inability to communicate, and disruptions in executive functioning (American Psychiatric Association, 2000; Weiner, 2003). As the disease progresses and individuals' condition declines, Alzheimer's disease patients become increasingly reliant on others for assistance with activities of daily living. According to the Alzheimer's Association and National Alliance for Caregiving (2004), 87% of individuals diagnosed with Alzheimer's disease are cared for by nonprofessional kin. With a heavy burden of responsibility, caregivers of persons with Alzheimer's disease may experience a myriad of psychological (Brummett et al., 2006), physiological (Mausbach, Patterson, Rabinowitz, Grant & Schulz, 2007), financial (Ory, Hoffman, Yee, Tennstedt, & Schulz, 1999), and relational ramifications (Spitznagel, Tremont, Davis, & Foster, 2006). Simultaneously, caregiving can be rewarding, gratifying, and satisfying for those providing care (Boerner, Schulz, & Horowitz, 2004).

Drawing on the physiological model of stress (Cohen, Kessler, & Underwood Gordon, 1995), caregiving responsibilities can be characterized as environmental stressors. An environmental stressor is a condition that poses a challenge to a person and tests that individual's capacity to cope with the situation. If the caregiver evaluates providing care as potentially burdensome, taxing, or strenuous (McNamara, 2000), and the external demands of caregiving exceed the individual's internal adaptive capacity to adapt to the demands, a stress response is initiated (Dohrenwend & Shroul, 1985). Research suggests, however, that individuals vary considerably in their experiences of caregiving and their evaluation of their caregiving responsibilities. As a result of the variability, some caregivers experience few negative effects of providing care for an individual with Alzheimer's disease and others suffer long-term personal and relational consequences.

The extent to which caregivers evaluate their caregiving responsibilities as stressful may be influenced by childhood experiences of stress. According to developmental programming approaches, stressful environmental conditions in early life, such as repeated or chronic childhood adversities, can recalibrate an individual's stress response system (Ellis & Del Giudice, 2014; Sih, 2011). Two alternative explanations linking childhood experiences of stress to adult responses are prominent within the literature. A sensitization perspective suggests that individuals become sensitized to potentially taxing stimuli, such that less demanding provocations are required to precipitate a stress response (Post, 1992). An alternative account submits that persons develop desensitized reactions to cues that normally trigger a cognitive, emotional, and ultimately, behavioral response (Rule & Ferguson, 1986). Whereas a sensitization perspective explains effects of early stress as increasing vulnerability to the effects of stressful events in adulthood, a desensitization explanation suggests childhood stressors can attenuate or eliminate responses to anxiety-inducing stimuli later in life.

Scholars have found empirical evidence to support both excessive and insufficient responses to stressors; however, the extent to which sensitization and desensitization provide complementary or competing explanations for caregiving outcomes remains unclear. Accordingly, the goal of this chapter is to examine caregiver distress as a function of both time invested in caregiving and history of family verbal aggression in childhood. In the sections that follow, we first review research that positions a history of family verbal aggression in childhood as a stressor. Then, we highlight how childhood stressors can sensitize individuals to adult responsibilities. Next, we examine literature addressing the association between childhood adversities and decreased reactivity to stressors in adulthood. Finally, we pose research questions to investigate the moderating effect of history of family verbal aggression on the relationship between time invested in caregiving and caregiver stress.

FAMILY VERBAL AGGRESSION IN CHILDHOOD AS A STRESSOR

Verbal aggression is defined as a communication behavior in which a person purposefully uses language to attack the self-concept of another person (Infante, 1987; Renfrew, 1997; Straus, 1979). Family violence researchers have identified nine distinct types of verbally aggressive messages, including (a) character attacks, (b) competence attacks, (c) background attacks, (d) physical appearance attacks, (e) maledictions, (f) teasing, (g) ridicule, (h) threats, and (i) swearing (Infante, Chandler, Rudd, & Shannon, 1990). Although verbal aggression is considered a destructive form of communication, individuals frequently deploy aggressive messages directed toward family members. Relative to other relationship types, adults report the greatest amount of conflict, criticism, and verbal aggression in their marital, sibling, and parent–child relationships (Argyle & Furnham, 1983).

Although the experience of family conflict and verbal aggression is ubiquitous, it is an unsettling, stressful aspect of family relationships. Researchers have consistently found that intense, negative conflict within the nuclear family threatens a child's sense of security and safety both in and beyond the home (Gordis, Margolin, & John, 2001). For example, Cummings, Goeke-Morey, Papp, and Dukewich (2002) found that young children respond to the expression of adult anger with a variety of negative emotions, such as anger, distress, fear, and sadness. The experience of family conflict also plays a critical role in predicting somatic symptoms, including trembling hands, headaches, and difficulty sleeping (Bi, Moos, Timko, & Cronkite, 2015). In extreme circumstances, children who witness verbally aggressive messages within the family system may suffer traumatic arousal symptoms and posttraumatic stress symptoms (Graham-Bermann & Levendosky, 1998).

Accordingly, the experience of frequent and repeated exposure to family verbal aggression in early life is posited as a stressful environmental condition that can recalibrate an individual's stress response system (Ellis & Del Giudice, 2014; Sih, 2011).

This recalibration during childhood is subsequently hypothesized to influence how an individual evaluates and responds to a stress-inducing stimuli in adulthood. In the following sections, we examine two alternative explanations linking childhood experiences of stress caused by family verbal aggression exposure to adult evaluations of caregiving responsibilities.

STRESS SENSITIZATIONS

A sensitization perspective posits that early life stressors heighten individuals' awareness to life events that stimulate anxiety, such that less weight is required to incur a stress response (Post, 1992). Accordingly, inconsequential stressors may induce reactivity because childhood adversities encourage hyperarousal to the environment. Given that minor triggers occur at a higher base rate than threatening events, individuals with sensitized stress response systems are susceptible to overtaking emotional, cognitive, and metabolic resources (Hertzman, 1999; Hertzman & Wiens, 1996).

Sensitization is an explanatory mechanism used to link negative childhood dynamics to psychological, cognitive, and physiological dysfunction in adulthood. More specifically, stress response system dysregulation reflected in excessive reactivity to environmental cues encourages pathogenic processes that eventuate in psychological issues such as anxiety disorders (Norman,

Byambaa, De, Butchart, Scott, & Vos, 2012), borderline personality traits (Braver, Bumberry, Green, & Rawson, 1992), depression (Mazzeo & Espelage, 2002; Norman et al., 2012), and dissociation (Teicher, Samson, Sheu, Polcari, & McGreenery, 2010). In addition, children develop cognitive biases that include selective attention to threat and hypervigilance for risk (Ford & Kidd, 1998). Exposure to violence in childhood also increases activity in the sympathetic nervous system and hypothalamic–pituitary–adrenal (HPA) axis (Saltzman, Holden, & Holahan, 2005).

Building upon this work, sensitization to stress may account for diversity in caregivers' accounts and consequences of providing care. Exposure to verbally aggressive messages in childhood may heighten emotional awareness to potential triggers. Furthermore, individuals may increase attention to potential threats and develop a cognitive processing bias toward information related to stress. Experiences of early stress may also heighten physiological reactivity, such as body temperature, heart rate, blood pressure, and skin conductivity. Because experiences of stress in childhood are likely to lay the foundation for an individual's threshold for stress in adulthood, a history of verbal aggression is likely to be related to the experience of stress associated with caregiving in adulthood.

DESENSITIZATION TO STRESSORS

Albeit a sensitization perspective suggests childhood adversities decrease an individual's tolerance for stress and encourage responsivity, a desensitization framework proposes a higher threshold for stress and diminished reactions to triggers that would normally prompt a response. *Desensitization* is defined as the attenuation or elimination of psychological, cognitive, physiological, and ultimately, behavioral responses to a stimulus (Rule & Ferguson, 1986). Diminished reactivity can be laboriously directed and controlled. In cognitive behavioral therapy, for example, desensitization is used to reduce or eradicate affective reactions through contact with emotionally provocative stimuli (Wolpe, 1973). Cognitive behavioral therapy treatments are effective in altering children psychologically and behaviorally (Weersing & Weisz, 2002).

Desensitization is recognized as a key mechanism in determining the effects of childhood exposure to chronic violence and aggression. More specifically, desensitization suggests that youth adapt to violence through recalibration in their psychological, cognitive, and physiological systems (Cooley-Quille & Lorion, 1999; Fitzpatrick & Boldizar, 1993). This adjustment is reflected in numbed or blunted emotional reactions to cues that would typically elicit a strong affective response (Ng-Mak, Salzinger, Feldman, & Stueve, 2002). Furthermore, children develop cognitions that violence is mundane, inevitable, and expected (Funk, Bechtoldt Baldacci, Pasold, &

Baumgardner, 2004). Exposure to aggression in childhood also attenuates stress reactivity during conflict in adulthood (Aloia & Solomon, 2015).

Using a similar logic, desensitization may explain the considerable variation in caregivers' experiences and evaluations of their responsibilities. Exposure to verbally aggressive messages in childhood can desensitize the cues that normally trigger a stress response. Furthermore, individuals may form cognitions about the normalcy and regularity of stress emerging from childhood experiences. Experiences of early stress may also mitigate physiological responsivity. Although providing care for a person with Alzheimer's disease is demanding, enduring exposure to verbal aggression in childhood may increase an individual's tolerance for the stress of caregiving in adulthood.

CAREGIVERS OF ALZHEIMER'S PATIENTS

Caregivers of persons with Alzheimer's disease endure a heavy burden of responsibility, reflected in psychological, physiological, financial, and relational ramifications. There is a robust association between caregiving for dementia patients and psychological problems such as anxiety (Dura, Stukenberg, & Kiecolt-Glaser, 1991), depression (Thompson, Spira, Depp, McGee, & Gallagher-Thompson, 2006), dysphoria (Dura et al., 1991), and distress (Adams, 2007). In addition to psychological difficulties, caregivers are also more likely to develop physiological consequences such as lower immunologic strength (Kiecolt-Glaser, Glaser, Gravenstein, Malarkey, & Sheridan, 1996), greater cardiovascular reactivity (Lee, Colditz, Berkman, & Kawachi, 2003), and higher cortisol levels (Gallagher-Thompson et al., 2006). Many caregivers also make significant financial sacrifices to provide care, including persistent out-of-pocket expenses and reduced earnings (Alzheimer's Association and National Alliance for Caregiving, 2004). Finally, dementia caregivers report relational strain and reduced leisure time with partners, family members, and friends (Ory et al., 1999). Our hypotheses reflect the assumption that time invested in caregiving corresponds with magnified adverse outcomes. Accordingly, we advance the following hypotheses:

H1: Duration of caregiving role is positively associated with (a) stress and (b) burnout.

H2: Time spent providing care is positively associated with (a) stress and (b) burnout.

In addition, we propose that the effect of time invested in caregiving on stress and burnout is moderated by history of family verbal aggression. Researchers offered two alternative explanations linking childhood experiences of stress to adult responses, and empirical evidence supports both perspectives. A sensitization perspective explains heightened responses to stress in adulthood through childhood adversities. Accordingly, we reason that childhood stress induced by a history of family verbal aggression may be relevant to the experience of adult caregiver stress. More specifically, the burden of caregiver responsibility is likely to be more salient for individuals with a sensitive stress response system calibrated by a history of family verbal aggression. The heightened impact of caregiving obligations, in turn, may elicit greater perceptions of stress and increased rates of burnout. Drawing from a sensitization framework, we would predict that the association between time invested in caregiving and (a) stress and (b) burnout is greater for individuals with a greater history of family verbal aggression.

A second explanation posits that childhood stress desensitizes individuals to burdensome, taxing, or strenuous demands, promoting a higher tolerance for stress in adulthood. A desensitization perspective, then, suggests that caregivers who experienced a history of family verbal aggression in childhood are more resilient to the weight of caregiver commitments. Moreover, individuals with a history of family verbal aggression are less attuned to the cues of stress associated with caregiver responsibilities. Diminished reactivity to the imposition of caregiving, therefore, limits the experience of stress and burnout for the care provider. Using desensitization as a foundation, we would predict that the association between time invested in caregiving and (a) stress and (b) burnout is lower for individuals with a greater history of family verbal aggression. Owing to the striking duality posited by both perspectives, we advance the following research question to investigate the moderating effect of history of family verbal aggression on the relationship between time invested in caregiving and (a) stress and (b) burnout.

RQ1: Is there an interaction between duration of caregiving role and history of family verbal aggression in predicting (a) stress and (b) burnout?

RQ2: Is there an interaction between time spent providing care and history of family verbal aggression in predicting (a) stress and (b) burnout?

METHOD

Participants were recruited from multiple support groups designed for adult caregivers of individuals suffering from Alzheimer's disease. Participants were emailed a URL that directed them to an online survey hosted by Qualtrics. The survey collected demographic information and items to capture the variables of interest. The survey was available to participants for a 6-month period.

Participants

One hundred and twenty individuals were recruited to participate in the study. The sample was composed of 88 females and 32 males. Ages ranged from 29 to 81 years old (M = 53.68, SD = 12.76). The majority of the sample identified as white (70.83%), but also included individuals who identified as Hispanic (19.17%), black (6.67%), and Asian (3.33%). The greater part of the sample indicated that they were currently married (66.67%); however, individuals also designated that they were divorced (18.33%), never married (10.83%), and widowed (4.17%). Finally, the largest portion of the sample reported having received a bachelor's degree (51.67%), but also included individuals who received a high school degree (28.33%), associate's degree (16.67%), master's degree (1.67%), and professional degree (1.67%).

Measures

Participants provided responses to closed-ended, multi-item self-report measures of stress, burnout, and history of family verbal aggression. We conducted a confirmatory factor analysis of the measurement model for the three variables simultaneously, with items representing each scale loaded on separate factors and all factors allowed to covary. To assess the confirmatory factor analysis, we used the following criteria: χ^2/df test > 3, comparative fit index (CFI) > 0.85, and root mean square error of approximation (RMSEA) < 0.10 (Brown & Cudeck, 1993; Kline, 1998). The data appropriately fit the measurement model: χ^2/df = 2.34, CFI = 0.91, RMSEA = 0.07.

Duration of caregiving role. An open-ended question measured the length of time participants reported caregiving. Specifically, individuals responded to, "How long have you been responsible for caring for your loved one with dementia?" Participants responded to the question by indicating the number of months/years individuals denoted a caregiving role (M = 12.15 months, SD = 13.95).

Time spent caregiving. To evaluate the amount of time individuals had invested in providing care, participants replied to an open-ended question. In particular, participants responded to, "How many hours a week are you responsible for caring for your loved one with dementia?" (M = 15.08 hours, SD = 7.50).

Stress. Cohen, Kamarck, and Mermelstein's (1983) Global Measure of Perceived Stress Scale assessed participants' experiences of anxiety, apprehension, and concern in the last month. Fourteen items, such as "In the last month, how often have you felt nervousness and stress?" and "In the last month, how often have you felt difficulties were piling up so high that you could not overcome them?" were included. Participants responded to questions using a 5-point Likert-type scale on which higher numbers reflected more frequent experiences of stress (1 = *Never*, 2 = *Almost never*, 3 = *Sometimes*, 4 = *Fairly often*, 5 = *Very often; M* = 2.76, *SD* = 1.12, α = 0.92).

Burnout. Seven items were used from Maslach's Burnout Inventory (Maslach, Jackson, & Leiter, 1997) to evaluate fatigue, exhaustion, and frustration from providing care for an individual suffering from Alzheimer's disease. Items such as "I feel emotionally drained from providing care" and "I feel like I am at the end of my rope" were included. Participants responded to statements using a 5-point Likert-type scale on which higher numbers reflected higher levels of burnout (1 = *Strongly disagree*, 2 = *Disagree*, 3 = *Uncertain*, 4 = *Agree*, 5 = *Strongly agree; M* = 2.80, *SD* = 1.58, α = 0.94).

History of family verbal aggression. Aloia and Solomon's (2015) History of Family Verbal Aggression Scale was used to assess the participants' receipt of verbally aggressive communication from family members during middle childhood (i.e., third, fourth, fifth, and sixth grades). This period of life was selected because the development of cognitive abilities, such as concentration and memory, render experiences during middle childhood easier to recall than experiences in early childhood (Burnett Heyes, Zokaei, van der Staaij, Bays, & Husain, 2012). Ten items, such as "A family member personally attacked my character" and "A family member criticized my shortcomings" were included. Participants responded to statements using an 8-point Likert-type scale on which higher numbers indicated more frequent perceived verbal aggression (0 = *This has never happened*, 1 = *Not during middle childhood, but it did happen before*, 2 = *Once during a typical year in middle childhood*, 3 = *Twice during a typical year in middle childhood*, 4 = *3–5 times during a typical year in middle childhood*, 5 = *6–10 times during a typical year in middle childhood*, 6 = *11–20 times during a typical year in middle childhood*, 7 = *More than 20 times during a typical year in middle childhood; M* = 3.06, *SD* = 1.32, α = 0.91).

RESULTS

Evidence of stress sensitization effects is primarily based on clinical samples and female populations (McLaughlin, Conron, Koenen, & Gilman, 2010). As a result, the applicability of the stress sensitization hypothesis to males remains unclear. Accordingly, we ran our analyses separately for female and male participants. Table 15.1 reports the correlations among all of our measures of interest for female and male participants. Results for female participants appear above the diagonal and the correlations for male participants are below the diagonal.

   Duration of caregiving role was significantly and negatively associated with time spent caregiving for both sexes. Consistent with H1, duration of caregiving role was significantly and positively associated with (a) stress and (b) burnout for female and male participants. Relevant to RQ1, duration of

TABLE 15.1 *Correlations among variables in the study*

Measure	1	2	3	4	5
1. Duration of caregiving role	—	−0.31**	0.24*	0.32**	0.27*
2. Time spent caregiving	−0.44**	—	0.24*	0.23*	−0.16
3. Stress	0.54***	0.03	—	0.87***	0.17
4. Burnout	0.41*	0.14	0.84***	—	0.19*
5. History of family verbal aggression	−0.08	0.29*	−0.10*	0.07	—

Note. Correlations for females are above the diagonal. Correlations for males are below the diagonal.
$*p < 0.05; **p < 0.01; ***p < 0.001.$

caregiving role was significantly and positively associated with history of family verbal aggression for females; duration of caregiving role was not significantly associated with history of family verbal aggression for males. As predicted by H2, time spent providing care was significantly and positively associated with (a) stress and (b) burnout for female participants. For males, time spent providing care was not significantly associated with (a) stress or (b) burnout (H2). Related to RQ2, time spent caregiving was not significantly associated with history of family verbal aggression for females; however, time spent caregiving was significantly and positively associated with history of family verbal aggression for males. In addition, stress was significantly and positively associated with burnout for both sexes. Stress was not significantly associated with history of family verbal aggression for females; however, stress was significantly and negatively associated with history of family verbal aggression for males. Finally, burnout was significantly and positively asso ciated with history of family verbal aggression for females; burnout was not significantly associated with history of family verbal aggression for males.

To test our hypotheses and research questions, we employed two hier- archical multiple regression analyses. In the first analysis, we entered stress as the dependent variable (see Table 15.2). The second analysis evaluated burn- out as the dependent variable (see Table 15.3). In both analyses, we entered duration of caregiving role, time spent caregiving, and history of family verbal aggression on the first steps. The second steps evaluated three product terms that represented the two-way interactions between all pairs of independent variables, and the third steps included a product variable representing their three-way interaction.

On the first step of the analysis that evaluated stress as the dependent variable, we observed significant positive coefficients for duration of caregiv- ing role and time spent caregiving for female and male participants; the coefficients for history of family verbal aggression were not significant for either sex. On the second step of the analysis, results revealed a significant

TABLE 15.2 *The regression of stress onto duration of caregiving role, time spent caregiving, and history of family verbal aggression*

	Unstandardized Slopes	R^2	R^2 Change	F Change
Step 1:				
Duration of caregiving role	**0.03**** (0.52***)	**0.18** (0.38)	**0.18** (0.38)	**6.09***** (6.22***)
Time spent caregiving	**0.05***** (0.46**)			
History of family verbal aggression	**0.12** (−0.08)			
Step 2:				
Duration × Time spent	**0.01** (0.01)	**0.26** (0.50)	**0.80** (0.12)	**2.87*** (1.98)
Duration × History of VA	**0.02**** (0.02)			
Time spent × History of VA	**−0.01** (−0.03)			
Step 3:				
Duration × Time spent × History of VA	**0.01** (−0.01)	**0.27** (0.51)	**0.01** (0.01)	**1.12** (0.01)
$F_{(7,85)} = 4.18, p < 0.001, R^2 = 0.27$ $(F_{(7,33)} = 3.77, p < 0.01, R^2 = 0.51)$				

Note. Results for females are in boldface. Results for males are in parentheses.
*$p < 0.05$; **$p < 0.01$; ***$p < 0.001$.

interaction between duration of caregiving role and history of family verbal aggression for female participants. Neither of the other two-way interactions was significant for either sex, and the three-way interactions tested on step three were also not significant for female and male participants. To determine the form of the significant two-way interaction, we plotted the regression of stress on duration of caregiving role at different levels of history of family verbal aggression for female participants (see Figure 15.1). Relevant to H1, duration of caregiving role was positively associated with stress at only moderate and high levels of history of family verbal aggression for female participants. Consistent with a sensitization perspective, this association increased for female caregivers as history of family verbal aggression increased from low (−1 SD, *ns*), to moderate ($p < 0.05$), to high (+1 SD, $p < 0.01$) levels.

On the first step of the analysis that evaluated burnout as the dependent variable, we observed significant positive coefficients for duration of the caregiving role and time spent caregiving for female and male participants; the coefficients for history of family verbal aggression were not significant for

TABLE 15.3 *The regression of burnout onto duration of caregiving role, time spent caregiving, and history of family verbal aggression*

	Unstandardized Slopes	R^2	R^2 Change	F Change
Step 1:				
Duration of caregiving role	**0.05***** (0.06*****)	**0.24** (0.29)	**0.24** (0.29)	**8.75***** (4.15**)
Time spent caregiving	**0.09***** (0.08**)			
History of family verbal aggression	**0.17** (–0.02)			
Step 2:				
Duration × Time spent	**0.01** (–0.01)	**0.28** (0.40)	**0.04** (0.11)	1.41 (1.61)
Duration × History of VA	**0.02** (0.01)			
Time spent × History of VA	**–0.02** (–0.05*****)			
Step 3:				
Duration × Time spent × History of VA	0.01 (–0.01)	**0.29** (0.40)	**0.01** (0.00)	**0.30** (0.07)
$F(7,85) = 4.42, p < 0.001, R^2 = 0.29$ $(F(7,33) = 2.50, p < 0.05, R^2 = 0.40)$				

Note. Results for females are in boldface. Results for males are in parentheses.
*$p < 0.05$; **$p < 0.01$; ***$p < 0.001$.

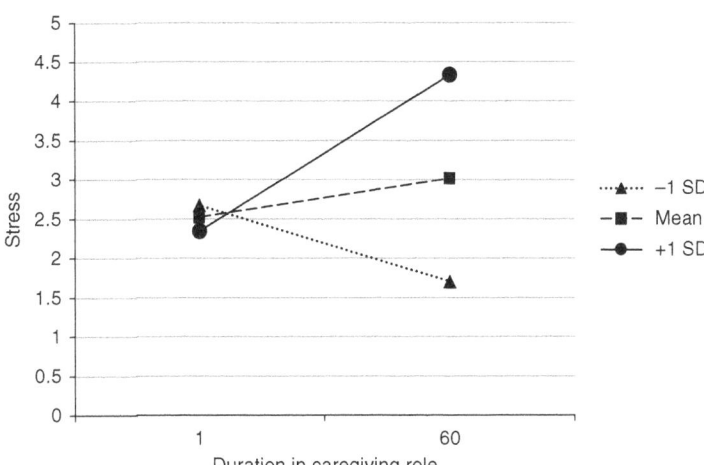

FIGURE 15.1 Duration in caregiving role as a predictor of stress moderated by history of family verbal aggression for female participants.

either sex. On the second step of the analysis, results revealed a significant interaction between time spent caregiving and history of family verbal aggression for male participants. Neither of the other two-way interactions was significant for either sex, and the three-way interactions tested on step three were also not significant for female and male participants. To determine the form of the significant two-way interaction, we plotted the regression of burnout on time spent caregiving at different levels of history of family verbal aggression for male participants (see Figure 15.2). Related to H2, time spent caregiving was positively associated with burnout at low levels of history of family verbal aggression for male participants (–1 SD, *ns*). Consistent with a desensitization perspective, however, time spent caregiving was negatively associated with burnout at high levels of history of family verbal aggression for male caregivers (+1 SD, *p* < 0.10).

DISCUSSION

Building on previous research that demonstrated that stressful environmental conditions in early life can recalibrate an individual's stress response, this study examined caregiver distress as a function of both time invested in caregiving and history of family verbal aggression in childhood. Earlier findings that link childhood stressors to caregiving in adulthood were established using primarily female populations. As a result, the fitness of the sensitization perspective and desensitization explanation was uncertain for male caregivers. According to the National Alliance for Caregiving and American Association for Retired Persons (2004), caregivers of individuals with

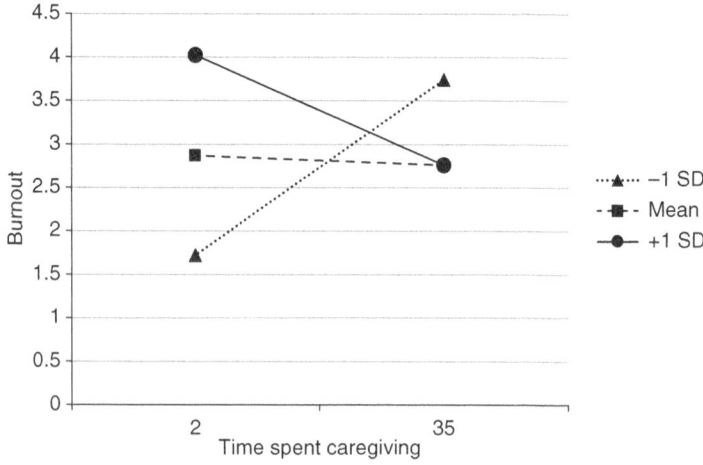

FIGURE 15.2   Time spent caregiving as a predictor of burnout moderated by history of family verbal aggression for male participants.

dementia are predominantly female. Consistent with previous research, our sample was composed of largely female care providers (73.33%). Furthermore, the majority of caregivers indicated that they were currently married (66.67%). This is also congruent with research that addresses the competing demands of multiple roles, such as wife, mother, employee, and care provider, for women caring for an individual with Alzheimer's disease (Norton, Gupta, Stephens, Martire, & Townsend, 2005).

Care providers expend an abundance of time to meet the caregiving demands of an individual with Alzheimer's disease. On average, participants reported enduring the responsibility of caregiving for 12.15 months. Furthermore, caregivers reported spending 15.08 hours per week on average providing care. Interestingly, we observed a negative relationship between duration of caregiving role and time spent providing care. This association suggests that caregivers spend less time providing care during an average week as the duration of their caregiving role progresses. Perhaps caregivers more clearly recognize the psychological, physiological, financial, and relational risks associated with providing care as the duration of providing care extends and, subsequently, reduce time spent caregiving to buffer against the consequences.

Bearing grave responsibility, caregivers of persons with Alzheimer's disease can experience psychological distress (e.g., Brummett et al., 2006). Both the zero-order correlations and the regression analyses indicated that duration of the caregiving role was positively associated with both stress and burnout for female and male caregivers. As the length of time during which individuals are responsible for providing care continues, caregivers are more likely to experience anxiety, apprehension, fatigue, and frustration. Furthermore, the regression analyses indicated that time spent providing care was also positively associated with stress and burnout; this relationship was replicated in the zero-order correlations for female caregivers. Considering that life expectancies continue to grow and population longevities are increasing (Salomon et al., 2013), this merits attention and concern. Previous research demonstrates that social support can operate as a protective factor against the detrimental effects of caregiving stress on psychological well-being (Brummett et al., 2006). Researchers should continue to move beyond documenting the deleterious effects of caregiving and consider the protective factors that may reduce adverse outcomes. For example, researchers may consider the buffering effects of social support on the adverse consequences of caregiving (Bodie, 2011). In addition, temperament or disposition may ameliorate the adverse effects of caregiving for an individual with Alzheimer's disease (Garmezy, 1985).

Drawing from our findings, caregiving responsibilities are burdensome and test caregivers' capacities to cope. We argued that the extent to which caregivers evaluate their caregiving responsibilities as stressful may be influenced by childhood experiences of stress. A sensitization perspective suggests that individuals become attuned to potentially taxing stimuli, such that less demanding provocations are required to encourage a stress response. Consistent with a sensitization account, the positive association between duration of caregiving role and stress increased as history of family verbal aggression increased for female caregivers. Experiences of early life stressors appear to amplify female caregivers' experiences of stress. Moreover, this result supports previous research that found that female caregivers are more susceptible to the negative outcomes associated with caregiving than are male care providers (Atienza, Collins, & King, 2001). Taken together, these findings endorse a sensitization perspective that explains heightened responses to the stress of caregiving in adulthood through childhood adversities.

Whereas a sensitization account explains effects of early stress as increasing responsivity, a desensitization explanation suggests childhood stressors attenuate reactions to anxiety-inducing stimuli in adulthood. Corresponding to a desensitization framework, time spent caregiving was negatively associated with burnout at high levels of history of family verbal aggression for male caregivers. This finding suggests that males who report being exposed to verbal aggression in childhood habituate to the experience of stress and perceive stress as less adverse. This desensitization can lead males to be more resilient to the negative psychological ramifications of caregiving. This finding adds strength to the argument that desensitization is an adaptive response to chronic environmental stress (Del Giudice, Ellis, & Shirtcliff, 2010).

Taken together, the results of this study further demonstrate that individuals vary considerably in their experiences of caregiving and their evaluation of their caregiving responsibilities. As a result, contemporaneous efforts to protect caregivers from stress and burnout must be multidimensional. More specifically, caregivers of persons with Alzheimer's disease require individual emotional, cognitive, and physical protective capacities, and family protective resources. Caregivers of persons with Alzheimer's disease necessitate emotional fortitude, including affective regulation and operative emotional arousal mechanisms (Thompson, 1994). In addition to emotional capacities, caregivers benefit from cognitive aptitudes, such as knowledge of Alzheimer's disease (Werner, 2001) and self-awareness of obligations (Mitnick, Leffler, & Hood, 2010). Individuals must also be physically able to adequately perform caregiver responsibilities (De Frias, Tuokko, & Rosenberg, 2005). Finally, family protective resources, such as adequate emotional (Penrod, Kane, Kane, & Finch, 1995) and financial support (Sharpe, Butow, Smith, McConnell, & Clarke, 2004), may help to mitigate the adverse consequences of caregiving for an individual afflicted by Alzheimer's disease.

This study examined Alzheimer's caregiver distress in adulthood as a function of both time invested in caregiving and history of family verbal aggression in childhood. Duration of caregiving role was positively associated with stress and burnout for both sexes. In addition, time spent caregiving was positively related with stress and burnout for female and male caregivers. In support of the sensitization perspective, the positive association between duration of caregiving role and stress increased as history of family verbal aggression increased for female caregivers. Consistent with a desensitization framework, time spent caregiving was negatively associated with burnout at high levels of history of family verbal aggression for male care providers. As we look to the future, we see potential for research that considers other childhood adversities, such as community violence, family economic adversity, and parental maladjustment, to evaluate the link between early life stressors and adult experiences of caregiving. In addition, we encourage researchers to consider factors that may buffer against the negative psychological, physiological, financial, and relational ramifications of providing care in adulthood.

REFERENCES

Adams, K. B. (2007). Specific effects of caring for a spouse with dementia: Differences in depressive symptoms between caregiver and non-caregiver spouses. *International Psychogeriatrics, 20,* 508–520. doi: 10.1017/S1041610207006278

Aloia, L. S., & Solomon, D. H. (2015). Conflict intensity, family history, and physiological stress reactions to conflict within romantic relationships. *Human Communication Research, 41,* 367–389. doi: 10.1111/hcre.12049

Alzheimer's Association and National Alliance for Caregiving. (2004). *Families care: Alzheimer's caregiving in the United States 2004.* Washington, DC: National Alliance for Caregiving.

American Psychiatric Association. (2000). *Diagnostic and statistical manual of mental disorders* (4th ed.). Washington, DC: American Psychiatric Association.

Argyle, M., & Furnham, A. (1983). Sources of satisfaction and conflict in long-term relationships. *Journal of Marriage and Family, 45,* 481–493. doi: 10.2307/351654

Atienza, A. A., Collins, R., & King, A. C. (2001). The mediating effects of situational control on social support and mood following a stressor: A prospective study of dementia caregivers in their natural environments. *Journal of Gerontology Series B: Psychological Sciences and Social Sciences, 56,* 129–139. doi: 10.1093/geronb/56.3.S129

Bi, X., Moos, R. H., Timko, C., & Cronkite, R. C. (2015). Family conflict and somatic symptoms over 10 years: A growth matrix model analysis. *Journal of Psychosomatic Research, 78,* 459–465. doi: 10.1016/j.jpsychores.2015.01.013

Bodie, G. D. (2011). The active-empathic listening scale (AELS): Conceptualization and evidence of validity within the interpersonal domain. *Communication Quarterly, 59,* 277–295. doi: 10.1080/01463373.2011.583495

Boerner, K., Schulz, R., & Horowitz, A. (2004). Positive aspects of caregiving and adaptation to bereavement. *Psychology and Aging, 19,* 668–675. doi: 10.1037/0882-7974.19.4.668

Braver, M., Bumberry, J., Green, K., & Rawson, R. (1992). Childhood abuse and current psychological functioning in a university counseling center population. *Journal of Counseling Psychology, 39*, 252–257. doi: 10.1037/0022-0167.39.2.252

Brown, M. W., & Cudeck, R. (1993). Alternative ways of assessing model fit. In K. A. Bollen & J. S. Long (Eds.), *Testing structural equation models* (pp. 136–162). Newbury Park, CA: SAGE.

Brummett, B. H., Babyak, M. A., Siegler, I. C., Vitaliano, P. P., Ballard, E. L., Gwyther, L. P., & Williams, R. B. (2006). Association among perceptions of social support, negative affect, and quality of sleep in caregivers and noncaregivers. *Health Psychology, 25*, 220–225. doi: 10.1037/0278-6133.25.2.220

Burnett Heyes, S., Zokaei, N., van der Staaij, I., Bays, P. M., & Husain, M. (2012). Development of visual working memory precision in childhood. *Developmental Science, 12*, 528–539. doi: 10.1111/j.1467-7687.2012.01148.x

Centers for Disease Control and Prevention. (2016, March). Caregiving for person with Alzheimer's disease or a related dementia. Retrieved from: www.cdc.gov/aging/caregiving/alzheimer.htm

Cohen, S., Kamarck, T., & Mermelstein, R. (1983). A global measure of perceived stress. *Journal of Health and Social Behavior, 24*, 385–397. Retrieved from: www.jstor.org/stable/2136404

Cohen, S., Kessler, R., & Underwood Gordon, L. (1995). Strategies for measuring stress in studies of psychiatric and physical disorders. In S. Cohen, R. Kessler, & L. Underwood Gordon (Eds.), *Measuring stress: A guide for health and social scientists* (pp. 3–26). New York, NY: Oxford University Press.

Cooley-Quille, M., & Lorion, R. (1999). Adolescents' exposure to community violence: Sleep and psychophysiological functioning. *Journal of Community Psychology, 27*, 367–375. doi: 10.1002/(SICI)1520-6629(199907)27:4<367::AID-JCOP1>3.0.CO;2-T

Cummings, E. M., Goeke-Morey, M. C., Papp, L. M., & Dukewich, T. L. (2002). Children's responses to mothers' and fathers' emotionality and tactics in marital conflict in the home. *Journal of Family Psychology, 16*, 478–492. doi: 10.1037/0893-3200.16.4.478

De Frias, C. M., Tuokko, H., & Rosenberg, T. (2005). Caregiver physical and mental health predicts reactions to caregiving. *Aging Mental Health, 9*, 331–336. doi: 10.1080/13607860500089674

Del Giudice, M., Ellis, B. J., & Shirtcliff, E. A. (2010). The Adaptive Calibration Model of stress reactivity. *Neuroscience and Biobehavioral Reviews, 35*, 1562–1592. doi: 10.1016/j.neubiorev.2010.11.007

Dohrenwend, B. P., & Shrout, P. E. (1985). "Hassles" in the conceptualization and measurement of life stress variables. *American Psychologist, 40*, 780–785. doi: 10.1037/0003-066X.40.7.780

Dura, J. R., Stukenberg, K. W., & Kiecolt-Glaser, J. K. (1991). Anxiety and depressive disorders in adult children caring for demented parents. *Psychology and Aging, 6*, 467–473. doi: 10.1037//0882-7974.6.3.467

Ellis, B. J., & Del Giudice, M. (2014). Beyond allostatic load: Rethinking the role of stress in regulating human development. *Development and Psychopathology, 26*, 1–20. doi: 10.1017/S0954579413000849

Fitzpatrick, K. M., & Boldizar, J. P. (1993). The prevalence and consequences of exposure to violence among African American youth. *Journal of the American Academy of Child and Adolescent Psychiatry, 32*, 424–430. doi: 10.1097/00004583-199303000-00026

Ford, J. D., & Kidd, P. (1998). Early childhood trauma and disorder of extreme stress as predictors of treatment outcome with chronic posttraumatic stress disorder. *Journal of Traumatic Stress, 11,* 743–761. doi: 10.1023/A:1024497400891

Funk, J. B., Bechtoldt Baldacci, H., Pasold, T., & Baumgardner, J. (2004). Violence exposure in real-life, video games, television, movies, and the internet: Is there desensitization? *Journal of Adolescence, 27,* 23–39. doi: 10.1016/j.adolescence.2003.10.005

Gallagher-Thompson, D., Shurgot, G. R., Rider, K., Gray, H. L., McKibbin, C., Kraemer, H., . . . Thompson, L. W. (2006). Ethnicity, stress, and cortisol function in Hispanic and non-Hispanic White women: A preliminary study of family dementia caregivers and noncaregivers. *American Journal of Geriatric Psychiatry, 14,* 334–342. doi: 10.1097/01.JGP.0000206485.73618.87

Garmezy, N. (1985). Stress-resistant children: The search for protective factors. In J. E. Stevenson (Ed.), *Recent research in developmental psychopathology: Journal of child psychology and psychiatry book supplement, no. 4* (pp. 213–233). Oxford: Pergamon.

Gordis, E. B., Margolin, G., & John, R. S. (2001). Parents' hostility in dyadic marital and triadic family settings and children's behavioral problems. *Journal of Consulting and Clinical Psychology, 69,* 727–734. doi: 10.1037/0022-006X.69.4.727

Graham-Bermann, S. A., & Levendosky, A. A. (1998). Traumatic stress symptoms in children of battered women. *Journal of Interpersonal Violence, 13,* 111–128. doi: 10.1177/088626098013001007

Hertzman, C. (1999). The biological embedding of early experience and its effects on health in adulthood. *Annals of the New York Academy of Science, 896,* 85–95. doi: 10.1111/j.1749-6632.1999.tb08107.x

Hertzman, C., & Wiens, M. (1996). Child development and long-term outcomes: A population health perspective and summary of successful interventions. *Social Science and Medicine, 43,* 1083–1095. doi: 10.1016/0277-9536(96)00028-7

Infante, D. A. (1987). Aggressiveness. In J. C. McCroskey & J. A. Daly (Eds.), *Personality and interpersonal communication* (pp. 157–192). Newbury Park, CA: SAGE.

Infante, D. A., Chandler, T. A., Rudd, J. E., & Shannon, E. A. (1990). Verbal aggression in violent and nonviolent marital disputes. *Communication Quarterly, 38,* 361–371. doi: 10.1080/01463379009369773

Kiecolt-Glaser, J. K., Glaser, R., Gravenstein, S., Malarkey, W. B., & Sheridan, J. (1996). Chronic stress alters the immune response to influenza virus vaccine in older adults. *Proceedings of the National Academy of Sciences of the USA, 93,* 3043–3047.

Kline, R. B. (1998). *Principles and practices of structural equation modeling.* New York, NY: The Guildford Press.

Lee, S., Colditz, G. A., Berkman, L. F., & Kawachi, I. (2003). Caregiving and risk of coronary heart disease in U.S. women: A perspective study. *American Journal of Preventive Medicine, 24,* 113–119. doi: 10.1016/S0749-3797(02)00582-2

Maslach, C., Jackson, S. E., & Leiter, M. P. (1997). Maslach burnout inventory. In C. P. Zalaquett & R. J. Wood (Eds.), *Evaluating stress: A book of resources* (pp. 191–218). Lanham, MD: Scarecrow Education.

Mausbach, B. T., Patterson, T. L., Rabinowitz, Y. G., Grant, I., & Schulz, R. (2007). Depression and distress predict time to cardiovascular disease in dementia caregivers. *Health Psychology, 26,* 539–544. doi: 10.1037/0278-6133.26.5.539

Mazzeo, S. E., & Espelage, D. L. (2002). Association between childhood physical and emotional abuse and disordered eating behaviors in female undergraduates: An investigation of the mediating role of alexithymia and depression. *Journal of Counseling Psychology, 49*, 86–100. doi: 10.1037//0022–0167.49.1.86

McLaughlin, K. A., Conron, K. J., Koenen, K. C., & Gilman, S. E. (2010). Childhood adversity, adult stressful life events, and risk of past-year psychiatric disorder: A test of the stress sensitization hypothesis in a population-based sample of adults. *Psychological Medicine, 40*, 1647–1658. doi: 10.1017/S0033291709992121

McNamara, S. (2000). *Stress in young people.* New York, NY: Continuum.

Mitnick, S., Leffler, C., & Hood, V. L. (2010). Family caregivers, patients, and physicians: Ethical guidance to optimize relationships. *Journal of General Internal Medicine, 25*, 255–260. doi: 10.1007/s11606-009-1206-3

National Alliance for Caregiving and American Association for Retired Persons. (2004). Caregiving in the U. S. Retrieved April 1, 2015 from www.caregiving.org/data/04finalreport.pdf.

Ng-Mak, D. S., Salzinger, S., Feldman, R., & Stueve, A. (2002). Normalization of violence among inner-city youth: A formulation for research. *American Journal of Orthopsychiatry, 72*, 92–101. doi: 10.1037/0002–9432.72.1.92

Norman, R. E., Byambaa, M., De, R., Butchart, A., Scott, J., & Vos, T. (2012). The long-term health consequences of child physical abuse, emotional abuse, and neglect: A systematic review and meta-analysis. *PLOS Medicine, 9*(11), e1001349. doi: 10.1371/journal.pmed.1001349

Norton, T. R., Gupta, A., Stephens, M. A. P., Martire, L. M., & Townsend, A. L. (2005). Stress, rewards, and change in the centrality of women's family and work roles: Mastery as a mediator. *Sex Roles, 52*, 325–335. doi: 10.1007/s11199-005-2676-3

Ory, M. G., Hoffman, R. R., Yee, J. L., Tennstedt, S., & Schulz, R. (1999). Prevalence and impact of caregiving: A detailed comparison between dementia and nondementia caregivers. *The Gerontologist, 39*, 177–185. doi: 10.1093/geront/39.2.177

Penrod, J. D., Kane, R. A., Kane, R. L., & Finch, M. D. (1995). Who cares? The size, scope, and composition of the caregiver support system. *The Gerontologist, 35*, 489–497. doi: 10.1093/geront/35.4.489

Post, R. M. (1992). Transduction of psychosocial stress into the neurobiology of recurrent affective disorder. *American Journal of Psychiatry, 149*, 999–1010. doi: 10.1176/ajp.149.8.999

Renfrew, J. W. (1997). *Aggression and its causes: A biopsychosocial approach.* New York, NY: Oxford University Press.

Rule, B. K., & Ferguson, T. J. (1986). The effects of media violence on attitudes, emotions, and cognitions. *Journal of Social Issues, 42*, 29–50. doi: 10.1111/j.1540–4560.1986.tb00241.x

Salomon, J. A., Wang, H., Freeman, M. K., Vos, T., Flaxman, A. D., Lopez, A. D., & Murray, C. J. L. (2013). Healthy life expectancy for 187 countries, 1990–2010: A systematic analysis for the Global Burden Disease Study 2010. *The Lancet, 380*, 2144–2162. doi: 10.1016/S0140-6736(12)61690–0

Saltzman, K. M., Holden, G. W., & Holahan, C. J. (2005). The psychobiology of children exposed to marital violence. *Journal of Clinical Child and Adolescent Psychology, 34*, 129–139. doi: 10.1207/s15374424jccp3401_12

Sharpe, L., Butow, P., Smith, C., McConnell, D., & Clarke, S. (2004). The relationship between available support, unmet needs and caregiver burden in patients with advanced cancer and their carers. *Psycho-Oncology, 14*, 102–114. doi: 10.1002/pon.825

Sih, A. (2011). Effects of early life stress on behavioral syndromes: An integrate adaptive perspective. *Neuroscience and Biobehavioral Reviews, 35*, 1452–1465. doi: 10.1016/j.neubiorev.2011.03.015

Spitznagel, M. B., Tremont, G., Davis, J. D., & Foster, S. M. (2006). Psychosocial predictors of dementia caregiver desire to institutionalize: Caregiver, care recipient, and family relationship factors. *Journal of Geriatric Psychiatry and Neurology, 19,* 16–20. doi: 10.1177/0891988705284713

Straus, M. A. (1979). Measuring intrafamily conflict and violence: The conflict tactics scales. *Journal of Marriage and the Family, 41,* 75–88. doi: 10.2307/351733

Teicher, M. H., Samson, J. A., Sheu, Y. S., Polcari, A., & McGreenery, C. E. (2010). Hurtful words: Association of exposure to peer verbal abuse with elevated psychiatric symptom scores and corpus callosum abnormalities. *American Journal of Psychiatry, 167,* 1464–1471. doi: 10.1176/appi.ajp.2010.10010030

Thompson, R. A. (1994). Emotion regulation: A theme in search of definition. *Monographs of the Society for Research in Child Development, 59*(2–3), 25–52. doi: 10.1111/j.1540-5834.1994.tb01276.x

Thompson, L. W., Spira, A. P., Depp, C. A., McGee, J. S., & Gallagher-Thompson, D. (2006). The geriatric caregiver. In M. E. Agronin & G. J. Maletta (Eds.), *Principles and practice of geriatric psychiatry* (pp. 37–46). Philadelphia, PA: Lippincott Williams & Wilkins.

Weersing, V. R., & Weisz, J. R. (2002). Mechanisms of action in youth psychotherapy. *Journal of Child Psychology and Psychiatry, 43,* 3–29. doi: 10.1111/1469-7610.00002

Weiner, M. F. (2003). Clinical diagnosis of cognitive dysfunction and dementing illness. In M. F. Weiner & A. M. Lipton (Eds.), *The dementias: Diagnosis, treatment, and research* (pp. 1–48). Washington, DC: American Psychiatric Publishing.

Werner, P. (2001). Correlates of family caregivers' knowledge about Alzheimer's disease. *International Journal of Geriatric Psychiatry, 16,* 32–38. doi: 10.1002/1099-1166(200101)16:1<32::AID-GPS268>3.0.CO;2-2

Wolpe, J. (1973). *The practice of behavior therapy.* New York, NY: Pergamon Press.

16

Depression and Sexual Intimacy: Layered Challenges and Communication Strategies

AMY L. DELANEY

Depression is a prevalent mental illness that both affects and is affected by patients' close relationships, particularly their romantic relationship (Hames, Hagan, & Joiner, 2013; Rehman, Gollan, & Mortimer, 2008). One specific effect of depression is a diminished ability to establish and maintain a fulfilling sexual relationship with one's partner (Eklund & Ostman, 2010; Laurent & Simons, 2009). Couples coping with depression encounter decreased sexual desire, difficulties with physical function, and lowered sexual satisfaction (Baldwin, 2001; Frohlich & Meston, 2002; Kennedy, Dickens, Eisfeld, & Bagby, 1999).

Prior research has emphasized how an individual's libido is hindered by depression, but emerging findings hint at a broad array of unique sexual intimacy challenges for couples coping with depression (e.g., Knobloch & Delaney, 2012; Ostman, 2008; Sharabi, Delaney, & Knobloch, 2016). The sexual relationship can be difficult for any couple to talk about, and communication about sex influences relationship outcomes for couples (Baxter & Wilmot, 1985; Byers, 2005; Theiss & Solomon, 2007). Yet, depressed couples are particularly prone to communication problems (Coyne, 1976a; Beach, Sandeen, & O'Leary, 1990; Segrin, 2000), making their sexual communication worthy of additional inquiry. This study draws on Goldsmith's (2001; 2004) normative perspective to highlight communication strategies depressed couples use to navigate conversations about their sex lives.

The purpose of this chapter is to shed light on the experiences of depressed individuals and their partner as they grapple with difficulties in their sexual relationship. The present investigation is an interview study with 33 individuals in relationships in which one or both partners reports depression, and the findings give insight into sexual intimacy challenges and communication strategies for depressed couples. The discussion supplements the literature by (a) offering an organizing framework for future investigations of sexual intimacy challenges for depressed couples, (b) extending the use of the normative perspective into the literatures on depression and sexual communication, and (c) offering pragmatic insight for the treatment of depression from a dyadic perspective.

DEPRESSION AND SEXUAL INTIMACY

Studies of depression in romantic relationships have established that negative sexual effects are common. For both men and women, depression is associated with physical function problems, decreased satisfaction, and wanting but struggling to reach a more intimate relationship with a partner (Frohlich & Meston, 2002; Kennedy et al., 1999; Ostman, 2008). Laurent and Simons (2009) assert that depressed individuals are five times more likely to experience a sexual desire disorder than nondepressed individuals. Research also shows that antidepressant medications contribute to decreased drive and increased dysfunction among individuals with depression, but even nonmedicated individuals report a reduced interest in sex (Baldwin, 2001; Kennedy et al., 1999). Clearly, the depression experience can include struggles with sexual drive, function, and satisfaction.

The existing literature, however, does not fully explain the effects of depression on the sexual relationship. Sexual dysfunction is documented both as a symptom of depression and as a side effect of its medication (Baldwin, 2001; Higgins, Nash, & Lynch, 2010; Kennedy et al., 1999). By examining only drive and function, scholars overlook other issues in the sexual relationship. Additionally, prior research in this area overwhelmingly has addressed experiences of depressed individuals but has failed to take into account effects for nondepressed partners. Accordingly, scholars have called for further research looking at sexuality within the context of the relationship (e.g., Eklund & Ostman, 2010; Reynaert, Zdanowicz, Janne, & Jacques, 2010).

A few studies have illuminated relational dimensions of sexual difficulties for depressed couples. Knobloch and Delaney (2012) pointed to sex as a source of both relational uncertainty (i.e., a lack of confidence in perceptions of the relationship; Solomon & Knobloch, 2004) and interference from partners (i.e., disruptions to one's ability to reach day-to-day goals). Ostman (2008) noted aspects within the patient, within the partner, and within the relationship as factors contributing to sexual troubles. Additionally, one's depressive symptoms can influence his or her partner's perceptions of sexual satisfaction (Bodenmann & Ledermann, 2007). Sharabi and colleagues (2016) documented sexual intimacy as a salient effect of depression, as patients and partners both cited decreased frequency and desire for sex as outcomes of depression. These studies hint at ways sexual problems appear in couples coping with depression.

A gap remains in scholars' knowledge of the range of sexual intimacy challenges depressed couples might face. Although findings on drive and function are established, more research is needed on relational aspects of sexual intimacy challenges (Baldwin, 2001; Bodenmann & Ledermann, 2007; Ostman, 2008). Existing literature (e.g., Bodenmann & Ledermann, 2007; Knobloch & Delaney, 2012) implies that other, more relational challenges exist for couples, but an inventory of those sexual difficulties is needed. A full explication of the sexual intimacy challenges associated with depression will make three important contributions to the literature by (a) augmenting existing perspectives on how depression can impact romantic relationships, (b) contributing to contemporary theory and research examining depression from a systemic perspective, and (c) aiding practitioners in isolating the negative effects of depression to better help couples navigate mental illness. Thus, RQ1 asks:

RQ1: What sexual intimacy challenges do depressed individuals and their partner experience?

COMMUNICATING ABOUT THE SEXUAL RELATIONSHIP

Prior investigations have emphasized the importance of communication in sexual relationships. Close ties exist between sexual satisfaction and relationship satisfaction (Byers, 2005; Sprecher & Cate, 2004). More specifically, several scholars have posited that *communication* is what drives the associations between the sexual relationship and other relationship outcomes (Byers, 2005; Hess & Coffelt, 2012; Theiss & Solomon, 2007). Satisfying conversations about sex might have positive relational and sexual outcomes because partners are better able to understand each other's sexuality (Faulkner & Lannutti, 2010). Alternately, fostering a productive communication environment might improve perceptions of sexual and relationship satisfaction (MacNeil & Byers, 2005). Although the importance of communication about sex is established, less is known about the nature of those associations and about the dynamics of communication about sex.

A second goal of this study is to call on communication scholarship to examine how depressed couples navigate sexual intimacy challenges. In any relationship (regardless of depression status), sexual communication can seem taboo or threatening because it might put partners at risk of rejection, threaten their self-confidence, be embarrassing, or endanger the relationship (Baxter & Wilmot, 1985; Montesi, Fauber, Gordon, & Heimberg, 2011; Theiss & Estlein, 2013). For depressed couples, communication about sex could be particularly intimidating because depressed individuals are prone to diminished social skills (Segrin, 2000, 2001). Individuals with depression often seek reassurance or negative feedback from their partner, which can be frustrating for both people (Coyne 1976a, 1976b; Joiner & Metalsky, 1995). Further, depression is associated with increases in stress and hostility between partners, decreases in supportive behaviors, and heightened reactivity to marital stressors (Beach & O'Leary, 1993; Beach et al., 1990). In sum, depression can impede couples' communication about their relationship, making discussing sex particularly challenging for these partners.

One communication theory that may be useful in this context is Goldsmith's (2001, 2004) normative perspective, which argues that interpersonal interactions are burdened by communication challenges and dilemmas. The normative approach is rooted in the multiple goals tradition (c.f. Caughlin, 2010; Clark & Delia, 1979), as Goldsmith assumes individuals use communication to achieve several potentially conflicting instrumental, identity, and relational objectives. Normative theory asserts that communication challenges are situated within a particular context, and communicators are strategic in how they approach challenging conversations (Goldsmith, Bute, & Lindholm, 2012). Normative theory is useful for answering questions about why some communication events are likely to be more "effective and appropriate" than others (Goldsmith, 2001, p. 518). Scholars must consider what partners say, how they say it, and meanings ascribed to those interactions (Goldsmith, 2004; Goldsmith, Lindholm, & Bute, 2006). The normative approach has proven useful in examining strategies used to manage difficult conversations about health. In contexts such as cardiac care, lung cancer, and organ transplant, research points to integrating humor, giving positive feedback, avoiding conversations, and managing uncertainty as strategic for both patients and network members (Caughlin, Mikucki-Enyart, Middleton, Stone, & Brown, 2011; Goldsmith et al., 2012; Scott, Martin, Stone, & Brashers, 2011). Given its utility for studying communication in difficult health circumstances, the normative approach stands to contribute to studies of depression.

The normative approach suggests that the particular communication techniques depressed couples use will be strategic and situated within the relationship. Individuals might purposefully communicate to manage the taboo around sexual conversations (Baxter & Wilmot, 1985), to account for frustrations with the depression and the relationship (Coyne 1976a; Joiner & Metalsky, 1995), and to attempt to fix physical and relational challenges to their sexual relationship (Baldwin, 2001; Knobloch & Delaney, 2012). The normative perspective posits that meeting these and other goals requires careful navigation of conversations. A record of the strategies individuals use will bolster theorizing about sexual communication and contribute to interventions helping depressed couples tackle sexual intimacy challenges. To explore the sexual communication strategies used by depressed couples, RQ2 is advanced:

RQ2: What strategies do depressed individuals and their partner use to communicate about their sexual relationship?

METHOD

The present study answered the aforementioned research questions with interview techniques rooted in grounded theory methods (Charmaz, 2006; Corbin & Strauss, 2008). Data collection and analyses were sensitized by the normative approach (Goldsmith, 2001, 2004; see Bowen, 2006 for a discussion of sensitizing concepts). All recruitment and interview procedures were approved by the corresponding university's Institutional Review Board.

Procedure

The study was advertised through nationwide depression support organizations (e.g., the Depression and Bipolar Support Alliance), a Facebook page dedicated to the research, and wesearchtogether.org, a database connecting depressed individuals with research opportunities. Participants were invited to schedule an interview if they met the criteria of being (a) 18 years of age or older and (b) currently involved in a romantic relationship, where (c) one or both partners have a professional depression diagnosis. In-person interviewees ($n = 8$) were provided with an informed consent document and asked to fill out a brief demographic questionnaire. Telephone interviewees ($n = 25$) completed a consent document and questionnaire online before the interview. Results did not differ based on medium of interview.

The semistructured interview protocol was identical for in-person and telephone interviews, and was similar for depressed and nondepressed partners. Questions asked participants how depression had impacted their relationship (e.g., "In what ways has depression been a stressor on your relationship with your partner?"), about their sexual relationship (e.g., "How do you feel like depression makes it challenging to be sexually intimate with your partner?"), and how they have approached these challenges to the relationship (e.g., "Can you describe a recent conversation you and your partner have had about your sexual relationship?"). Each participant received a $20 gift card to a national retailer in exchange for her or his time and participation.

Sample

The full sample included 33 individual interviews (31 transcribed verbatim audio recordings, two analyzed from extensive notes because participants requested not to be audio recorded). Seven couples participated in the study ($n = 14$), and 19 individuals participated without a partner also being interviewed. Each partner was interviewed individually. All 33 participants described their race as Caucasian/white, and the mean age was 39 years old (range 21–69). Eight males and 25 females participated. Individuals described their relationships as dating (n = 3), cohabiting but not engaged (n = 11), engaged but not cohabiting (n = 2), engaged and cohabiting (n = 1), or married (n = 16). Two female same-sex couples participated in the study. The mean reported relationship length was 6.92 years (range 3.5 months to 21 years).

Eighteen participants were the only depressed partners in the relationship, while 11 reported that both partners had been diagnosed. The remaining four participants were in a relationship with a depressed partner. Of the seven couples, three involved both partners with a depression diagnosis, and four had one partner diagnosed. Participants reported diagnoses of major depression (n = 21), chronic mild depression (n = 4), postpartum depression (PPD; n = 4), seasonal affective disorder (SAD; n = 3), psychotic depression (n = 3), or other (n = 5; bipolar disorder, generalized depression, and agitated depression). Participants completed the Center for Epidemiologic Studies Depression Scale (Radloff & Locke, 2008). The mean score for the full sample was 26.14 (SD = 15.75), with a significantly higher mean for participants who reported that they were depressed (M = 28.16, SD = 15.45) than for nondepressed respondents (M = 11.50, SD = 9.68; $t(31)$ = 2.08, p = 0.05). Twenty-four participants reported currently receiving treatment (medication or counseling) for depression.

RESULTS

Transcripts (369 single-spaced pages) and notes were analyzed through a multiphase, abductive process during and after data collection, including the composition of detailed memos after each interview. Memos reflected on emerging findings, lingering questions, and trends across participants. These memos allowed for identification of initial codes and prompted revisions in the interview protocol. After data collection and transcription, open, line-by-line coding was conducted on 10 interview transcripts. This coding was characterized by constant comparison within and among participants (Glaser & Strauss, 1967). Following Charmaz (2006), the line-by-line coding involved short, action-focused labels that maintained close links to the data itself.

Next, the most significant and frequent codes were extracted to construct a scheme for focused coding, which involved comparing the data to the codes and applying codes in a way that refined the understanding of the data (Charmaz, 2006). A next analytical step was focused coding, which meant reading each interview and labeling passages with the appropriate category. Finally, axial coding (Corbin & Strauss, 2008) allowed for alignment of categories in meaningful ways. The following pages include an overview of these findings, with exemplars of each category in participants' own words. All names are replaced with pseudonyms.

Sexual Intimacy Challenges

Participants' responses indicated that they perceive challenges to their sexual relationship as *layered*. A primary layer of challenges centered on the impact on libido and desire. Beyond sex drive or desire, though, participants described secondary sets of challenges. These secondary challenges highlighted *cognitive* and *interactive* processes as additional hindrances to couples' goals for a satisfying sexual relationship.

Primary challenges. Participants cited troubles with drive and libido as their main sexual intimacy challenges. Mark (33, married, major depression) opened his interview by asserting that his sexual relationship with his wife was "dead" as a result of his major depression. Jesse (21, cohabiting with girlfriend with major depression and SAD, nondepressed) described his girlfriend's decreased interest as affected by her symptoms, saying, "When she gets sad, she just doesn't have any interest in sex." Kathryn (30, engaged, major depression) noted the change in her interest, explaining she used to be a very sexual person, but now has "no sexual urge."

The *loss* of libido is not the only way depressed couples encountered this primary challenge. James (34, married, major depression) described that as his treatment started to work, his desire for sex returned. This did not solve the problems in his sexual relationship, though, as his wife was no longer interested. He recalled, "It really hurt when I felt my libido came back and my wife didn't particularly feel responsive to it." His wife, Hilary (38, married, nondepressed), recounted the same issue, and noted the frustrating loss and later return of his sex drive. In this case, it was the return of James's libido (even more than the loss of it) that challenged the couple. Broadly, participants identified changes to libido as a primary challenge to their sexually intimate partnership.

Secondary challenges. Beyond frequently mentioned troubles with libido, participants noted several additional barriers to a close sexual connection. *Cognitive* and *interactive* challenges pose a second layer of sexual difficulties for depressed couples.

Cognitive challenges. Cognitive challenges are barriers to sexual intimacy that stem from issues with *self-esteem* and feelings of *isolation*.

Self-esteem. Participants described a diminished view of themselves as linked to difficulties with physical intimacy. Brooke (31, engaged, major depression) and Patrice (53, married, major depression) both described how their own self-doubt made them feel less interested in sex. Mark (33, married, major depression) felt as though his lack of self-confidence was at the root of both his depression and his sexual challenges with his wife: "I think it was a confidence thing. It was performance and confidence, you know my lack of and my embarrassment and apologizing for performance." Wendy (46, cohabiting, major depression) articulated how her self-esteem troubles made her hesitant to connect sexually with her partner: "When I'm feeling really heavy with my depression, I don't like myself. I think, why do I want to share myself if I don't even like myself?"

Whereas the aforementioned participants cited ways decreased self-esteem made them less interested in sex, others perceived self-esteem issues as making them less desirable to their partners. Renee (30, married, major depression) felt as though her behaviors while depressed made her unattractive to her husband. Paula (43, dating, major depression) also noticed how diminished self-esteem drove a wedge between her and her partner, saying, "I complain a lot that I don't like myself. So I know that that, it can get draining, she can get annoyed." Taken together, these participants' accounts suggest depression's effect on self-esteem can encumber a couple's sexual connection.

Isolation. Participants also described how feelings of isolation impact the sexual relationship. Hannah (28) and Cassandra (26) are a dating couple, both diagnosed with major depression, and each described how they "felt closed off" and "don't want to even be touched" when coping with feelings of depression. Peter (34, dating, psychotic depression) described how depression makes him push his partner away: "So when she tries to express affection for me, I pull back and I just can't receive it as an act of love from another person. . . . I'm very stand-offish and cold." Similarly, Ruth (30, married, PPD) believed feelings of seclusion from her husband challenged their physical relationship. In her words:

> It's just that feeling of being separated from each other. Whether it's from one of us pushing the other one away or just from not understanding. . . . feeling very much like I've messed up the relationship and just wanting to be sort of alone and separate from it.

When a depressed partner wants to be alone, the couple cannot connect physically. Together, issues with self-esteem and feelings of emotional and physical isolation represent a cognitive layer of sexual intimacy challenges for depressed couples.

Interactive challenges. Interactive challenges are obstacles to sexual intimacy that are manifest in *conversations* and in trouble with *initiation*.

Conversations. Depressed couples experienced barriers to productive conversations about sex. Luke (56, married to a partner with PPD, nondepressed) described his wife as willing to talk about sexual issues, but in his words, "I'm not quite there yet in talking of how to handle it." In her interview, his wife, Ruth (30, married, PPD), corroborated Luke's take: "It's not something that, that he's, that he has any real comfort level discussing. . . . It makes it almost impossible." Peter (34, dating, psychotic depression) wanted to talk to his partner about their sexual challenges, but reported not having the conversational skills to do so: "I didn't know how to intellectualize it . . . I felt like I had limited resources, like, tools to deal with this." Several participants lamented lacking the ability or skills to discuss sex with their partner.

Another conversational difficulty appeared in descriptions of conversations about sex as futile. Todd (68, married to a partner with major depression, nondepressed) explained: "We talk, and she gets it off her chest, and it goes nowhere, which I think to the both of us in that sense is frustrating you know." His wife, Patrice (53, married, major depression), described her own exasperation at ineffectual conversations: "I'm tired of always having to explain things again and again and then come back and explain them again and again." Similarly, Renee (30, married, major depression) explained, "I just feel like it would be a pointless conversation, and we have enough of those as it is."

Clearly, conversations about sex can be tricky for depressed couples to navigate. Rachel (50, married, both partners suffer from major depression) shared her frustration with trying to talk with her husband about her desire for an improved sexual connection:

You know, like we go camping a lot, so I said, "You can't set a fire in the woods and come back ten hours later and expect it to still be burning. You know, you have to tend the fire. You know this isn't just about the sex, it's about the intimacy." And he'll respond like, "Well, I don't know what to tell you. You're just going to have to take care of yourself until this gets fixed." You know? So I'm always up against a wall, and I don't know what's driving that because he won't talk about it.

Yet, when asked about the best part of their relationship, her husband, Benjamin, immediately responded with "communication." Rachel and Benjamin illustrate that conversations about sex for depressed partners are difficult, but both partners might not be in tune to how important and/or difficult those conversations are.

Initiation. Participants also cited difficulties getting started in intimate situations and rekindling a struggling sexual relationship. For example, Mark (33, married, major depression) explained that a couples' counselor had given him some literature about reinitiating physical contact, but his wife was uncomfortable with even reading that information, let alone following its advice. Similarly, Luke (56, married to a wife with PPD, nondepressed) explained that both partners were struggling with picking up their physical relationship. Challenges with initiation occur when partners struggle to relate in ways that start a sexual encounter.

Partners might be interested in sexual activity but unable to start that interaction with a partner. Ruth (30, married, PPD) desired more affection from her partner to help initiate sexual activity, saying:

A lot of times, I find myself thinking, you know, if he would be more physically affectionate, again that I, that I would be able to be a lot of it, a lot of what he needs to happen with us is me wanting him to sort of meet me halfway.

Partners also struggle with initiating interactions because of the risk of rejection, such as James (34, married, major depression), who said, "I just can't initiate it. You know and risk getting rebuked." Joseph (52, cohabiting, major depression) described rejection as a major difficulty in initiating sex, as most interactions about sex start with him trying to engage and his girlfriend shutting him down. Cassandra (26, cohabiting with a depressed partner, depressed) described herself as "very timid and very shy about approaching those kinds of things because I don't want to be turned down by my own partner. . . . And so for most of the time, I wait for her to instigate anything."

Initiation interactions can be daunting owing to difficulty with sending and receiving cues. Karen (29, cohabiting, agitated depression) described her preference for a direct, verbal initiation as opposed to a subtle or indirect one. Renee (30, married, major depression) reflected on how she and her husband were often not on the same page when it came to initiating sexual activity:

I don't even know! Because later on he's like, "Well I tried to" but I'm like, "You tried to how? What do you mean you tried to?" A few times I notice it, but it's um, it's not a physical thing because he's not a physical person. And it's usually some kind of comment about blow jobs!

Couples can struggle with initiation cues so vague that a partner does not notice them, or cues so blunt that they are actually a turn off for one partner.

In sum, several layers characterize depressed couples' experiences of sexual intimacy challenges. Most couples experience difficulty with decreased libido, but many also encounter secondary challenges – cognitive, interactive, or both – creating further barriers to couples' goals to improve or maintain a sexual connection.

Communication Strategies

A second research question inquired into ways partners communicate strategically about sexual intimacy. Participants described five communication strategies, but maintained conflicting accounts about the utility of those strategies.

Humor. Participants described how humor facilitated interactions about sex and made discussions more comfortable for partners. Luke (56, married to a wife with PPD, nondepressed) shared that his wife's humor helps them during sexual conversations: "I am kind of witless and not particularly funny about anything, but, um, I think that her sense of humor in those conversations and, and being able to laugh at ourselves has helped us a great deal."

Wendy (46, cohabiting, major depression) also explained that keeping the conversation "light" helped broach uncomfortable conversations. Cassandra (26, cohabiting with a partner with SAD, major depression) shared that conversations about sex typically involve some giggles. In her words, "you don't wanna make being intimate super serious, you know?" Humor appears to be an effective strategy in two ways. First, it helps partners cope with cognitive challenges related to isolation. Laughing together helps partners connect and reminds them that they are coping with depression (and its relational effects) as a team. Second, humor helps partners cope with conversational challenges. If lightening the mood helps participants feel at ease talking about sex, they may be able to then communicate further to cope with sexual intimacy issues.

Yet, humor did not appear to be a universally effective strategy. April (25, cohabiting, major depression), for example, said, "One of his things that drives me nuts is he can't always be serious . . . more times not . . . he's not serious." Her partner only initiated and participated in conversations about sex by making jokes about oral sex. April described how his jokes made her feel misunderstood and as if she could not talk about her serious relationship concerns. April's situation suggests that humor can also be off-putting for partners, especially if jokes drive a further wedge between loved ones. If an attempt to lighten the mood is perceived as inappropriate or insensitive, it might actually exacerbate problems. In sum, participants described humor as a strategy for conversations about sexual intimacy, but not an entirely effective one.

Planning. Participants also described conversations focusing on collaborating to address sexual problems. These conversations prioritized the future and ways to address their difficulties. Caroline (38, married, bipolar disorder with depressive episode(s)) approached her husband after a marriage retreat and said, "Let's make sure to have sex at least three times a week." Cassandra (26, cohabiting with a partner with SAD, major depression) and her partner scheduled sex after her therapist recommended it. Planning conversations centered on many ways to establish or increase intimacy, not just scheduling sex. Ruth (30, married, PPD) explained that when she or her husband voiced concerns about intimacy, they worked together to develop a plan, such as to hold hands every time they are out. Others described planning time to snuggle or to make sure to kiss before bed each night. As couples planned ways to increase intimacy, they were collaborating to meet a goal of a more fulfilling sex life. The planning strategy is helpful for setting the tone to initiate a sexual connection, and thus helps couples grapple with interactive challenges.

Not every participant perceived planning conversations to be particularly helpful in tackling the sexual intimacy challenges in their relationship. Ruth's husband, Luke, explained, "I mean, we both come up with a lot of great suggestions, but they don't always work for us. Yeah . . . fixing it is a bigger issue." Luke's description implies that although planning helps partners confront some conversational challenges, it may fall short of helping address the other layers of sexual intimacy challenges. A planning conversation does not necessarily give partners tools to cope with self-esteem and isolation, and may not improve partners' libidos. Planning ways to improve the sexual relationship seems to be a strategy that could address some challenges, but may not actually help to address the more primary layers of sexual difficulties.

Timing of conversations. Timing of conversations about sex was also strategic. Some preferred talking about sex while in bed or in another intimate situation, whereas others preferred a nonsexual setting. Alison (39, engaged, generalized depression) shared that talking was more effective if she waited for a comfortable moment outside of a sexual situation, explaining, "I mean, it's not immediately after we've been intimate. But, sometime in the day or two afterwards." Other participants felt the setting of the bedroom made it easier to approach the subject of sex, such as Kathryn (30, engaged, major depression), who said, "Maybe if we're laying in bed already, and the lights are off, and we're just talking to each other. . . . Then it's just a lot easier for me." These differing accounts illustrate how there may not be a specific time or place best suited for discussing sex, but finding a comfortable time is one way couples communicate strategically about sex. Different approaches to timing may help partners cope with different sexual intimacy challenges. Talking about sex in a nonsexual context could be effective when partners prioritize protecting self-esteem or having a conversation about depression's libido effects. Alternatively, timing a conversation about sex in a more intimate setting might mitigate partners' discomfort with talking about a sensitive subject.

This strategy could involve making some unsuccessful attempts. Cassandra (26, cohabiting, major depression) attempted to talk about sex with her partner, Hannah (28, cohabiting, SAD), in bed, but found this was "probably the worst time, cause it's like you spring it up on someone. At least that's how she felt." She later talked to her partner in a nonintimate situation, while having a cigarette on the porch. In her words,

I was like, "This is casual enough." Um, in the daylight and under the trees and what have you, I was like, "I would like to be intimate, or I would like to do so and so." And she's like, "Oh, okay." So that was a pleasant conversation. Nothing happened, um, but that's alright 'cause we talked about it and it was a good step.

For this couple, trial-and-error helped them figure out when and where to talk about sex in a comfortable and productive way. Timing conversations could be an ineffective strategy when the timing meets one partner's needs (e.g., Cassandra's wish to have a conversation in a comfortable setting), but violates the other's (e.g., Hannah feeling pressured into a difficult interaction). The timing of conversations strategy involves a careful balance of addressing layers of challenges and both partners' perceptions.

Avoiding conversations. Some participants circumvented difficult conversations altogether. Partners cited avoidance as a default strategy because previous attempts at conversations were too challenging or not productive, such as Julie (53, married, major depression), who said talking about sex "doesn't work because I'm scared and I just, you know, figure it's a lost cause." Similarly, Alison (39, engaged, generalized depression) noted that she stopped approaching her fiancé about the topic because "things don't ever get anywhere. . . . no matter how intense our conversation is about wanting something different, it doesn't change." Other participants side-stepped conversations about sex to avoid sex. Renee (30, married, major depression and SAD) shared that she would "default to the migraine excuse." She went on to explain that she did this because "I don't think he would understand, or because I feel guilty. I feel like I'm a bad wife. 'Cause a good wife would [want to have sex], or whatever." In these cases, avoidance is perceived as advantageous for participants who see conversations as overwhelming or futile. Avoidance also functions to cope with libido and self-esteem challenges. If partners avoid a conversation by claiming a migraine or changing the subject, they can elude confronting their issues with libido or self-esteem.

Participants also recounted ways avoidance was not a useful strategy. Some wanted to talk about sex, but their partner's avoidance precluded any beneficial interactions. In Julie's (53, married, major depression) words, "I wish we could, but there's just no talking to him about it." When asked about conversations that have gone badly, Hannah (28, cohabiting with a partner with SAD, major depression) cited avoidance, saying "Um, if one of us just sort of closes up and doesn't want to talk anymore." Avoidance could be a negative strategy in cases where it compounds difficulties with communication or exacerbates feelings of isolation.

Prioritizing intimacy. Depressed couples also communicated to prioritize intimacy over intercourse or other physically intimate contact. Through communication, participants tried to reframe intimacy in their relationship. Rachel (50, married, both partners with major depression) explained her focus on closeness: "Yeah, not just about sexuality. It's about the intimacy and feeling connected and feeling like we're in it together kind of thing." She went on to share how she would tell her husband: "It's not about the act of sex. It's about the intimacy. It's about the holding of the hands, the long kisses, the, you know, the brushing up against the small of my back when we're walking." Megan (52, married, diagnosed with psychotic depression, husband diagnosed with SAD) explained how prioritizing intimacy over sexual contact maintained some closeness in her marriage when her husband lost interest in sex. Monica (37, cohabiting, both partners with major depression) described how she and her boyfriend schedule "snuggle time" and make sure to spend close time together (talking, kissing, cuddling) each day, calling this time "really intentional." Partners believed prioritizing intimacy in the relationship was one way they could communicatively address the sexual intimacy challenges. Prioritizing intimacy may be most effective in addressing feelings of isolation. By placing intimacy at the forefront (instead of the act of sex), couples may be able to establish a connection that sustains the relationship as they address other challenges.

Several participants believed this strategy fell short of actually fixing their sexual problems. For some couples, prioritizing intimacy was intended to set the tone for the sexual relationship to pick back up, but reported it did not work. Rachel (50, married, both partners with major depression) communicated to her husband that intimacy was more important than sex, but lamented, "we still have our fundamental, underlying problem." Although prioritizing intimacy may be helpful in some ways, its downfall as a communication strategy may be that it does not fix the primary layer of libido problems. Thus, communicating to prioritize intimacy can help couples circumvent some sexual intimacy challenges, but falls short of addressing the core problem.

DISCUSSION

This study sheds light on experiences of depressed couples by, first, explicating the layered and complex sexual intimacy challenges in depression, and, second, outlining strategic ways partners communicate about sex. The following pages situate these findings within existing literature, discuss theoretical and practical implications, and propose areas to explore further.

Sexual Intimacy Challenges (RQ1)

Sexual intimacy challenges for depressed couples are multidimensional and layered. One participant's frustration illustrates the multilayered challenges that couples deal with in the depression context. Megan (52, married, both partners with depression) described how her husband's decreased libido was frustrating, but then her efforts to talk about that impact were shut down, which was even more trying. As she explained, her partner usually responds with "Don't even ask" or "I do not want to talk about that." Megan's experience exemplifies the layers of sexual intimacy challenges. First, her spouse is not interested in sex; then, he is not willing to converse about what this means for their relationship. Primary challenges with drive, function, and frequency are already noted in the literature (e.g., Baldwin, 2001; Kennedy et al., 1999) and were, indeed, reported by most participants in this sample. *Cognitive* barriers and *interactive* problems document additional ways depressed couples perceive sexual intimacy challenges as more complex than the effect on libido or the side effects of antidepressant medications. Couples who solve problems with libido could face other sexual issues, and couples who cope with secondary challenges may not be able to reverse or manage depression's effects on libido. This study answers calls for research examining the relational context of depression-related sexual intimacy challenges (e.g., Eklund & Ostman, 2010; Reynaert et al., 2010).

Sexual Communication Strategies (RQ2)

In response to the second research question, analyses revealed five communication strategies depressed couples turn to in conversations about sex. Individuals integrate *humor, planning, timing of conversations, avoidance,* and *prioritizing intimacy* into conversations about sex. Yet, these strategies were not perceived to be universally effective. Participants also discussed ways they had tried to communicate strategically but failed to address their challenges or meet their goals. Communication is not likely the only solution to sexual issues for depressed couples, but couples who communicate effectively are likely to have more satisfying sex lives (Byers, 2005).

These results corroborate previous findings pointing to relational communication as challenging for depressed couples (Beach et al., 1990; Joiner & Metalsky, 1995; Segrin, 2000) and sexual communication as difficult for romantic couples (Baxter & Wilmot, 1985). They also enhance these literatures by explicating specific strategies depressed couples turn to in these tough conversations. Although some scholars assert that open or direct communication about sex is most effective (e.g., Byers & Demmons, 1999; Theiss & Solomon, 2007), other scholars have pointed to less direct techniques as more appropriate (e.g., Miller-Ott & Linder, 2013). Accordingly, participants suggested that avoiding conversations or integrating humor was best in their given relationships and contexts. This aligns with other recent findings pointing to topic avoidance as a salient communication practice in depressed couples (Knobloch, Sharabi, Delaney, & Suranne, 2015). Further, although the depression literature highlights several ways depressed individuals communicate ineffectively (e.g., through destructive nonverbals or excessive reassurance seeking; Segrin, 2000; Joiner & Metalsky, 1995), the findings suggest depressed patients and their partners devise methods of communicating that help them to cope with inherent relational struggles accompanying depression.

Theoretical Implications

Depression and sexual intimacy. Results illuminating the layered nature of sexual intimacy challenges for depressed couples are an important step in theorizing about depression and sexual intimacy. Whereas previous work has categorized issues with sexual intimacy as a symptom of depression (e.g., Baldwin, 2001) or a side effect of its medication (e.g., Higgins et al., 2010), participants' accounts of libido difficulties, cognitive troubles, and interactive struggles offer a layered model of sexual intimacy challenges to set the stage for theorizing on sexual intimacy in depression. Next, scholars can turn to the dual control model (Bancroft, Graham, Janssen, & Sanders, 2009), which argues that both individual and interactive factors combine to enhance or inhibit sexual arousal. The dual control model calls attention to circumstances that contribute to increased inhibition and decreased excitation. Blending the current findings with the dual control model positions cognitive and interactive challenges as notable inhibiting factors and highlights the importance of the interactive challenges for depressed couples.

Communication strategies. The findings on communication strategies reflect and build upon previous work rooted in the normative approach to communication in the study of illness (Brashers, Goldsmith, & Hsieh, 2002; Scott et al., 2011). Participants were not asked directly about conversational challenges, but independently reported conversations about sex as a barrier to the sexual partnership. Their descriptions of not having the skills to talk about sex and of their frustration over unproductive conversations hint at Goldsmith's (2001, 2004) focus on conversational challenges when messages might carry multiple meanings and interactants balance discordant goals (Caughlin, 2010; Clark & Delia, 1979). Strategies uncovered in this study could allow for the management of competing interpersonal goals. *Planning* is useful because it prioritizes improving the couple's sexual relationship while preserving relational goals of both partners by encouraging collaboration. Similarly, the use of *humor* in conversations about sex allows individuals to protect their own and their partner's identity (e.g., Miller-Ott & Linder, 2013), but also raises the subject of the sexual relationship. Participant narratives of strategic communication also echoed the normative principle that strategies are not always effective but are situated within a specific context and carry specific meanings for partners (Goldsmith et al., 2006). Normative thinking frames evaluation of messages as the result of meanings attributed to those messages (Goldsmith, 2004). Indeed, these participants' accounts of conversations as both effective and ineffective point to ways that a communication strategy may be advantageous for some objectives and for some couples, but may carry risks for others.

These findings comport with previous normative research in illness settings in demonstrating the normative principle that the contexts shape communication challenges and strategies (Goldsmith et al., 2006; Middleton, McAninch, Pusateri, & Delaney, 2016). Couples coping with a cardiac event use humor, cooperation and problem solving/planning, and avoidance (Goldsmith et al., 2012). Avoidance of conversations can be functional within the lung cancer context (Caughlin et al., 2011). Timing of conversations is a strategy for partners in the cancer context, and framing of the illness and its effects occurs in parents discussing HIV with children (Donovan-Kicken, Tollison, & Goins, 2011; Edwards, Donovan-Kicken, & Reis, 2014). Together with the current findings, these studies suggest that some normative communication strategies are common to conversations across illness contexts.

Practical Implications

The current findings make two significant practical contributions. First, the layered nature of depression's sexual effects means that although physicians and psychiatrists have strategies for tackling libido problems (e.g., changes in medication), practitioners must also approach couples' sexual intimacy challenges in other ways. Couples could benefit from interventions targeted toward improving damaged self-esteem, connecting with each other despite feelings of isolation, tackling difficult conversations, and initiating intimate contact. Second, practitioners should call on the normative perspective to guide interventions with depressed couples. The depression treatment literature often prioritizes effective communication (e.g., Carr, 2009; Whisman & Beach, 2012), but does not delineate what constitutes *effectiveness*. Some encourage openness, while others suggest problem solving, emotional expression, and avoidance of criticism (Carr, 2009; Whisman & Beach, 2012). The normative principles outlined here imply that specific tactics might not be most advisable, instead encouraging communicators to negotiate competing demands of the specific circumstance (cf. Caughlin et al., 2011; Goldsmith, 2004). Practitioners should tailor treatment and communication strategies to individual couples in ways that acknowledge the complexities of each couple's situation.

Limitations and Directions for Future Research

These contributions should be considered in combination with the study's limitations. The nationwide sample was racially homogeneous. Thus, these findings do not speak to issues that may be related to culturally diverse experiences of depression or how culture may relate to conversations about sexual intimacy. Although several couples participated, the study primarily features one partner's perspective, and, thus, data were analyzed at the individual level. These data reflect participants' accounts of conversations and cannot reflect how strategic communication about sex unfolds in actual interactions.

Several directions for new scholarship exist. Future research should examine temporal facets of the layered nature of sexual intimacy challenges. How do challenges develop across the depression experience? Scholars can also delve into the strategies uncovered here. What factors influence use and perceived effectiveness of each sexual communication strategy? Finally, researchers should observe strategies in action as conversations happen between partners. What does each strategy look like in practice, and how do partners shape the sexual communication climate? This study has established a foundation for future research into how depressed couples communicate to navigate sexual intimacy challenges.

REFERENCES

Baldwin, D. S. (2001). Depression and sexual dysfunction. *British Medical Bulletin, 57,* 81–99. doi: 10.1093/bmb/57.1.81

Bancroft, J., Graham, C. A., Janssen, E., & Sanders, S. A. (2009). The dual control model: Current status and future directions. *The Journal of Sex Research, 46,* 121–142. doi: 10.1080/00224490902747222

Baxter, L. A., & Wilmot, W. W. (1985). Taboo topics in close relationships. *Journal of Social and Personal Relationships, 2,* 253–369. doi: 10.1177/0265407585023002

Beach, S. R. H., & O'Leary, K. D. (1993). Marital discord and dysphoria: For whom does the marital relationship predict depressive symptomatology? *Journal of Social and Personal Relationships, 10,* 405–420. doi: 10.1177/0265407593103007

Beach, S. R. H., Sandeen, E. E., & O'Leary, K. D. (1990). *Depression in marriage: A model for etiology and treatment.* New York, NY: Guilford Press.

Bodenmann, G., & Ledermann, T. (2007). Depressed mood and sexual functioning. *International Journal of Sexual Health, 19,* 63–73. doi: 10.1300/J514v19n04_07

Bowen, G. A. (2006). Grounded theory and sensitizing concepts. *International Journal of Qualitative Methods, 5,* 1–9.

Brashers, D. E., Goldsmith, D. J., & Hsieh, E. (2002). Information seeking and avoiding in health contexts. *Human Communication Research, 28,* 258–271. doi: 10.1111/j.1468-2958.2002.tb00807.x

Byers, E. S. (2005). Relationship satisfaction and sexual satisfaction: A longitudinal study of individuals in long-term relationships. *The Journal of Sex Research, 42,* 113–118. doi: 10.1080/00224490509552264

Byers, E. S., & Demmons, S. (1999). Sexual satisfaction and sexual self-disclosure within dating relationships. *The Journal of Sex Research, 36,* 180–189. doi: 10.1080/00224499909551983

Carr, A. (2009). The effectiveness of family therapy and systemic interventions for adult-focused problems. *Journal of Family Therapy, 31,* 46–74. doi: 10.1111/j.1467-6427.2008.00452

Caughlin, J. P. (2010). A multiple goals theory of personal relationships: Conceptual foundation and program overview. *Journal of Social and Personal Relationships, 27,* 824–848. doi: 10.1177/0265407510373262

Caughlin, J. P., Mikucki-Enyart, S. L., Middleton, A. V., Stone, A. M., & Brown, L. E. (2011). Being open without talking about it: A rhetorical/normative approach to understanding topic avoidance in families after a lung cancer diagnosis. *Communication Monographs, 78*, 409–436. doi: 10.1080/03637751.2011.618141

Charmaz, K. (2006). *Constructing grounded theory: A practical guide through qualitative analysis*. Thousand Oaks, CA: SAGE.

Clark, R. A., & Delia, J. G. (1979). Topoi and rhetorical competence. *Quarterly Journal of Speech, 65*, 187–206.

Corbin, J., & Strauss, A. (2008). *Basics of qualitative research*. Thousand Oaks, CA: SAGE.

Coyne, J. C. (1976a). Depression and the response of others. *Journal of Abnormal Psychology, 85*, 186–193. doi: 10.1037/0021-843X.85.2.186

Coyne, J. C. (1976b). Toward an interactional description of depression. *Psychiatry, 39*, 28–40. doi: 10.1080/00332747.1976.11023874

Donovan-Kicken, E., Tollison, A. C., & Goins, E. S. (2011). A grounded theory of control over communication among individuals with cancer. *Journal of Applied Communication Research, 39*, 310–330. doi: 10.1080/00909882.2011.585398

Edwards, L. L., Donovan-Kicken, E., & Reis, J. S. (2014). Communicating in complex situations: A normative approach to HIV-related talk among parents who are HIV+. *Health Communication, 29*, 364–374. doi: 10.1080/10410236.2012.757715

Eklund, M., & Ostman, M. (2010). Belonging and doing: Important factors for satisfaction with sexual relations as perceived by people with persistent mental illness. *International Journal of Social Psychiatry, 56*, 336–447. doi: 10.1177/0020764008101635

Faulkner, S. L., & Lannutti, P. J. (2010). Examining the content and outcomes of young adults' satisfying and unsatisfying conversations about sex. *Qualitative Health Research, 20*, 375–385. doi: 10.1177/1049732309354274

Frohlich, P., & Meston, C. (2002). Sexual functioning and self-reported depressive symptoms among college women. *The Journal of Sex Research, 39*, 321–325. doi: 10.1080/00224490209552156

Glaser, B. G., & Strauss, A. L. (1967). *The discovery of grounded theory*. Chicago, IL: Aldine.

Goldsmith, D. J. (2001). A normative approach to the study of uncertainty and communication. *Journal of Communication, 51*, 514–533. doi: 10.1111/j.1460-2466.2001.tb02894.x

Goldsmith, D. J. (2004). *Communicating social support*. New York, NY: Cambridge University Press.

Goldsmith, D. J., Bute, J. J., & Lindholm, K. A. (2012). Patient and partner strategies for talking about a lifestyle change following a cardiac event. *Journal of Applied Communication Research, 40*, 65–86. doi: 10.1080/00909882.2011.636373

Goldsmith, D. J., Lindholm, K. A., & Bute, J. J. (2006). Dilemmas of talking about lifestyle changes among couples coping with a cardiac event. *Social Science & Medicine, 63*, 2079–2090. doi: 10.1016/j.socscimed.2006.05.005

Hames, J. L., Hagan, C. R., & Joiner, T. E. (2013). Interpersonal processes in depression. *Annual Review of Clinical Psychology, 9*, 355–377. doi: 10.1146/annurev-clinpsy-050212-185553

Hess, J. A., & Coffelt, T. A. (2012). Verbal communication about sex in marriage: Patterns of language use and its connection with relational outcomes. *Journal of Sex Research, 49*, 603–612. doi: 10.1080/00224499.2011.619282

Higgins, A., Nash, M., & Lynch, A. M. (2010). Antidepressant-associated sexual dysfunction: Impact, effects, and treatment. *Drug, Healthcare and Patient Safety*, 2, 141–150. doi: 10.2147/DHPS.S7634

Joiner, T. E., & Metalsky, G. I. (1995). A prospective test of an integrative interpersonal theory of depression: A naturalistic study of college roommates. *Journal of Personality and Social Psychology*, 69, 778–788. doi: 10.1037/0022-3514.69.4.778

Kennedy, S. H., Dickens, S. E., Eisfeld, B. S., & Bagby, R. M. (1999). Sexual dysfunction before antidepressant therapy in major depression. *Journal of Affective Disorders*, 56, 201–208. doi: 10.1016/S0165-0327(99)00050-6

Knobloch, L. K., & Delaney, A. L. (2012). Themes of relational uncertainty and interference from partners in depression. *Health Communication*, 27, 750–765. doi: 10.1080/10410236.2011.639293

Knobloch, L. K., Sharabi, L., Delaney, A. L., & Suranne, S. (2015). The role of relational uncertainty in topic avoidance among couples with depression. *Communication Monographs*, 83, 25–48. doi: 10.1080/03637751.2014.998691

Laurent, S. M., & Simons, A. D. (2009). Sexual dysfunction in depression and anxiety: Conceptualizing sexual dysfunction as part of an internalizing dimension. *Clinical Psychology Review*, 29, 573–585. doi: 10.1016/j.cpr.2009.06.007

MacNeil, S., & Byers, E. S. (2005). Dyadic assessment of sexual self-disclosure and sexual satisfaction in heterosexual dating couples. *Journal of Social and Personal Relationships*, 22, 169–181. doi: 10.1177/0265407505050942

Middleton, A. V., McAninch, K. M., Pusateri, K. B., & Delaney, A. L. (2016). "You just gotta watch what you say in those situations": A normative approach to confidant communication surrounding sexual assault disclosure. *Communication Quarterly*, 64, 232–250. doi: 10.1080/01463373.2015.1103290

Miller-Ott, A. E., & Linder, A. (2013). Romantic partners' use of facework and humor to communicate about sex. *Qualitative Research Reports in Communication*, 14, 69–78. doi: 10.1080/17459435.2013.835344

Montesi, J. L., Fauber, L. R., Gordon, E. A., & Heimberg, R. G. (2011). The specific importance of communicating about sex to couples' sexual and overall relationship satisfaction. *Journal of Social and Personal Relationships*, 28, 591–609. doi: 10.1177/0265407510386833

Ostman, M. (2008). Severe depression and relationships: The effect of mental illness on sexuality. *Sexual and Relationship Therapy*, 23, 355–363. doi: 10.1080/14681990802419266

Radloff, L. S., & Locke, B. Z. (2008) Center for Epidemiologic Studies depression scale (CES-D). In A. J. Rush, Jr., M. B. First, & D. Blacker (Eds.), *Handbook of psychiatric measures* (2nd ed., pp. 506–508). Washington, DC: American Psychiatric Publishing.

Rehman, U. S., Gollan, J., & Mortimer, A. R. (2008). The marital context of depression: Research, limitations, and new directions. *Clinical Psychology Review*, 28, 179–198. doi: 10.1016/j.cpr.2007.04.007

Reynaert, C., Zdanowicz, N., Janne, P., & Jacques, D. (2010). Depression and sexuality. *Psychiatria Danubina*, 22, 111–113.

Scott, A. M., Martin, S. C., Stone, A. M., & Brashers, D. E. (2011). Managing multiple goals in supportive interactions: Using a normative theoretical approach to explain social support as uncertainty management for organ transplant patients. *Heath Communication*, 26, 393–403. doi: 10.1080/10410236.2011.552479

Segrin, C. (2000). Social skills deficits associated with depression. *Clinical Psychology Review*, 20, 370–403. doi: 10.1016/S0272-7358(98)00104-4

Segrin, C. (2001). *Interpersonal processes in psychological problems*. New York, NY: Guilford Press.

Sharabi, L., Delaney, A. L., & Knobloch, L. K. (2016). In their own words: How clinical depression affects romantic relationships. *Journal of Social and Personal Relationships*, *33*, 421–448. doi: 10.1177/0265407515578820

Solomon, D. H., & Knobloch, L. K. (2004). A model of relational turbulence: The role of intimacy, relational uncertainty, and interference from partners in appraisals of irritations. *Journal of Social and Personal Relationships*, *21*, 795–816. doi: 10.1177/0265407504047838

Sprecher, S., & Cate, R. M. (2004). Sexual satisfaction and sexual expression as predictors of relationship satisfaction and stability. In J. H. Harvey, A. Wenzel, & S. Sprecher (Eds.), *The handbook of sexuality in close relationships* (pp. 235–256). Mahwah, NJ: Lawrence Erlbaum Associates.

Theiss, J. A., & Estlein, R. (2013). Antecedents and consequences of the perceived threat of sexual communication: A test of the relational turbulence model. *Western Journal of Communication*, *78*, 404–425. doi: 10.1080/10570314.2013.845794

Theiss, J. A., & Solomon, D. H. (2007). Communication and the emotional, cognitive, and relational consequences of first sexual encounters between partners. *Communication Quarterly*, *55*, 179–206. doi: 10.1080/01463370601036663

Whisman, M. A., & Beach, S. R. H. (2012). Couple therapy for depression. *Journal of Clinical Psychology*, *68*, 526–535. doi: 10.1002/jclp.21857

Epilogue: The Important Role of Relationship Research in Promoting Healthy Individuals and Relationships

JENNIFER A. THEISS AND KATHRYN GREENE

The scholarship that is showcased in this volume highlights the dynamic ways in which people's health and relationships are intertwined. Several studies pointed to the ways that health diagnoses – such as cancer, Alzheimer's disease, diabetes, and mental health conditions – can shape the nature and quality of people's close relationships with regard to interdependence, uncertainty, information management, support, and communication. Other research summarized in this volume highlights the ways that families, friends, and romantic partners can influence people's health behavior, including the adoption of healthy diet and exercise routines, encouragement to schedule visits with health care providers, adherence to illness treatment plans, and the management of stress. Taken together, these studies demonstrate the central role that close relationships play in the pursuit of both individual and relational health and wellness. In particular, the scholarship in this volume is organized around several interpersonal processes in close relationships that are especially relevant to health contexts, including interpersonal influence, information management, uncertainty, support and caregiving, and communication. Thus, in this epilogue, we take stock of the contributions that relationship researchers can make toward enhancing people's health and relationships, and we offer recommendations for moving this literature forward in theoretically significant and pragmatically important ways.

RELATIONSHIP PROCESSES VITAL TO HEALTH AND WELLNESS

There are a variety of relationship processes involved in health contexts that have become cornerstones of research on relationships, health, and wellness. In this volume, we privileged five aspects of close relationships that can shape and reflect people's health and wellness, including attempts at interpersonal influence, decisions about information and privacy management, appraisals of contextual and relational uncertainty, efforts to provide support and coping, and patterns of communication behavior. The chapters in this book point to the ways that these relationship processes can be affected by diagnoses of health or illness, as well as the ways they might shape the health and wellness of individuals and their relationships.

Interpersonal influence reflects the ways that relationship partners and family members are involved in people's health behaviors and the strategic efforts they employ to encourage their loved ones to make healthy choices. The chapters in this book that highlight the communication strategies and health outcomes of interpersonal influence focus primarily on the attempts of spouses and romantic partners to influence health behaviors such as obtaining cancer screenings (Birmingham & Reblin, Chapter 1), sharing relevant personal information with health care providers (Haas, Chapter 2), and encouraging healthy diet and exercise (Burke, Chapter 3). Although romantic partners can exert considerable influence on one another's health behavior given their prominence and significance in people's lives, interpersonal influence can come from many different people in a variety of social contexts. Peer influence from friends, for example, can encourage individuals to engage in unhealthy and potentially risky behaviors such as smoking, drug use, excessive alcohol consumption, and unprotected sexual encounters. Families also have the potential to influence individuals' health behaviors, such as parents attempting to control the food environment to shape children's choices for healthy eating, or adult children asserting influence over health care decisions and end-of-life care for their elderly parents. Thus, there are countless opportunities for researchers seeking to explore the nature and impact of interpersonal influence across a diverse set of relational and health contexts.

The ways that people manage information with regard to their health is another fruitful avenue for relationship researchers. Two chapters in this volume focused on perceptions of privacy surrounding personal health information and the conditions or factors that prompt individuals to disclose or withhold their health information with relationship partners. Leustek and Theiss (Chapter 4) focused on the health-related topics that individuals with type 2 diabetes avoid discussing with their romantic partner, whereas Venetis, Gettings, and Chernichky-Karcher (Chapter 5) examined the relationship conditions that shape people's decisions to disclose information about their mental health. These chapters are representative of a growing body of research on the ways that individuals share information about stigmatized illnesses. Considerations of privacy and disclosure are important for individuals grappling with a wide range of health conditions across a diverse set of relationship contexts. Information management also involves examinations of the ways that people seek information about health. For example, Scheinfeld, Nelson, and Crook (Chapter 6) explored the ways that parents seek information about nutrition and fitness and the strategies they employ to communicate this information to their children. Notably, these chapters are just a small cross section of the rich and vibrant body of research on the ways that people manage information, disclosure, and privacy when it comes to seeking and sharing health-related information with relationship partners. There is a relatively large literature, for instance, on the information practices related to sexual health, especially information seeking and disclosure of HIV and other sexually transmitted infections (e.g., Brashers et al., 2000; Greene, Derlega, Yep, & Petronio, 2003). Across a variety of contexts, relationship researchers have established a firm foundation for grounding researching on issues related to privacy and information management.

A third feature of health and relationships that was highlighted in this volume involves experiences of uncertainty related to illness or to the relationship. People can experience uncertainty with regard to their health or a particular illness, as well as uncertainty about how a relationship might be affected by a partner's health condition. Some of the chapters in this volume focus on the uncertainties that arise in close relationships as a result of illness or severe health conditions, such as Catona's (Chapter 7) research on the ways that Alzheimer's disease can raise questions about how to relate to a partner with this condition, or Keeler's (Chapter 8) study on the uncertainties that arise between siblings who are co-managing an aging parent's health care. Other chapters emphasize the uncertainties that stem from illness or other health contexts, such as the study by Carpenter, Greene, Catona, and Checton (Chapter 9) on health uncertainty stemming from a cardiac condition, or the work by Frisby, Matig, and Harris (Chapter 10) on the uncertainties that parents have about how to help their children cope with bereavement. The literature on uncertainty in close relationships is robust and scholars have identified the antecedent conditions that can give rise to uncertainty for individuals, as well as the consequences of uncertainty for relationship quality (Theiss, 2018). Health contexts provide a unique backdrop for investigating experiences of uncertainty because they raise important questions about the vitality and longevity of one's self and the implications of that for the wellbeing of people's close relationships.

The field of relationship research is also rich with studies on the interpersonal qualities of support and coping. Family, friends, and romantic partners are an important source of social support in any context that can elicit distress. In health contexts, in particular, close relationships are essential for helping individuals cope with stressful circumstances. Along these lines, this volume highlighted research by Tao, Randall, and Totenhagen (Chapter 11) on the ways that same-sex romantic partners can support one another through the potential stress and depression resulting from family rejection. The study by Steuber-Fazio, Moran, McNair, and Cogland (Chapter 12) described the support needs of men whose wives were experiencing postpartum depression. The clinical work conducted by Banerjee, Manna, and Parker (Chapter 13) examined the strategies that oncology nurses employ to provide proper support and care for their patients. Social support can take a variety of forms, including emotional, instrumental, informational, esteem, and network support (e.g., Cutrona & Russell, 1990). Given that the chapters in this volume focused predominantly on the provision of emotional support, there are a number of opportunities for relationship researchers to expand this body of work to examine how relationship partners enact other types of social support in response to distressing health conditions and how the quality of that support influences outcomes for both individuals and their relationships.

This volume also included research on the ways that communication can shape and reflect relationship conditions in the context of challenging health conditions. Haverfield and Theiss (Chapter 14) focused on the ways that parental alcoholism can influence family communication patterns and the outcomes of those interpersonal dynamics for the psychological well-being of children into adulthood. Similarly, research by Aloia and Stone (Chapter 15) examined how patterns of family verbal aggression in childhood can buffer the stress associated with caring for a parent with Alzheimer's disease later in life. Finally, Delaney's study (Chapter 16) demonstrated the various ways that depressive symptoms can undermine sexual intimacy and the communication strategies that relationship partners use to navigate these challenging circumstances. As a set, the chapters in this section, as well as others in this volume, highlight the influential role of communication behavior in the context of health and wellness. On the one hand, some studies have shown that effective communication may be compromised in the face of health conditions that elicit stress or are considered taboo. People are often reluctant to disclose information about stigmatizing mental or physical health conditions, they may avoid conversations that are perceived as embarrassing or face-threatening, or they might attempt to assert control or dominance in an effort to change a partner's health behavior in the face of illness. On the other hand, research has also highlighted the potential for communication to serve as a catalyst for behavior change or as a tool of relationship maintenance for individuals coping with negative health outcomes. For example, interpersonal communication can be beneficial for encouraging a relationship partner to adopt healthier diet and exercise habits, for expressing solidarity and support for a partner who is undergoing treatment for illness, or for bolstering relational intimacy despite potentially devastating health conditions. Thus, communication dynamics mark an important area of inquiry for scholars who are interested in the interplay between health and relationships, as well as a fruitful target for practitioners looking to develop programs designed to improve health and relational outcomes.

Beyond the relationship processes that are privileged in the chapters in this volume, there are several other features of close relationships that are worthy of exploration with regard to their associations with people's health and wellness. One body of research that has seen significant growth and shows great potential for enhancing health and wellness is the literature on affection. A number of studies have shown that sending and receiving expressions of affection are associated with physiological responses, such as a reduction in cholesterol (Floyd, Mikkelson, Hesse, & Pauley, 2007), lower resting heart rate (Floyd et al., 2007), and reduced levels of the stress hormone cortisol (Floyd & Riforgiate, 2008). Taken together, these studies highlight the importance of expressed and received affection for people's physical well-being, which can have long-term implications for promoting positive health outcomes. Along these lines, there is a growing body of research that considers the connections between relationship dynamics and physiological markers of health. For example, the dynamics of interpersonal conflict have been linked to various biomarkers, with demand/withdraw conflict patterns contributing to increased cortisol (Hefner et al., 2006) and more hostile conflict behaviors slowing wound recovery (Kiecolt-Glaser et al., 2005). Similarly, social support tends to buffer stress, resulting in decreased cortisol and more rapid cortisol recovery following stressful events (Faw, 2018; Priem & Solomon, 2015). Thus, future research on the associations between relationship processes and biomarkers may be fruitful for enhancing people's health and wellness.

FUTURE DIRECTIONS FOR RESEARCH ON RELATIONSHIPS, HEALTH, AND WELLNESS

Although many of the studies included in this volume drew on well-established theory to ground their investigations, including attachment theory (Bowlby, 1969), the disclosure decision-making model (Greene, 2009), family communication patterns theory (Koerner & Fitzpatrick, 2002), uncertainty management theory (Brashers, 2001), privacy management theory (Petronio, 2002), problematic integration theory (Babrow, 2001), and relational turbulence theory (Solomon, Knobloch, Theiss, & McLaren, 2016), much of the existing research on relationships, health, and wellness adopts a variable analytic approach to testing associations among key relationship processes and health constructs. In addition, given that applications of relationship research to health contexts are still relatively new, much of the existing research in this field tends to be exploratory in nature. As the field continues to mature, we hope to see the results of exploratory investigations transformed into the articulation of new theory that can formally ground questions about the ways that health and relationships are interdependent. Moreover, to the extent that existing theories can be used to inform the questions that scholars are asking about these associations, we encourage them to apply relevant theory whenever possible. Given the theoretically rich foundations of relationship research, scholars who employ theory to guide their research are poised to make significant contributions to this emerging body of work on relationships, health, and wellness.

Another important consideration for scholars in the field of health and relationships is increased attention to issues of diversity and inclusion. Much of the existing research on relationships, health, and wellness examines largely homogeneous samples that are predominantly white, cis-gendered, and middle to upper class. We applaud the work being done by Haas (Chapter 2) and Tao, Randall, and Totenhagen (Chapter 11), in particular, for exploring health concerns and stressors among same-sex couples, and we are proud to include their scholarship in this volume, but considerably more research is required to better understand the health needs and relational implications of health and wellness for more marginalized, stigmatized, and underserved populations. The health disparities that have been documented among individuals from racial, ethnic, and sexual minority groups (e.g., Collins, Hall, & Neuhaus, 1999), as well as economically disadvantaged individuals from urban and rural communities (e.g., Hartley, 2004), point to the need for increased research on the relational and health outcomes that characterize these groups.

A third avenue for development going forward is for relationship scholars to devise strategies for translating their research into practice. The practical implications of this body of research for improving people's health and relationships cannot be overlooked. The communication skills training module for oncology nurses that was developed and tested by Banerjee, Manna, and Parker (Chapter 13) is a positive step in the direction of translating the theoretical and empirical richness of relationship research into concrete skills and strategies that can be implemented to improve care. Beyond the practical implications of this research for health care contexts, there is tremendous potential for the development of science-based programs and interventions designed to help people navigate some of the relational challenges that arise when coping with adverse health conditions. Relationship researchers should be thinking of ways to translate their empirical findings into concrete recommendations for helping siblings co-manage elder care, helping spouses adjust to a partner's dementia or depression, or helping parents introduce healthy choices for their children. Several chapters in this volume lay the foundation for developing practical guidelines for coping with these challenging circumstances and we look forward to the continuation of this important translational work.

Along these lines, we are hopeful that this volume will also help open a dialogue between relationship researchers and health care professionals that leads to increased partnerships and interdisciplinary collaborations. Relationship researchers are engaged in scholarship that can inform the ways that health care professionals engage with patients around the treatment of illness and the incorporation of partners and families in health maintenance and decision-making. Thus, health care providers stand to benefit and improve their practice by implementing the findings of relationship research. For their part, relationship researchers would benefit from opportunities to interface with health care professionals to improve their understanding of the relationship influences in health care and to identify fruitful avenues for future exploration. Encouraging more conversations and collaborations between social scientists and health care professionals has the potential to enhance the research and practice in both fields.

CONCLUSION

Close relationships are one of the cornerstones of the human experience. As such, close friends, family members, and romantic partners are involved and influential in a variety life events and circumstances. The research contained in this volume showcases the variety of ways in which relationship processes are relevant to conditions of health and wellness. Some studies demonstrate that the quality of close relationships is shaped by the health and vitality of the individuals in those relationships. Other perspectives highlight the ways that relationship partners can influence one another's healthy or unhealthy behaviors. Some scholars point to the ways that relationships are responsive to conditions of illness or hardship, while others consider the ways that partners can buffer against negative consequences. Regardless of their particular orientation or perspective, all of the studies included in this volume demonstrate that relationships and health go hand in hand. Although the contribution of this research contained in this volume is notable for the ways in which it advances theory and practice, it merely scratches the surface of what is possible when relationship scholars apply their expertise to the problem of improving health and wellness. Opportunities exist to continue to expand this work in ways that can make a significant impact on people's lives and relationships, which is a contribution worth exploring.

REFERENCES

Babrow, A. S. (2001). Uncertainty, value, communication, and problematic integration. *Journal of Communication, 51*, 553–573. doi: 10.1111/j.1460-2466.2001.tb02896.x

Bowlby, C. (1969). *Attachment and loss* (Vol. 1). New York, NY: Basic Books.

Brashers, D. E. (2001). Communication and uncertainty management. *Journal of Communication, 51*, 477–497. doi: 10.1111/j.1460-2466.2001.tb02892.x

Brashers, D., E., Neidig, J. L., Haas, S. M., Dobbs, L. K., Cardillo, L. W., & Russell, J. A. (2000). Communication and the management of uncertainty: The case of persons living with HIV or AIDS. *Communication Monographs, 67*, 63–84. doi: 10.1080/03637750009376495

Collins, K. S., Hall, A., & Neuhaus, C. (1999). *U.S. minority health: A chartbook*. New York, NY: Commonwealth Fund.

Cutrona, C. E., & Russell, D. W. (1990). Type of social support and specific stress: Toward a theory of optimal matching. In B. R. Sarason, I. G. Sarason, & G. R. Pierce (Eds.), *Social support: An interactional view* (pp. 319–366). New York, NY: John Wiley & Sons.

Faw, M. H. (2018). Supporting the supporter: Social support and physiological stress among caregivers of children with disabilities. *Journal of Social and Personal Relationships, 35*, 202–223. doi: 10.1177/0265407516680500

Floyd, K., Mikkelson, A. C., Hesse, C., & Pauley, P. M. (2007). Affectionate writing reduces total cholesterol: Two randomized, controlled trials. *Human Communication Research, 33*, 119–142. doi: 10.1111/j.1468-2958.2007.00293.x

Floyd, K., Mikkelson, A. C., Tafoya, M. A., Farinelli, L., La Valley, A. G., Judd, J., . . . Wilson, J. (2007). Human affection exchange: XIV. Relational affection predicts resting heart rate and free cortisol secretion during acute stress. *Journal of Behavioral Medicine, 32*, 151–156. doi: 10.3200/BMED.32.4.151–156

Floyd, K., & Riforgiate, S. (2008). Affectionate communication received from spouses predicts stress hormone levels in healthy adults. *Communication Monographs, 75*, 351–368. doi: 10.1080/03637750802512371

Greene, K. (2009). An integrated model of health disclosure decision making. In T. D. Afifi & W. A. Afifi (Eds.), *Uncertainty, information management, and disclosure decisions: Theories and applications* (pp. 226–253). New York, NY: Routledge.

Greene, K., Derlega, V. J., Yep, G. A., & Petronio, S. (2003). *Privacy and disclosure of HIV in interpersonal relationships: A sourcebook for researchers and practitioners.* Mahwah, NJ: Lawrence Erlbaum Associates.

Hartley, D. (2004). Rural health disparities, population health, and rural culture. *American Journal of Public Health, 94*, 1675–1678. doi: 10.2105/AJPH.94.10.1675

Hefner, K. L., Loving, T. J., Kiecolt-Glaser, J. K., Himawan, L. K., Glaser, R., & Malarkey, W. B. (2006). Older spouses' cortisol responses to marital conflict: Associations with demand/withdraw communication patterns. *Journal of Behavioral Medicine, 29*, 317–325. doi: 10.1007/s10865-006-9058-3

Kiecolt-Glaser, J. K., Loving, T. J., Stowell, J. R., Malarkey, W. B., Lemeshow, S., Dickinson, S. L., & Glaser, R. (2005). Hostile marital interactions, proinflammatory cytokine production, and wound healing. *Archive of General Psychiatry, 62*, 1377–1384. doi: 10.1001/archpsyc.62.12.1377

Koerner, A. F., & Fitzpatrick, M. A. (2002). Toward a theory of family communication. *Communication Theory, 12*, 70–91. doi: 10.1111/j.1468–2885.2002.tb00260.x

Petronio, S. (2002). *Boundaries of privacy: Dialectics of disclosure.* Albany, NY: SUNY Press.

Priem, J. S., & Solomon, D. H. (2015). Emotional support and physiological stress recovery: The role of support matching, adequacy, and invisibility. *Communication Monographs, 82*, 88–112. doi: 10.1080/03637751.2014.971416

Solomon, D. H., Knobloch, L. K., Theiss, J. A., & McLaren, R. M. (2016). Relational turbulence theory: Explaining variation in subjective experiences and communication within romantic relationships. *Human Communication Research, 42*, 507–532. doi: 10.1111/hcre.12091

Theiss, J. A. (2018). *The experience and expression of uncertainty in close relationships.* Cambridge: Cambridge University Press.

INDEX